£48 —

**This book is to be returned on or before
the last date stamped below.**

HENRY, Kristin

# A Colour Atlas of
# Thymus and Lymph Node Histopathology
# with Ultrastructure

Copyright © K. Henry & G. Farrer-Brown, 1981
Published by Wolfe Medical Publications Ltd, 1981
Printed by Royal Smeets Offset b.v., Weert, Netherlands
ISBN 0 7234 0743 6

This book is one of the titles in the series of
Wolfe Medical Atlases, a series which brings
together probably the world's largest systematic
published collection of diagnostic colour
photographs.
For a full list of Atlases in the series, plus
forthcoming titles and details of our surgical,
dental and veterinary Atlases, please write to
Wolfe Medical Publications Ltd, Wolfe House,
3 Conway Street, London W1P 6HE.

General Editor, Wolfe Medical Atlases:
G. Barry Carruthers, MD(Lond)

A Colour Atlas of
# Thymus and Lymph Node Histopathology
## with Ultrastructure

## Kristin Henry
MBBS, MRCP, FRCPath

Reader in Pathology, Westminster Medical School,
Honorary Consultant Pathologist, Westminster Hospital,
London SW1

## Geoffrey Farrer-Brown
MA, MB, BChir, MD, FRCPath

Consulting Pathologist at the Nightingale BUPA and
Fitzroy Nuffield Hospitals, London NW1

Wolfe Medical Publications Ltd

*To*
*K.F.W.H. and A.C.T.*

# Contents

# Acknowledgements

Much of the material used in this Atlas results from research projects supported by the Cancer Research Campaign and the Muscular Dystrophy Group of Great Britain, and from our many colleagues participating in the British National Lymphoma Investigation Trial: to all of them we extend our thanks. We should also like to thank the following friends and colleagues for allowing us to photograph their slides/specimens – Professor J. G. Azzopardi, **819**, **820**; Dr M. H. Bennett, **16**, **165**; Professor A. H. Cameron, **292**, **293**, **670**, **671**; Dr K. M. Cameron, **813**, **814**; Dr Jonathan Gluckman, **821**, **822**; Professor M. S. R. Hutt, **329**, **330**, **364**, **365**, **638**, **641**, **823**; Dr G. Frizzera, **277**, **278**; Dr B. C. Morson, **334**, **335**, **336**; Dr K. Namba, **791**, **792**; Professor K. G. Naik, **288**, **289**; Dr G. Slavin, **184**; Professor A. C. Thackray, **344**, **345**, **346**, **347**; for providing photographs from their collections – Dr N. Byrom, **860**; Professor M. A. Epstein, **861**, **862**; Professor D. A. G. Galton, **579**; Dr P. D. James, **790**; to Dr B. Achong for the electronmicrograph, **643**. Diagrams **0** and **50** are reproduced from The Lymphocyte by K. Henry and J. Goldman in *Recent Advances in Pathology, 9* (1975), Ed. C. V. Harrison and H. K. Weinbren, by kind permission of the publishers, Churchill Livingstone. Figure **714** is reproduced from *Primary lymphomas of the gastrointestinal tract* by K. Henry and G. Farrer-Brown, Histopathology I Ed. R. E. Cotton, by kind permission of Blackwell Scientific Publications Ltd.

We gratefully acknowledge the expert help of Medical Laboratory Scientific Officers in our respective Histopathology Departments, particularly those at the Westminster Hospital and Medical School, who prepared the majority of the sections. We especially wish to thank Miss Phyl Brock and Mr J. Patel for their dedication in the provision of the wide range of special stains and enzyme/immunocytochemical preparations, and Mr S. J. Kee for his expertise in the printing of the electronmicrographs. The photographs of the macroscopic specimens were largely prepared by members of the Department of Medical Photography at the Westminster Hospital and we gratefully acknowledge their help.

We thank also past and present colleagues at the Royal Postgraduate Medical School, London, the Bland-Sutton Institute of Pathology, Middlesex Hospital Medical School and the Westminster Medical School and Hospital. Finally, we owe a very great debt of gratitude to Mrs Norma Jackson and Miss Joan Carter for their patience in typing and retyping the text, and to Mrs Shirley Jones for her meticulous preparation of the Index.

# Preface

This colour Atlas is intended as a visual aid to the interpretation of the difficult field of thymus and lymph node histopathology, and is designed for use by both practising and trainee pathologists, final year clinical students, research workers and clinicians active in this field.

The sections on thymus pathology include involution, aplasia, thymitis (inflammation) and neoplasia; with the emphasis on the thymitis associated with myasthenia gravis and on thymic tumours including thymomas. The largest individual sub-sections on the lymph node are devoted to Hodgkin's disease, lymphomas other than Hodgkin's disease, and to infectious conditions. Other major sections are concerned with common reactive conditions and reactive processes with characteristic features, which may be confused with lymphomas. The histopathology of extra-nodal sites, such as spleen, skin and gastrointestinal tract are only included where they relate to lymph node pathology.

Since the interpretation of reactive and neoplastic lesions is helped by the understanding of the normal, we have considered it essential to describe and illustrate *normal* thymus and lymph node structure. Many sections also include examples of plastic processed material and electronmicrographs since they, too, greatly facilitate the interpretation and diagnosis of thymus and lymph node pathology. Technical aspects include a short description of the handling and processing of surgical material and the final illustrative section is devoted to routine and special staining techniques and certain immunocytological and histochemical reactions.

Essentially this Atlas is a synthesis of the authors' experience in this field. Information relating to clinical data and aetiology have either been extracted from recent publications or reflect the personal views of the authors. Introductory texts have been kept deliberately brief. However, it is hoped that the more comprehensive legends to the selected illustrations – labelled where appropriate – taken with the introductory texts, will describe adequately the salient features of the normal and pathological conditions covered. A short list of books for recommended reading and an extensive Index are included.

In compiling this Atlas one of the biggest problems dictated by space and cost has been the limitation of the number of colour illustrations considered necessary to cover all aspects of this large and important area of pathology. Also, it has not always been possible to provide consistency in colour because of the different origins of material, and the variability in the routine and special stains used. The colour illustrations represent a very wide range of magnifications; from × 3 for whole-section mounts, through × 30 for low power views and up to × 940 for the oil immersion (high power) fields. However, in view of the differences in absolute size induced by routine fixation and processing procedures, and because we consider it more important for the reader to assess cell size in relation to normal cellular constituents (e.g. small = red cells, large = endothelial or macrophage nuclei) magnifications are indicated only for the macroscopic specimens and the electronmicrographs.

The majority of photomicrographs were taken with a Wild M20 camera microscope using Agfachrome 50L, a minority being taken with a Zeiss Ultraphott II camera microscope with Kodachrome 2. The electronmicrographs were taken either with the Hitachi 12U or the AEI 801 electron microscopes.

# The Lymphoreticular and Mononuclear Phagocytic System (LRMPS)

The lymphoreticular and mononuclear phagocytic system of cells – collectively called the LRMPS – is now known to be of prime importance in immunological function, with the cells of the lymphoid series closely collaborating with those of the mononuclear phagocytic system. It has been shown that in the lymphoid series there are at least two classes of lymphocytes – the thymus (T), dependent lymphocytes, and the bursa/bone marrow (B), dependent lymphocytes – both of which derive initially from bone marrow precursors. There has been clarification of the anatomical and functional distribution of the mononuclear phagocytic cells which are a constant component of lymphoreticular tissues. Mononuclear phagocytic cells are given different names according to their site and, though they may function independently in a purely phagocytic capacity, they are extremely important in many immunological reactions. The LRMPS can be conveniently divided into three functional compartments, as shown in figure **0**.

1  Stem cell compartment represented by yolksac, foetal liver and bone marrow which is responsible for the generation of the various populations of stem cells.
2  Primary or central lymphoid organs responsible for the production and control of immunologically competent cells such as thymus.
3  The secondary or peripheral lymphoreticular tissues which function in an executive capacity. (See also page 78, 109.)

# The thymus gland

The thymus(s) arises from the entoderm of the third and possibly fourth branchial pouches during the sixth week of gestation. It is thus a paired structure sharing a common origin with the inferior parathyroid glands. With continued growth there is downward migration into the anterior mediastinum. Only the upper poles of the left and right thymuses remain in the neck and, unless the connective tissue investing the two portions of the thymus are dissected away, the organ appears as one. The two thymus (lobes) are, however, quite separate, (**1** and **2**). Failure of normal descent results in ectopic thymic tissue which may be found anywhere from the neck down to the diaphragm. The lymphoid nature of the thymus is not evident until around the ninth week of gestation when lymphocytes derived from bone marrow populate the epithelial thymus. At about the same time the thymus assumes a lobular configuration.

The thymus gland achieves its greatest weight proportional to body weight at birth and its greatest absolute weight at puberty. With increasing age there is involution with loss of thymic parenchyma and replacement with fat. This normal involutionary process is known as age or physiological involution (see **37–39**), and should be distinguished from the very rapid involution known as stress or accidental involution which can occur in response to a number of different agents (see **40–47**) and which is mediated through the pituitary adrenal axis and is better referred to as steroid-induced involution.

The thymus is a central or primary lymphoid organ responsible for the production, differentiation and direction of a population of small lymphocytes concerned primarily with cell-mediated immunity. Such thymus-dependent lymphocytes are known as T-lymphocytes in contrast to bone marrow dependent B-lymphocytes with which they intimately co-operate. There is thus a vertical division in the immune system dividing the thymus-dependent functions of cell-mediated immunity from that of the bone marrow function of controlling humeral antibody (immunoglobulin) production. Failure of development of the thymus and/or defective T-lymphocyte

9

function are recognised clinically by a number of immune-deficiency syndromes and histopathologically by the absence of T-lymphocytes in certain well-defined areas of lymph nodes, spleen or other extra-nodal lymphoreticular tissues.

The basic unit of the thymus is the thymic lobule composed of a lymphocyte-rich outer cortex and an inner medulla with numerous epithelial cells, fewer lymphocytes and the unique structures known as Hassall's corpuscles (see **8–11**). It is the epithelial component – in addition to secreting mucosubstances – which is responsible for the production of the thymic hormones including thymosine. Among other cell types which are a normal constituent of the thymus, are eosinophils, mast cells and the striated muscle or myoid cells (see **28–36**). In contrast to lymph nodes and other secondary (peripheral) lymphoid tissues, only occasional lymphoid follicles with germinal centres are found in the *normal* thymus. The frequency of these structures increases, however, in certain conditions such as myasthenia gravis (see **54–66**). The thymus is also an important site in neoplastic transformation, not because thymic tumours are common but because there is a very high incidence in these neoplasms of an associated immunologically orientated disease.

**0**

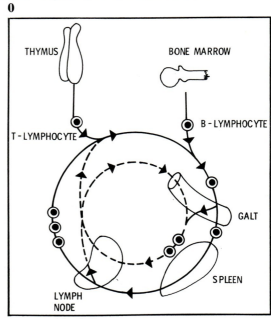

**1 and 2  Normal foetal thymus** During intrauterine life the left and right thymus glands migrate downward into the anterior mediastinum where they come to lie in apposition, simulating one organ. When the loose connective tissue has been dissected away the two distinct and separate parts are clearly visible, **1**. The upper portions of each gland represent the cervical extension which, when present, remains in the neck and is accessible to biopsy. The rest of the organ overlies the base and the greater vessels of the heart. Figure **2** shows the thymuses viewed from behind. The two glands have been artificially separated and it can be seen that the only point where there is communication is via the venous drainage (the great vein of Keynes). In some individuals there may be failure of normal descent of each part into the mediastinum or there may be over descent. Abnormalities of descent account for the finding of ectopic thymic tissue anywhere from the neck to the diaphragm.

**1**

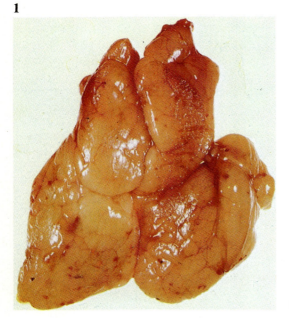

× 2

**2**

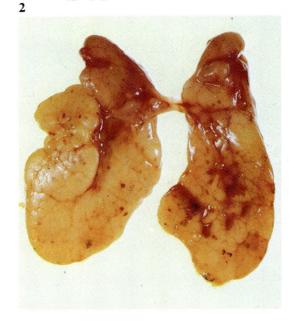

**3**

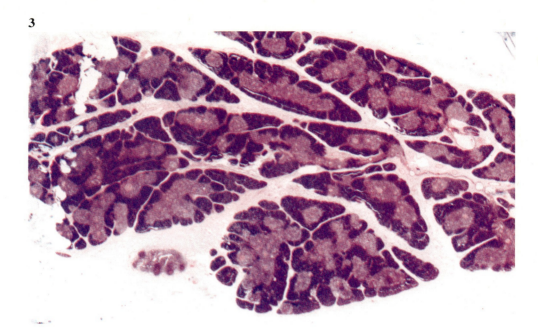

**3  Normal child's thymus** The thymus is derived from the entoderm of the third and probably fourth branchial arches, with a probable contribution from the cervical sinus. The thymus is, therefore, essentially an epithelial organ and may be viewed as a foregut derivative. The characteristic lobular structure as shown here is not evident until the third intrauterine month; until then the rudimentary thymus appears as an epithelial organ. The periphery of the lobules is bounded by a capsule from which are derived the connective tissue septa. Each lobule is composed of an outer darkly-staining cortex and an inner paler-staining medulla which is continuous throughout each half of the gland. *(H&E)*

**4  Normal child's thymus** The outer cortex is composed of numerous densely-packed small lymphocytes (thymocytes) and the inner medulla consists of fewer lymphocytes admixed with the thymic epithelial cells. The lymphocytes are derived from bone marrow (stem) cells which migrate to the thymus at about the third intrauterine month. Scattered throughout the medulla are elongated or rounded epithelial structures known as the Hassall's corpuscles which are unique to the thymus. The epithelial component is essential for the normal maturation and competence of the lymphoid component, and is the source of the various thymic hormonal/ humeral factors now being defined. *(H&E)*

**4**

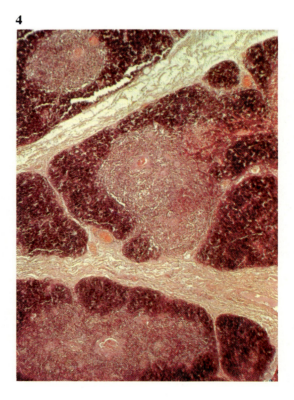

**5 Normal child's thymus** The inner part of the lobule, the medulla, consists of a loose cytoplasmic network formed from processes of the epithelial cells, among which are scattered the lymphocytes. Epithelial cells are also present in the cortex but are not usually evident because they are obscured by the closely-packed cortical lymphocytes and, at this site, they tend to be more attenuated. The rounded structure is a Hassall's corpuscle (*arrow*) which has undergone cystic change – a common finding. The red material seen at its centre consists of cell debris mixed with keratinous material. *(H&E)*

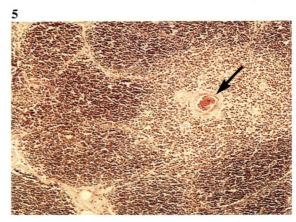

**6 Normal child's thymus, reticulin content** This figure demonstrates the sparse reticulin fibre pattern, which is in marked contrast to the rich reticulin network present in lymph nodes (see **194**). Fibres are confined to the capsule and vascular septa and to the small vessels which penetrate the parenchyma; in particular, there is an absence of reticulin fibre at the cortico-medullary junction (*arrow*). *(Gordon & Sweets)*

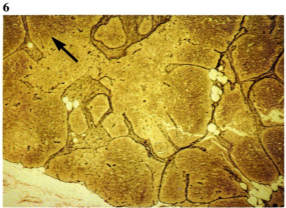

**7 Normal medullary epithelial cells** The processes of the thymic epithelial cells are shown here by a silver impregnation technique. This network of elongated branching and ramifying epithelial processes enclosing the lymphoid population is a normal characteristic of thymus. The darkly-staining bodies (*arrow*) are Hassall's corpuscles. This technique does not stain the reticulin fibre. *(Lithium carbonate)*

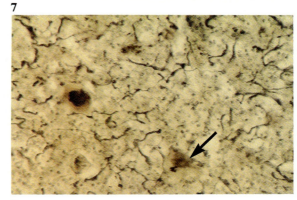

**8 Normal medulla, Hassall's corpuscles** Hassall's corpuscles are found in the medulla and are composed of aggregates of epithelial cells. These aggregates are not always rounded and may be elongated as shown here. Around the Hassall's corpuscles are a network of epithelial cells (*arrow*) and a population of lymphocytes showing some variation in size. The epithelial cell nuclei are pale and vesicular with a centrally placed nucleolus. The cytoplasm, though abundant, is poorly defined and forms communications with the cytoplasm of other epithelial cells. *(H&E)*

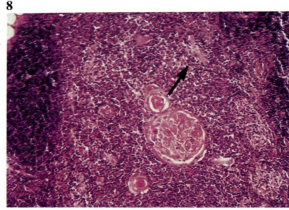

**9 Normal Hassall's corpuscles** Very often, the central portion appears cystic. The contents of the 'cyst' or lumen include degenerate, keratinised epithelial cells and other cellular elements such as myoid cells, lymphocytes and eosinophils. Trichrome stains are very useful in enhancing the different components of Hassall's corpuscles, and of the thymus gland in general. The keratin of the epithelium stains red as do some of the degenerate cells within the lumen, in contrast to the orange-brown granularity of the myoid cells (see **28–31**). *(Masson's trichrome)*

9

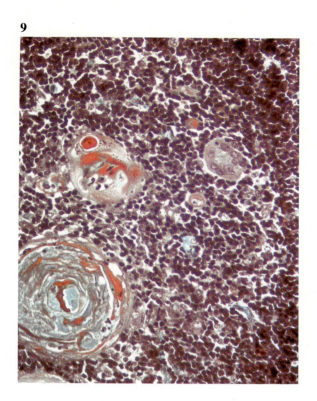

**10 Normal Hassall's corpuscles** The section has been specially stained to show the tonofibrils which are now seen as dark blue-staining fibres (*arrow*). The epithelial cell nucleoli of the Hassall's corpuscles and of the epithelial cell population in the surrounding medulla are also well demonstrated by this particular stain, and contrast with the lymphoid cells which show a densely aggregated chromatin pattern. *(Phosphotungstic acid/haematoxylin (PTAH))*

10

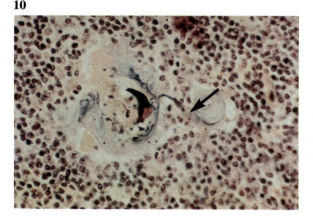

**11 Normal Hassall's corpuscles** In this section of resin-embedded material the features of a typical Hassall's corpuscle are emphasised. Note the concentric arrangement of the epithelial cells around the central cavity, and the dark blue staining keratinous material which consists of both tonofibrils and keratohyalin. *(Toluidine blue)*

11

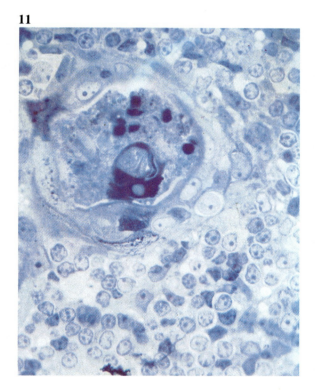

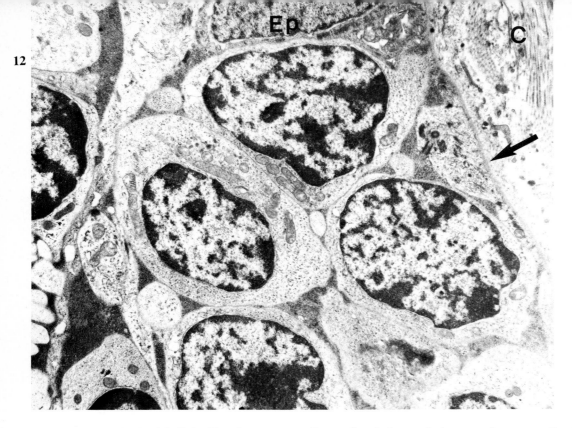

**12   Normal cortical epithelial cells, ultrastructure** Immediately beneath the capsular connective tissue (c) is a continuous network of thymic epithelial cells (Ep) enclosing groups of primitive lymphoid cells rich in RNA. These epithelial cells possess a basal lamina (*arrow*) where they abut on connective tissue whether this is of the capsule, septa or adventitia of blood vessels and they are continuous with the epithelial network of the medulla. Thus, there is an anatomical barrier formed by the epithelial cell network separating the lymphocytes from the vascular and connective tissue. *(× 6,500)*

**13   Normal cortico-medullary epithelial cells, ultrastructure** Elongated processes of epithelial cells pass between lymphocytes and contain prominent arrays of tonofilaments (*arrow* ). The epithelial cell nuclei often show the presence of nuclear bodies (Nb), structures which are increased in number in thymomas and in the active epithelial cells found in the thymuses of patients with myasthenia gravis. The cell (M) at the upper right field is a macrophage. *(× 12,200)*

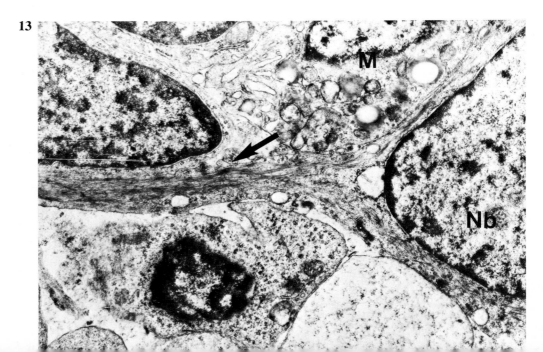

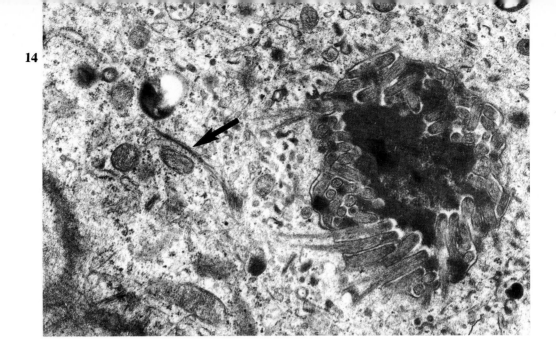

**14  Normal medullary epithelial cells, ultrastructure** Some medullary epithelial cells, in addition to showing the presence of tonofilaments (*arrow*), may show intracellular microcysts into which their cytoplasmic processes extend – in this case, cilia. Larger cysts (see **48**) may also be lined by ciliated epithelium. *(× 22,000)*

**15  Normal Hassall's corpuscle, ultrastructure** A portion of the luminal aspect of a Hassall's corpuscle is shown here. The epithelial cells contain much electron-dense fibrillar material (tonofilaments – t). Where the cytoplasm abuts on the central cavity or lumen, it shows numerous small villiform projections (microvilli) and encloses electron dense cellular debris. *(× 4,800)*

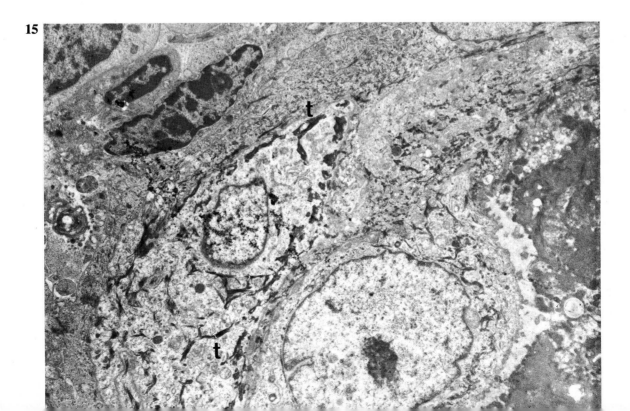

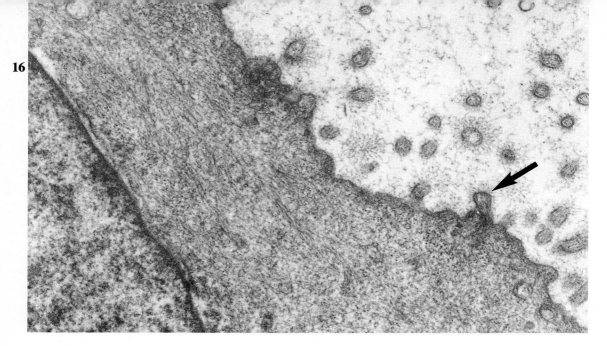

**16 Normal Hassall's corpuscle, ultrastructure**
Part of an epithelial cell forming a Hassall's corpuscle showing the microvilli lining the cavity is seen here. Note the glycocalyx coating (*arrow*) of the microvilli, which is similar in appearance to that coating glandular and absorptive cells in other anatomical sites. (× *68,000*)

**17 Normal Hassall's corpuscle, ultrastructure**
The cytoplasm of epithelial cells in the vicinity of Hassall's corpuscles often shows spherical membrane-bound dense core secretory granules (*arrow*). The precise nature of these granules is not known but they are considered to be related to the various thymic hormones currently being defined. (×*16,800*)

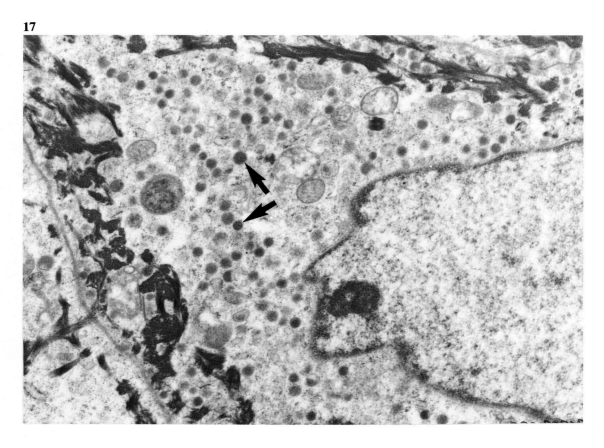

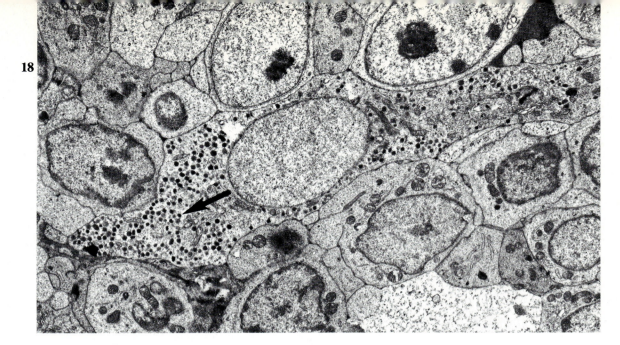

**18** Normal medulla, ultrastructure In some species (in this case, bird) scattered argentaffin cells are present in the medulla. At ultrastructural level these cells contain numerous dense core secretory granules (*arrow*) larger in size than those present in human epithelial cells. *(× 5,350)*

**19** Mucin secretion in foetal thymus The thymus from this still-born infant shows some involution and numerous active Hassall's corpuscles. Mucin secretion is evident both within the epithelial cells of the Hassall's corpuscles and in individual medullary epithelial cells. Much of the mucin is a sulphated acid mucopolysaccharide. *(Alcian blue/ neutral red)*

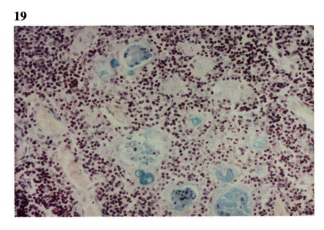

**20** Mucin secretion in normal adult thymus Mucin secretion is demonstrated here as a single globule of mucus within an aggregate of epithelial cells. It is a normal property of thymic epithelium but is not usually evident at light microscopical level unless there is hyperplasia of the epithelial component, or there is a defect of mucin secretion (see **24**), or unless special staining techniques have been employed. *(Mucicarmine/green filter)*

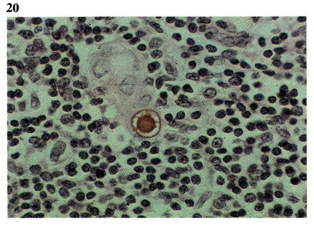

**21**

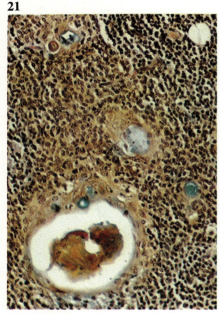

**22**

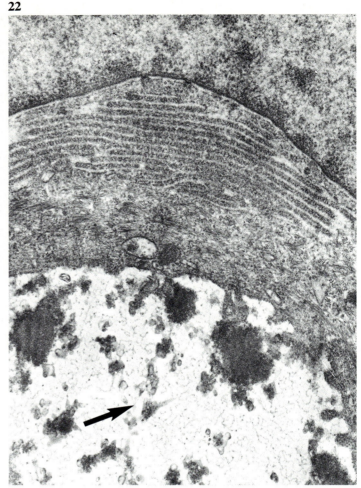

**21  Mucin secretion in normal child's thymus** Well-defined mucin droplets are seen in the Hassall's corpuscles and in adjacent epithelial cells. This active mucin production supports the concept of the Hassall's corpuscles as dynamic units rather than effete worn-out structures. The granular orange brown cell in the upper left-hand field is a thymic myoid cell. *(Alcian blue/phloxine tartrazine)*

**22  Mucin secretion in normal adult thymus, ultrastructure** Enclosed within the cytoplasm of this epithelial cell is a large mucus droplet aggregated into amorphous electron-dense material. Mucin in a more finely divided form (*arrow*) is also evident. *(× 33,000)*

**23  Mucin secretion in an abnormal adult thymus** This thymus was from a patient with rheumatic heart disease (see also **93**). The epithelial component is hyperplastic and mucus secretion (*arrow*) is abundant. Increased mucus secretion is also a feature of some thymuses in myasthenia gravis (see **81** and **82**). *(Periodic acid Schiff (PAS))*

**23**

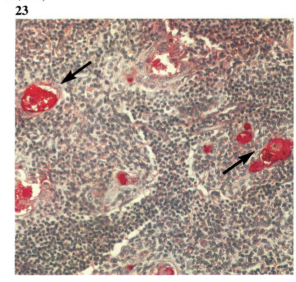

**24 Mucin secretion in abnormal infant thymus**
This thymus from a baby who died of cystic fibrosis of the pancreas shows abundant acid mucopolysaccharide secretion. Many of the Hassall's corpuscles are distended with mucin which, with this staining procedure, stains purple (*arrow*). No nuclear counter stain has been used. *(Alcian blue/periodic acid Schiff (AB/PAS))*

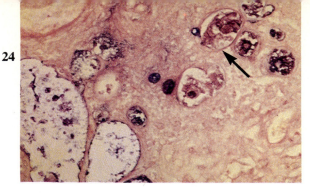

**25 Imprint from normal foetal thymus** By the imprint technique the lymphoid cells appear more variable in size than in conventional paraffin processed material, and range from small mature lymphocytes (thymocytes) to larger immature (blast) forms. Occasional eosinophils (*arrow*) are also present. *(May-Grünwald/Giemsa)*

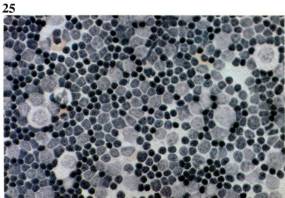

**26 Eosinophils in normal foetal thymus**
Eosinophils are a normal component of thymus, particularly in children and infants, when they may be very numerous. Often there is a predominance of immature cell forms (*arrow*). Such collections of eosinophils usually occur within the septal connective tissue. Mast cells are another normal cellular component of thymus. They are increased in inflammations of the thymus (thymitis) (see **74** and **75**) and in some species, such as dog, are numerous. *(H&E)*

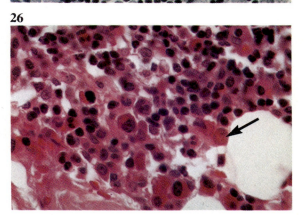

**27 Germinal centres in normal thymus** A lymphoid follicle with a well-defined germinal centre is present within the medulla of this thymic lobule. The thymus is a primary or central lymphoid organ concerned with the generation and control of immunologically competent T-lymphocytes acting outside the organ, and is not concerned with local immune reactions involving the B-cells series (see **0**). However, lymphoid follicles with germinal centres are occasionally present in the thymic medulla of apparently normal individuals; presumably, they reflect a low background response to antigenic material by immunologically competent B-lymphoid cells present within the thymus. *(H&E)*

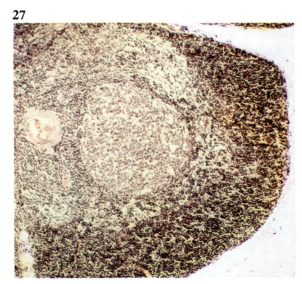

**28 Myoid cells in foetal thymus** The structures
shown here are thymic striated muscle – or myoid
cells. They range from infrequent elongated forms
with visible cross striations to more numerous
rounded cells resembling rhabdomyoblasts ( *blue* )
in which the myofilaments are arranged in a
haphazard manner. Myoid cells are a normal
component of thymus and can be found at all ages
if looked for. They are not recognised easily in
routine H&E preparations, being more readily
seen by special staining techniques. *(PTAH)*

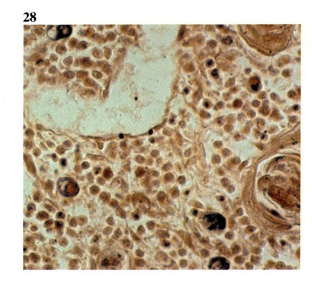

**29 Myoid cell in adult thymus** The well-
developed cross striations in this
elongated myoid cell are easily visible by
special staining. Such obvious cross striations are, however, uncommon. Myoid
cells occur most frequently at the cortico-
medullary junction and in the vicinity of
Hassall's corpuscles but are present, also,
in the cortex where they are even more
difficult to identify at light microscopical
level. They are very numerous and well-
formed in certain species, particularly
birds and reptiles. In all these locations
they are found in intimate contact with
epithelial cells, sometimes to such an
extent that the two types of cells appear
fused (see **33**). *(PTAH)*

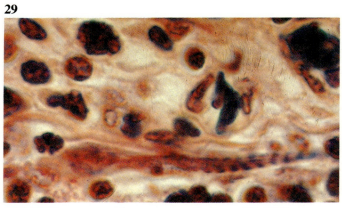

**30 Myoid cells in adult thymus** Myoid cells are
more conspicuous when they occur in
multinucleate form (*arrow*). The nuclei are
peripheral and the abundant granular cytoplasm is
here stained blue. They were termed 'myoidzellen'
by the German anatomists of the last century for,
although they noted the morphological
resemblance to striated muscle, they still
considered them to represent altered thymic
reticular (epithelial) cells. *(PTAH)*

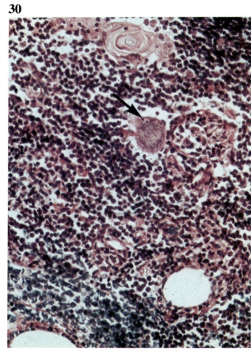

**31 Myoid cells in adult thymus** This resin-embedded binucleate myoid cell (*arrow*) shows nuclear irregularity and prominent nucleoli but no visible cross striations. As shown here, myoid cells are not only closely associated with the epithelium of Hassall's corpuscles, but even may be seen in degenerate form *within* the corpuscles (see **86**). *(Toluidine blue)*

**32 Immunofluorescent preparation of myoid cells in a child's thymus** The myoid antigen is similar to that of skeletal and cardiac muscle. Thus, when serum known to contain antibody to striated muscle (*myoid antibody*) is conjugated with fluorescein-isothyocyanate and then applied to a section of normal child's thymus, innumerable fluorescent cells are demonstrated. In this preparation none show visible cross-striations: the faintly stained structure seen at the extreme left is a Hassall's corpuscle. *(Fluorescein isothyocyanate)*

**33 Myoepithelial complex, ultrastructure** At ultrastructural level, myoid cells are seen frequently in close relation to epithelial cells including those of Hassall's corpuscles and with which there are desmosomal connections. The term 'myoepithelial complex' is suggested for these structures. As in this myoid cell (M), there is no orderly alignment of myofilaments (*arrow*), hence in light microscopic preparations regular cross-striations are rarely visible. *(× 12,000)*

31

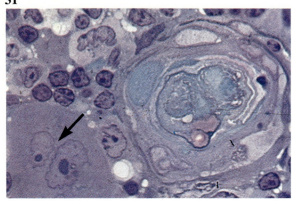

32

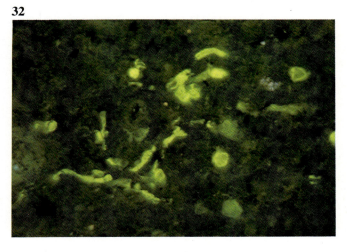

33

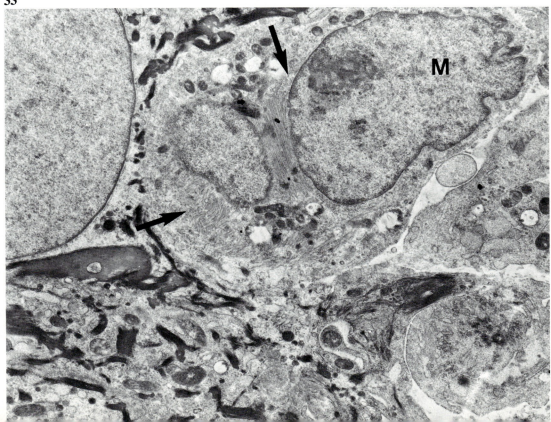

**34**

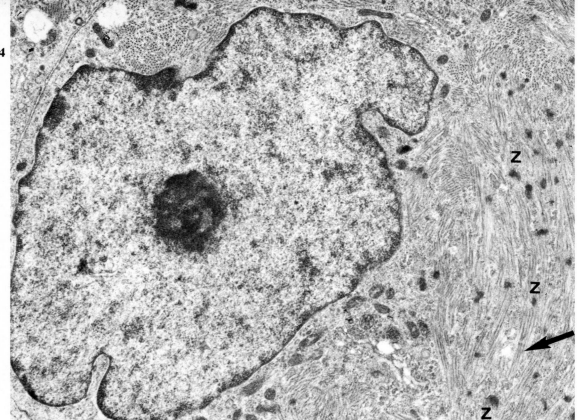

**34 Myoid cell in adult thymus, ultrastructure** In
this myoid cell both thick myosin and thin actin
filaments are present within the cytoplasm but
have been cut at various angles. In the upper field
most of the fibres are transversely sectioned while
to the right of the nucleus they are predominantly
sectioned longitudinally and appear as short runs
of myofilaments (*arrow* ) between primitive Z
lines (Z) and dense bodies (×4,300)

**35 Myoid cell, ultrastructure** Part of the periphery
of a myoid cell is seen with the presence of primitive sarcomeres consisting of both thick myosin
and thin actin filaments aligned between Z lines
(Z). There is abundant glycogen, a well-formed
basal lamina where the cell abuts on connective
tissue, and scattered triads (Tr) in relation to the
sarcoplasmic reticulum. (× 48,000)

**35**

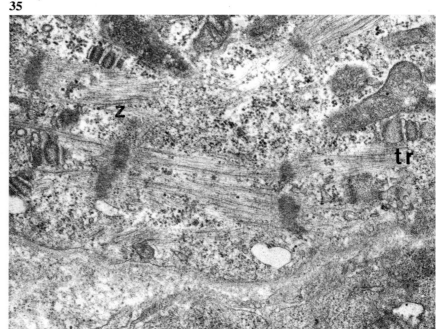

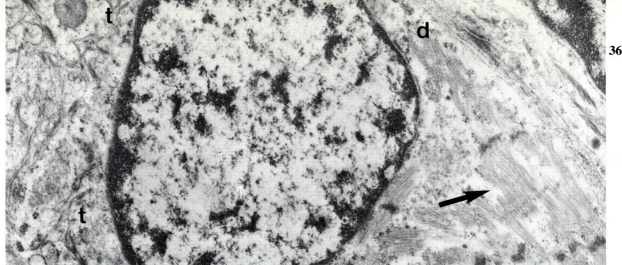

**36 Thymic myoid/epithelial cells, ultrastructure** In addition to myoid/epithelial complexes, there are in both normal and myasthenic thymuses occasional cells which apparently contain tonofilaments (t) in addition to thick and thin myofilaments (*arrow*) as shown here. No cytoplasmic membrane was visible between the two areas of specialisation. Because of the very close association of myoid cells to epithelium it is also possible that these apparently hybrid cells arise by fusion rather than representing dual differentiation of the embryonic thymic cells. Desmosome, d. *(× 19,600)*

**37 and 38 Thymus from young adults showing early age involution** With age the thymic parenchyma gradually shrinks in size and is replaced by fat. This process of involution is known as age or physiological involution and starts soon after puberty. In the thymus in **37** there is early involution but the thymic lobules between the adipose tissue show a normal architecture with a normal reticulin pattern (see also **6**). The thymus in **38** also shows early involution and fatty replacement but this patient had myasthenia gravis and there is a lymphoid follicle with a germinal centre in the medulla (see also **54–57**). *(37 Gordon & Sweets; 38 H&E)*

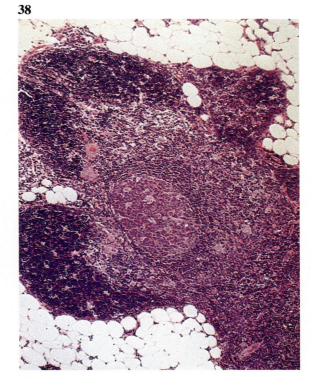

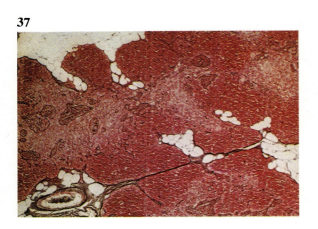

**39 Thymus from a middle-aged patient showing advanced age involution** Eventually, with further ageing, all that remains are small irregular strands of tissue composed of lymphocytes and shrunken epithelial cells, and occasional calcified Hassall's corpuscles (*arrow*). This age or physiological involution must be taken into account always when assessing thymic histopathology. Failure to identify atrophic thymic tissue also causes diagnostic difficulty as, for example, when such tissue is present in biopsy material taken during parathyroid exploration. *(H&E)*

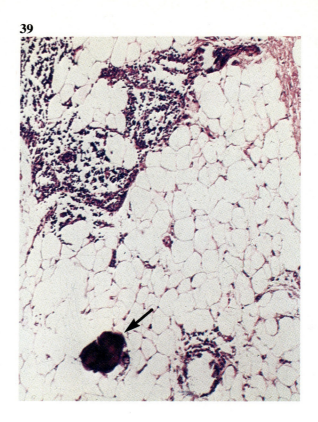

**40 Stress involution in stillborn infant's thymus** Early evidence of so-called stress or accidental involution of the thymus is aggregation or clumping of the cortical lymphocytes, accompanied by necrosis. This process, seen here, is known also as steroid-induced involution and acute lympholysis, and results in a rather mottled or moth-eaten appearance of the cortex, which is in marked contrast to the dense, closely-packed lymphocytic zone of normal thymic cortex. *(H&E)*

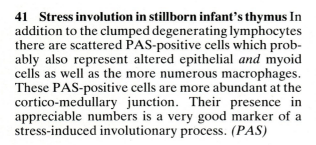

**41 Stress involution in stillborn infant's thymus** In addition to the clumped degenerating lymphocytes there are scattered PAS-positive cells which probably also represent altered epithelial *and* myoid cells as well as the more numerous macrophages. These PAS-positive cells are more abundant at the cortico-medullary junction. Their presence in appreciable numbers is a very good marker of a stress-induced involutionary process. *(PAS)*

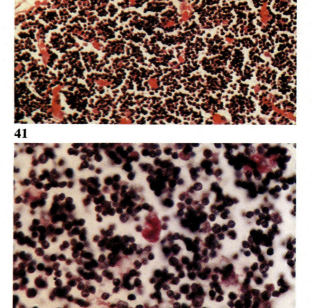

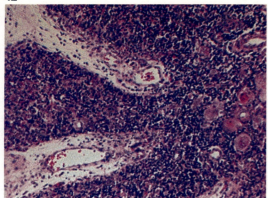

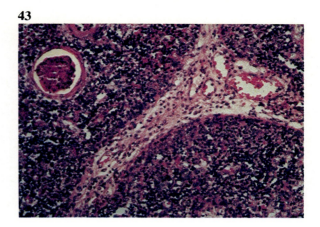

**42 and 43   Stress involution in neonatal thymuses**
If the involutionary process proceeds, there will be
a reduction in thymic volume. At first the lobular
pattern is retained, **42**, but the absence of the
darkly staining cortex results in a uniform appearance of the thymic parenchyma. At higher
magnification, **43**, this uniformity of staining can
be identified as a result of a reduction in the
numbers of cortical lymphocytes (thymocytes).
The cortical epithelial cells are now revealed and
the small veins and anterioles also appear
prominent. Note the palisade arrangement of the
cortical epithelial cells where they abut on the
connective tissue of the capsule. *(H&E)*

**44   Stress involution of the thymus in a young child**
The section includes both the left and right glands
(see **1** and **2**) and emphasises the marked
involution of this thymus with its shrunken thymic
lobules widely separated by increased amounts of
connective tissue. The cause of the involution in
this child was prolonged steroid administration; it
is seen also in a number of diseases characterised
by chronic wasting or infection, following X-rays
or radiomimetic drugs, in certain physiologic states
such as pregnancy or lactation, and in stillbirths as
already illustrated. *(PAS)*

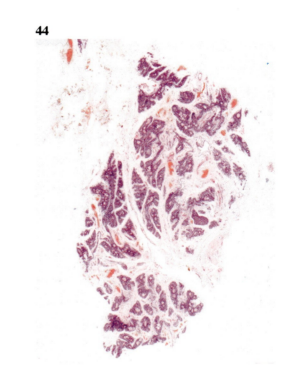

**45   Stress involution in the thymus of a young
child** There is a very marked reduction in the
thymic lymphocyte population particularly in
the cortex. The resultant irregular shrunken
lobules are composed of spindle-shaped
epithelial cells (*arrows*) and there is loss of demarcation between cortex and medulla. The
Hassall's corpuscles are often cystic and,
because they are crowded together,
appear increased in number. An alternative
term to stress or accidental involution, is
steroid-induced involution and acute
lympholysis, since the basis of this lesion is a
massive emigration/destruction of thymic
cortical lymphocytes mediated via the
pituitary adrenal axis. *(H&E)*

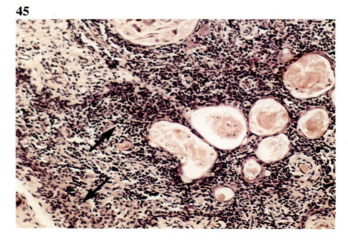

**46  Involution and cyst formation in a patient with a chronic debilitating disease** The thymic lobules are irregular and shrunken, and aggregation and fusion of Hassall's corpuscles has resulted in the formation of a cystic space lined by flattened epithelium, as seen on the left-hand side. Thus at least some forms of thymic cysts are considered to arise from dilatation and fusion of the Hassall's corpuscles. *(H&E)*

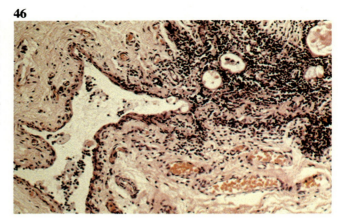

**47  Involution and cyst formation** This cyst is filled with red and blue-staining mucin, and is still in continuity with a moderately age-involuted thymus. Sometimes, however, thymic cysts attain a large size when their relationship to the thymus is not always appreciated. *(AB/PAS)*

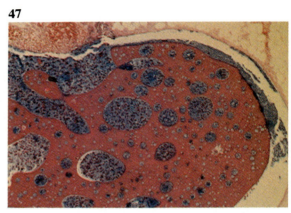

**48  Ciliated cysts** Another type of cyst occasionally seen is lined by ciliated respiratory-type epithelium *(arrow)*. This small cyst contains flocculent mucoid material and a few lymphocytes, and is present within a markedly involuted thymus. *(H&E)*

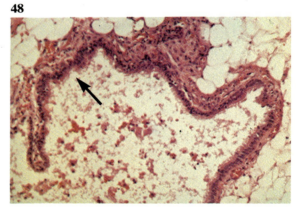

**49  Epithelial islands in thymus** A compact island of hyperplastic epithelial cells of variable morphology is shown here, adjacent to remnants of a calcified Hassall's corpuscle *(arrow)*. Such islands are a relatively common finding in age-involuted thymus, but may occur at any age in abnormal thymuses and it is possible that some such islands represent the earliest stage of thymoma formation. *(H&E)*

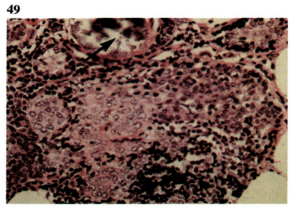

**50 Diagramatic representation of the sites of the defects in some of the immune deficiency syndromes** Defects of thymic development are shown in relation to both bone marrow and to the third branchial arch. Such defective development is mainly expressed morphologically as aplasia. Mesenchymal abnormalities may contribute also to some defects of thymic function. In adults, thymic neoplasms – thymomas – are sometimes associated with acquired immunological defects such as hypogammaglobulinaemia.

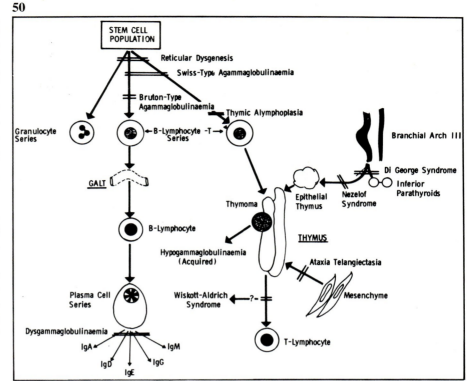

**51 Thymic aplasia in an infant** The thymic lobules are widely separated by fat and appear small and hypoplastic. There is no development of cortex and there is a striking absence of Hassall's corpuscles. Such aplastic thymuses often fail to descend into the mediastinum and remain in the neck as bilateral rudimentary structures. *(H&E)*

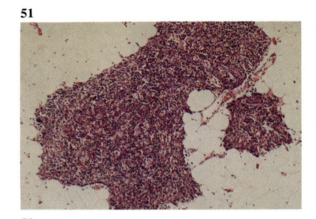

**52 Thymic aplasia in an infant** Part of an aplastic lobule, illustrating that the majority of cells are epithelial and that, while there are a few lymphocytes, there is no lymphoid aggregation to form a cortex; nor is there epithelial aggregation to form Hassall's corpuscles. *(H&E)*

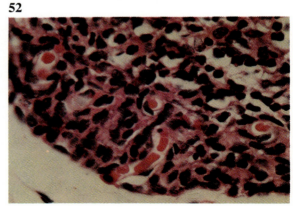

## The Thymus in myasthenia gravis

It has long been known that a relationship exists between myasthenia gravis and abnormalities of the thymus gland – either in the form of an inflammatory lesion or as a thymic tumour – thymoma. This relationship is emphasised still further by remission and even complete cure following thymectomy in some patients with myasthenia gravis, usually those without thymoma and in whom the duration of the disease has been short. The inflammatory lesion formerly described as thymic hyperplasia is found in 75–80 per cent of patients with myasthenia gravis without thymoma and is characterised by increased numbers of lymphoid cells within the medulla, together with the formation of lymphoid follicles and germinal centres, often in close association to hyperplastic epithelium and degenerate myoid cells. This inflammation is now generally interpreted as an auto-immune thymitis but the exact mechanism whereby thymitis results in the abnormality of the motor end plate (the site of the lesion in myasthenia gravis) has been understood rather poorly until recently. The myoid antibody occurring in patients with myasthenia gravis which reacts with the striated muscle cells of skeletal and cardiac muscle and to the myoid cells (see **84–89**) within the thymus is not the cause of the myasthenic symptoms; in particular, the myoid antibody is not directed at the motor end plate. Furthermore, it is present in patients with thymoma but without myasthenia gravis. Thus the recent finding that over 80 per cent of myasthenic patients possess an antibody reacting with the acetylcholine receptor (AChR) substance of the motor end plate is of extreme aetiological importance. The formation of this AChR antibody is still the subject of debate. The authors are in no doubt, however, that the myoid cells – ubiquitous to the thymus and which are so frequently found often in degenerate form in association with the inflammatory lesion of myasthenic thymitis – are a source of antigen, provoking the formation of the antibody: a belief supported by the finding of receptor substance to AChR on both epithelial and myoid cells, and the demonstration within thymus of apparently fused epithelial and myoid cells. The mechanism whereby thymomas result in myasthenia gravis is much less clear-cut since thymectomy is followed infrequently by remission and there is no good correlation between the existence of AChR antibody in these patients and their disease. However, residual thymic tissue around thymomas often shows similar abnormalities observed in non-thymomatous myasthenia gravis.

**53**

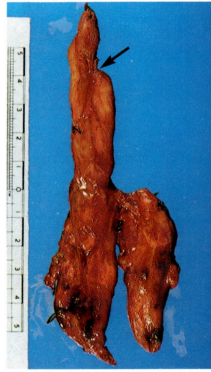

**53 Thymectomy specimen from a patient with myasthenia gravis** The two 'lobes' are quite distinct and do not show the degree of age or physiological involution appropriate to the 29-year-old patient. The right half of the organ has a prominent and elongated cervical portion (*arrow*).

**54 Myasthenia gravis without thymoma** This section of the thymus from a 33-year-old patient is typical of the pathological changes found in myasthenia gravis without thymoma. There is a relative absence of age involution and while lobular structure is maintained, the cortex (*arrow*) is reduced in size at the expense of a greatly widened medulla. Numerous lymphoid follicles with well-defined germinal centres are present within the medulla and represent the most easily recognised and characteristic thymic abnormality. (*H&E*)

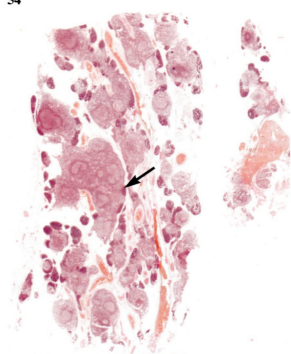

**55 Myasthenia gravis without thymoma** This expanded medulla contains several lymphoid follicles with well-demarcated germinal centres, and increased numbers of lymphoid cells. The epithelial component including Hassall's corpuscles is prominent, and the reduced cortex appears as an irregular rim of darkly-staining tissue. This appearance, formerly described as thymic hyperplasia, is now considered to represent an auto-immune inflammatory process – thymitis – and is seen in approximately 75–80 per cent of non-thymomatous myasthenic thymuses. Thymitis may be graded as mild (Grade I), moderate (Grade II) or severe (Grade III) according to the number and size of the germinal centres within a given area. (*H&E*)

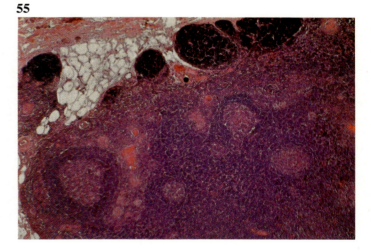

**56 Myasthenia gravis without thymoma** This example of severe thymitis (Grade III) in a patient with non-thymomatous myasthenia gravis shows prominent germinal centres. The epithelium is markedly hyperplastic and on the left-hand field forms well-demarcated irregular islands. Alteration in the epithelial component (in this case resulting in an archipelago-like appearance) with or without lymphoid follicles with germinal centres, is seen also in other diseases associated with thymic pathology – such as systemic lupus erythematosus. (*H&E*)

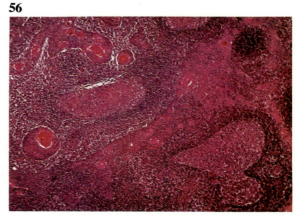

**57 Myasthenia gravis without thymoma** A conspicuous finding in this disease is the presence of Hassall's corpuscles and hyperplastic epithelium ranged around the lymphoid follicles with their germinal centres. This arrangement supports the concept that the source of the antigen provoking the germinal centre formation is related to the epithelial component and/or their associated myoid cells (see **84–89**). In this patient the thymus has undergone age involution. *(H&E)*

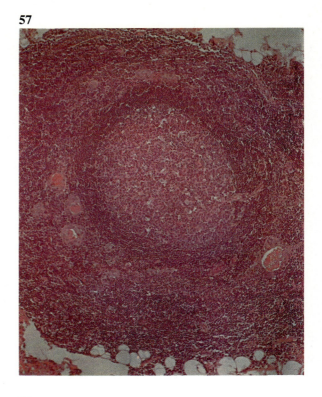

**58 Lymphoid follicles in myasthenia gravis** The lymphoid follicles and germinal centres which form within the medulla are morphologically comparable with those found in peripheral lymphoreticular tissue (see **197–200**). In this field the majority of follicle centre cells are small and irregular but there are some occasional large 'blast' cells (*arrow* ), and there is part of the surrounding mantle of small mature lymphocytes on the left. *(H&E)*

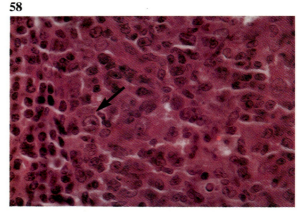

**59 Lymphoid follicles in myasthenia gravis** The reticulin content is also similar to follicles at other sites (see **226**) with the fibres mainly being external to the mantle zone. Note the closely associated Hassall's corpuscles (*arrow*) and the small vessels delineated by reticulin. *(Gordon & Sweets)*

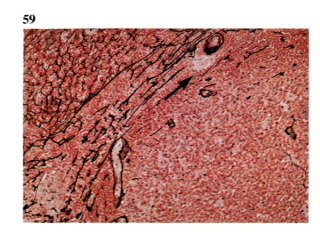

**60 Lymphoid follicles in myasthenia gravis** Like all reactive germinal centres there is a prominent component of pyroninophilic cells – stained red – which include both 'blast' forms and plasma cells. Plasma cells are also present in the cuff and surrounding parenchyma. *(Methyl green-pyronin (MGP))*

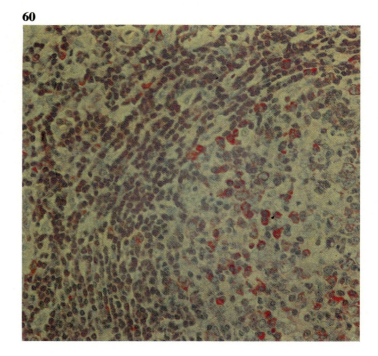

**61 Germinal centres in myasthenia gravis** Occasionally, there is a striking accumulation of immunoglobulin within the plasma cells of the germinal centres so that these cells are seen easily in routine preparations *(arrows)*. Such prominent B-cell proliferation with plasma cell differentiation is consistent with the view that the various antibodies associated with myasthenia gravis are produced locally within the thymus. *(H&E)*

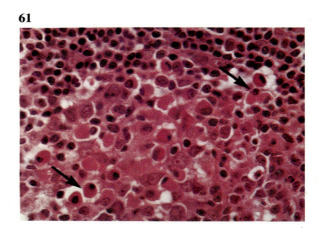

**62 Germinal centres in myasthenia gravis** Trichrome stains are very valuable in detecting stored immunoglobulin. In this germinal centre occasional plasma cells are seen with their cytoplasm staining the characteristic crimson of IgA or IgG. This staining procedure also clearly delineates the other cellular components of the germinal centre with the well-defined nuclear contours of the various cell types standing out sharply against the green background. *(Masson's trichrome)*

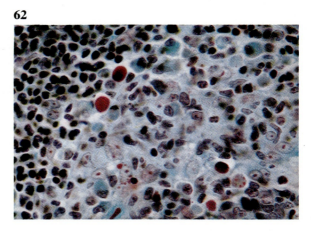

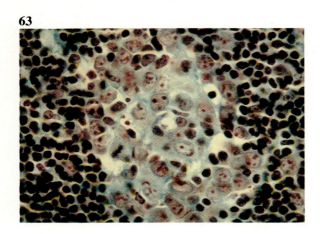

**63 Germinal centres in myasthenia gravis** In this very small, early, germinal centre, most of the cells present show the nuclear characteristics of centroblasts with finely dispersed chromatin and several nucleoli – often in relation to the nuclear membrane. Such small germinal centres are often overlooked or interpreted as groups of epithelial cells. *(Masson's trichrome)*

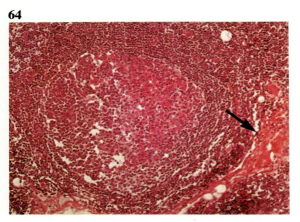

**64 and 65 Polarity of germinal centres in myasthenia gravis** Biphasic staining due to the different cellular components is a frequent finding in the germinal centres. The paler staining less cellular dendritic zone as seen in **64** contrasts with the darker staining zone rich in lymphoid cells and tingeable body macrophages. Figure **65** includes two germinal centres with prominent polarity. The paler staining dendritic zones are nearest the epithelial/myoid cell complexes (*arrows*), the putative source of antigen. Note the epithelial hyperplasia and the cystic Hassall's corpuscle. *(64 H&E; 65 Masson's trichrome)*

**66 Germinal centres in myasthenia gravis – post-reactive eosinophilic change** Just as in lymph nodes (see **233** and **234**), the germinal centres in myasthenic thymitis may occasionally appear eosinophilic due to the intercellular deposition of proteinaceous material. The cellular components of such centres appear inactive with little evidence of proliferation, and support the view that eosinophilic change is a post-reactive degenerative manifestation. *(H&E)*

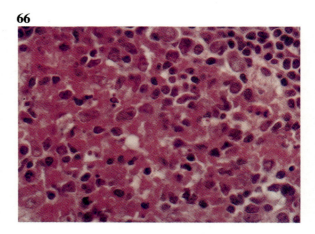

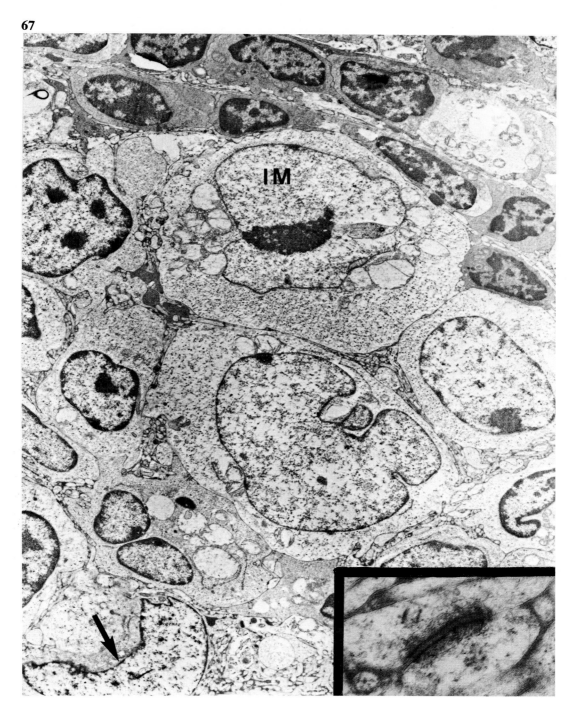

**67 Germinal centres in myasthenia gravis, ultrastructure** Part of a germinal centre is shown at the junction with the cuff of small lymphocytes. Variable-sized lymphoid cells are present and include an immunoblast (IM) rich in cytoplasmic RNA and with the characteristic large nucleolus in association with the nuclear membrane. The cell at the bottom (*arrow*) is a dendritic cell with complex cytoplasmic processes, between which are electron dense protein-aceous material. The inset shows a desmosomal contact between processes of dendritic cells. (× 5,800; inset × 37,200)

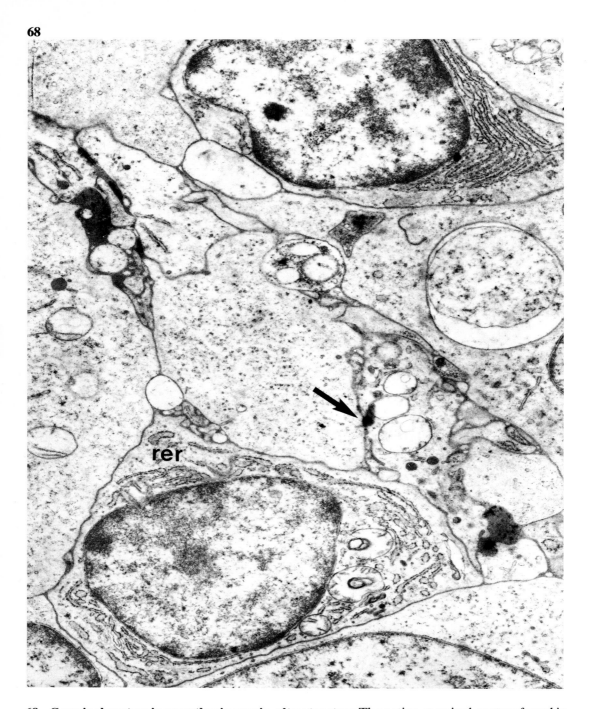

**68 Germinal centres in myasthenia gravis, ultrastructure** The active germinal centres found in myasthenic thymitis also resemble active lymph nodal germinal centres in that both contain plasma cells. Immunoglobulin can be seen within the rough endoplasmic reticulum (rer) in both the plasma cells shown here. Note the desmosome connecting dendritic cell processes (*arrow*). (× 12,800)

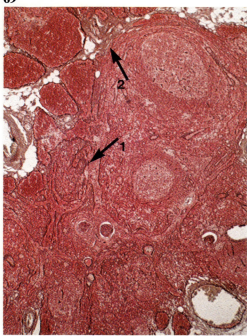

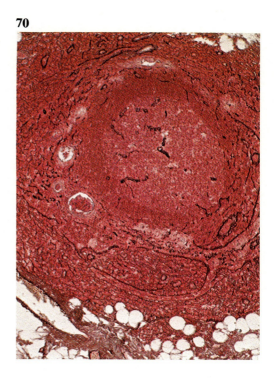

**69 Reticulin pattern in myasthenia gravis without thymoma** In contrast to the normal thymus with its sparse reticulin, the inflammatory process in myasthenia gravis is associated with a prominent reticulin network. Most of the reticulin is present in the medulla around the lymphoid follicles and at the cortico-medullary junction (*arrow 1*) and septa (*arrow 2*). (*Gordon & Sweets*)

**70 Reticulin pattern in myasthenia gravis without thymoma** It has been stated that in myasthenia gravis the lymphoid follicles with germinal centre formation are found within the septa (extraparenchymal compartment) and not in the medulla. This view is contrary to the authors' findings and, as shown here, reticulin preparations confirm that the lymphoid follicles are in direct continuity with the medulla and in intimate association with the Hassall's corpuscles. (*Gordon & Sweets*)

**71 Plasma cells in myasthenia gravis without thymoma** In the thymitis of non-thymomatous myasthenia gravis (myasthenic thymitis), in addition to an overall increase in the number of lymphocytes there is usually a striking increase in the number of plasma cells – stained reddish-pink – in the medulla and septa. In normal thymus only occasional plasma cells are present, though they may be increased in some involuted thymuses. (*MGP*)

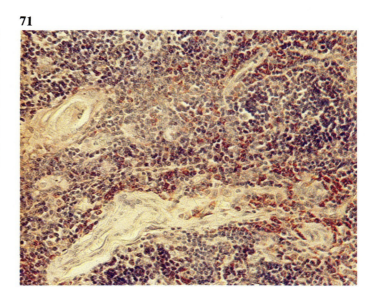

**72 Plasma cells in myasthenic thymitis** As in the germinal centres, the medulla also may contain plasma cells with cytoplasm distended with secretory products (Russell bodies) here stained red. *(Masson's trichrome)*

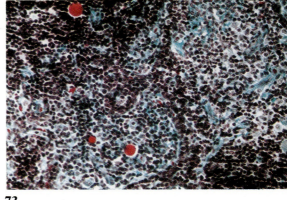

**73 Differentiation of medullary lymphoid cells in myasthenia gravis** This high-power field contains lymphocytes, a number of pyroninophilic plasma cells and an immunoblast *(arrow)* in close proximity to a group of epithelial cells on the right, and emphasises the range of 'differentiation' of the reactive lymphocytic infiltrate in myasthenic thymitis. *(MGP)*

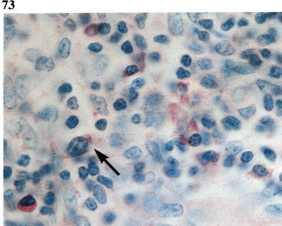

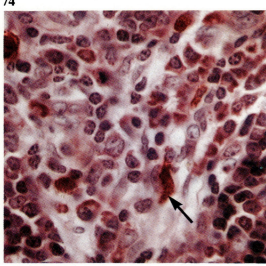

**74 Mast cells in myasthenia gravis** Mast cells are increased in number in thymitis, but are seen poorly in routine preparations. With pyronin staining, mast cells are seen easily; in contrast to the rose-pink of the cytoplasm of the plasma cells, mast cell granules are stained an intense orange-red colour *(arrow)*. *(MGP/Haematoxylin)*

**75 Perivascular spaces in myasthenia gravis** Perivascular spaces are not apparent in normal thymus glands. Occasionally, however, dilated perivascular spaces are conspicuous in myasthenic thymitis not associated with tumour (see **117–120**). In this thymus showing some age involution, the perivascular spaces contain not only lymphocytes but mast cells-here stained blue. *(AB/PAS)*

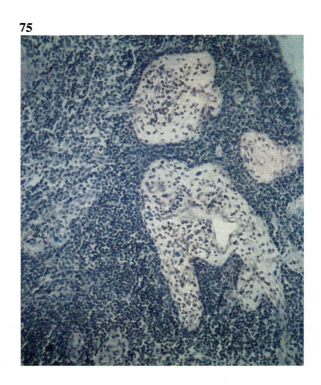

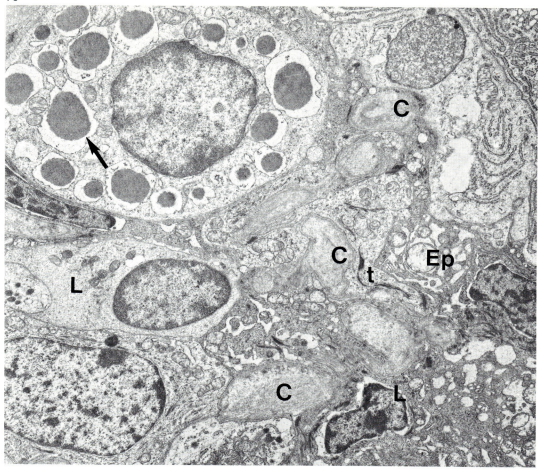

**76 Thymitis in myasthenia gravis, ultrastructure** A representative field in thymitis illustrating lymphocytes (L), actively secreting plasma cells containing immunoglobulin seen as electron dense material (*arrow*), and portions of hyperplastic epithelial cells (Ep).Between the cellular components are bundles of collagen (C). Tonofilaments = t. *(× 7,500)*

**77 Hyperplasia in myasthenia gravis** In addition to the lymphoid hyperplasia, the epithelial component may also be hyperplastic and form prominent islands as shown here. It is the epithelial cells which secrete the various thymic hormones – including thymosine – currently being defined. Note the abundant blue-staining fine tonofilaments in the epithelial cell cytoplasm. *(PTAH)*

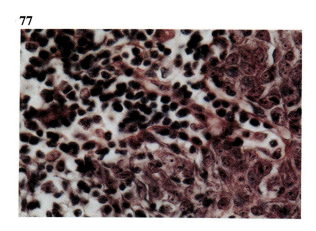

**78**

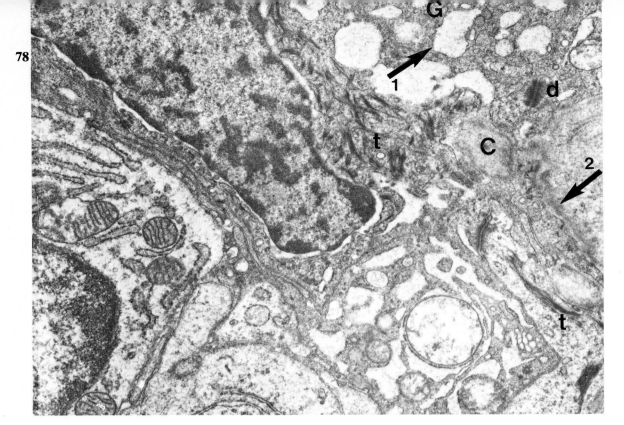

**78  Epithelial hyperplasia in myasthenia gravis, ultrastructure** At this level the hyperplastic epithelial cells contain distended endoplasmic reticulum (*arrow 1*) and a prominent Golgi apparatus denoting actively secreting cells. Branching tonofilaments (t) are numerous, there are well-formed desmosomes (d) and, where the epithelium adjoins connective tissue (C), there is a basal lamina (*arrow 2*). The cell on the left is a plasmablast. ( Golgi  - G )  *(× 18,150)*

**79**

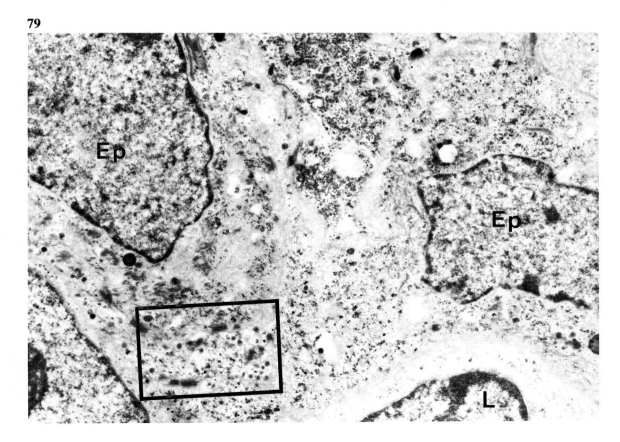

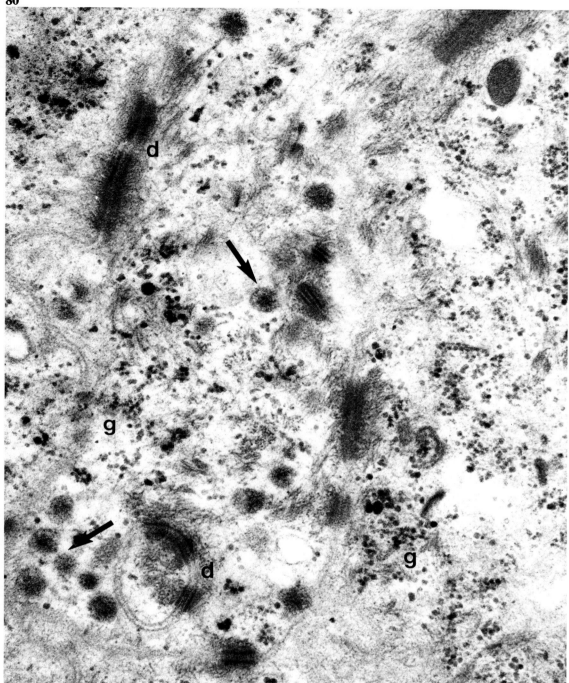

**79 and 80   Epithelial hyperplasia in myasthenia gravis, ultrastructure** Figure **79** shows parts of several hyperplastic epithelial cells (Ep) and a lymphocyte (L). The epithelial nuclei have large nucleoli and contain nuclear bodies. The cytoplasm contains much granular material and fine tonofilaments. Figure **80** shows the boxed field at higher magnification. The granular material consists both of glycogen (g) and membrane-bound secretory granules (*arrows*). Fine tonofilaments inserting into increased numbers of desmosomes (d) are prominent. *(**79** × 10,250; **80** × 52,800)*

39

**81**

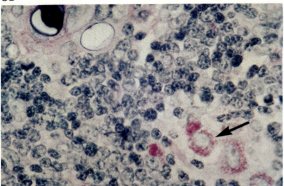

**82**

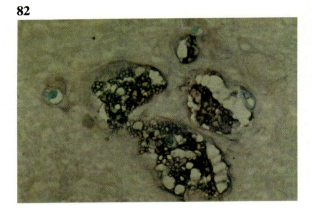

**81 Mucin secretion in myasthenia gravis** The epithelial component, including that of Hassall's corpuscles, may show increased mucin secretion. In this field the mucin is stained by alcian blue and PAS and thus appears as dark blue globules in contrast to the granular pink-staining of glycogen (*arrow*) which is stained only by the PAS technique. *(AB/PAS)*

**82 Mucin secretion in myasthenia gravis** This field shows a group of Hassall's corpuscles containing abundant mucin mainly in the form of brown-staining sulphated acid mucopolysaccharide. No nuclear counterstain has been used. *(High iron diamine (HID/AB))*

**83**

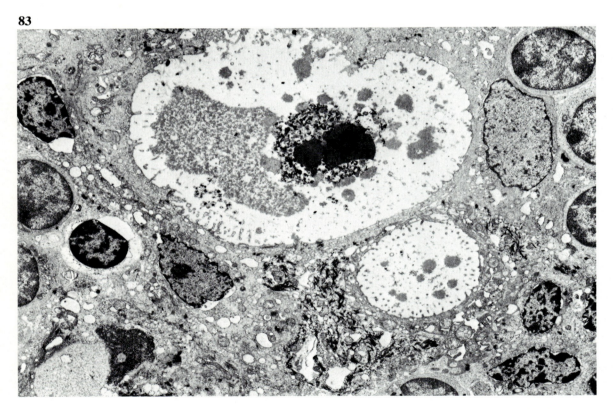

**83 Mucin secretion in myasthenia gravis, ultrastructure** In some examples of myasthenic thymitis, the epithelial component shows the formation of gland-like spaces lined by microvilli and containing mucin – similar to those found in normal thymus but more numerous. In this micrograph two such gland-like spaces are seen within a group of epithelial cells. *(× 4,800)*

**84**

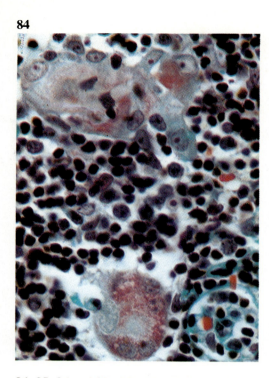

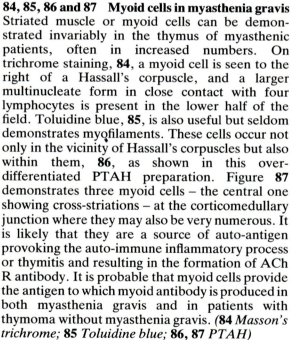

**85**

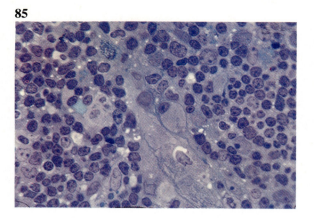

**86**

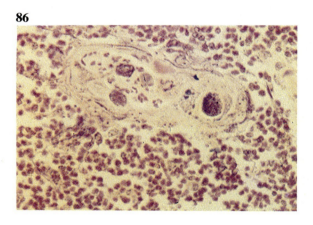

**84, 85, 86 and 87    Myoid cells in myasthenia gravis**
Striated muscle or myoid cells can be demonstrated invariably in the thymus of myasthenic
patients, often in increased numbers. On
trichrome staining, **84**, a myoid cell is seen to the
right of a Hassall's corpuscle, and a larger
multinucleate form in close contact with four
lymphocytes is present in the lower half of the
field. Toluidine blue, **85**, is also useful but seldom
demonstrates myofilaments. These cells occur not
only in the vicinity of Hassall's corpuscles but also
within them, **86**, as shown in this over-
differentiated PTAH preparation. Figure **87**
demonstrates three myoid cells – the central one
showing cross-striations – at the corticomedullary
junction where they may also be very numerous. It
is likely that they are a source of auto-antigen
provoking the auto-immune inflammatory process
or thymitis and resulting in the formation of ACh
R antibody. It is probable that myoid cells provide
the antigen to which myoid antibody is produced in
both myasthenia gravis and in patients with
thymoma without myasthenia gravis. (**84** *Masson's
trichrome;* **85** *Toluidine blue;* **86, 87** *PTAH*)

**87**

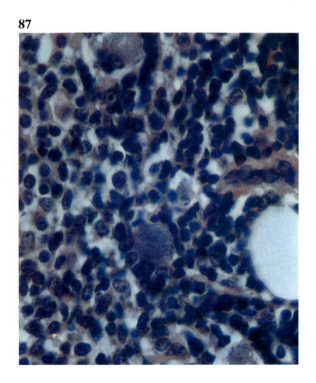

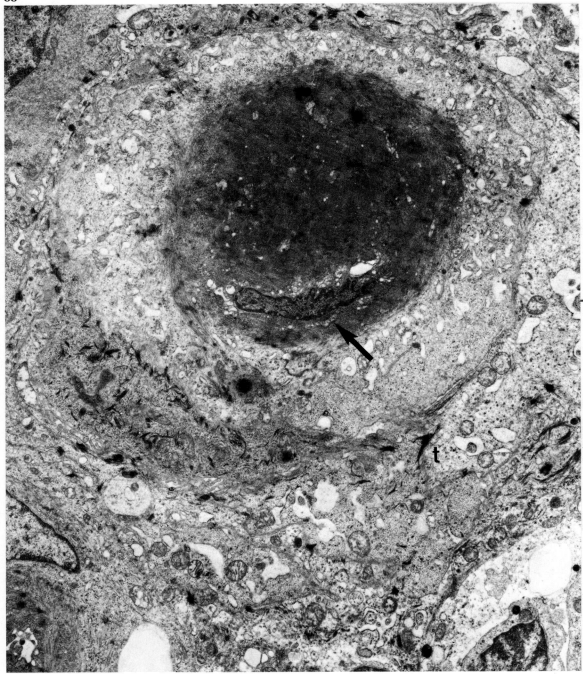

**88 and 89   Myoid/epithelial complex in myasthenia gravis, ultrastructure** Figure **88** shows a degenerate myoid cell closely surrounded by the cytoplasm of epithelial cells rich in tonofilaments (t), forming a myoid/epithelial complex. The myofilaments are condensed and form a large central electron dense body in which the nucleus (*arrow*) can be just discerned. The cell in the lower left corner is another myoid cell showing early degenerative changes including vacuolation. At higher magnification, **89**, the myofilaments at the periphery of the dense body are well preserved and are seen in both longitudinal (*arrow 1*) and transverse (*arrow 2*) sections. The very close contact between the cytoplasm of the myoid cell and that of the epithelial cell is striking. (**88** × *9,900;* **89** × *28,700*)

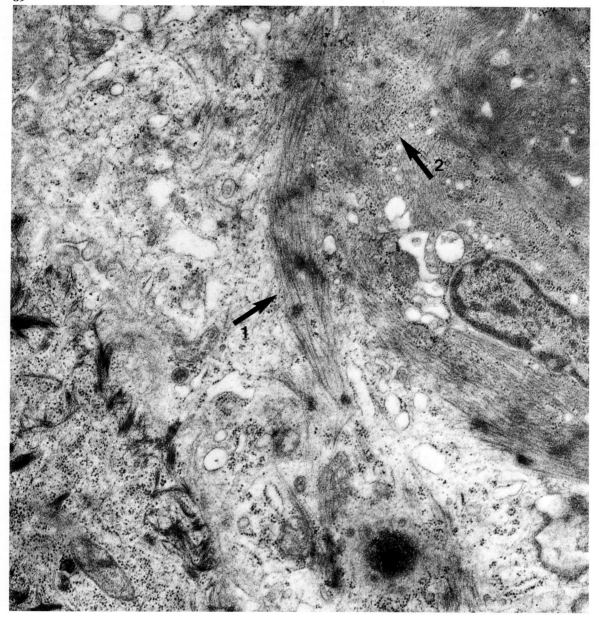

**90**

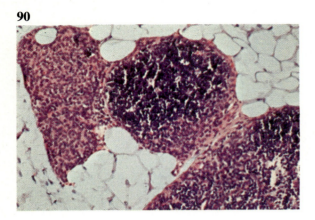

**91**

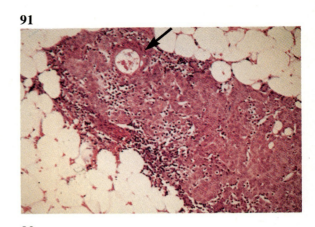

**92**

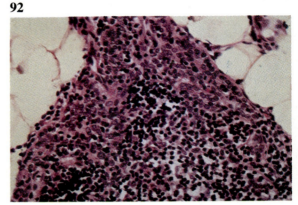

**90, 91 and 92 Epithelial islands in myasthenia gravis** In some myasthenic patients without tumour there are no medullary lymphoid follicles or light microscopic evidence of inflammation in the thymus. It is, therefore, of interest that in such thymuses occasional small islands of epithelium may be found, which may represent the earliest stages in the development of a thymoma. Figure **90** shows a small epithelial island *(left)* in which the component cells closely resemble those seen in a predominantly epithelial thymoma. Figure **91** shows an epithelial island with a distinct organoid pattern reminiscent of a carcinoid tumour (see **164**) which is in continuity with a Hassall's corpuscle-like structure *(arrow)*. Figure **92** demonstrates epithelial proliferation in the superficial cortical epithelium with the component cells assuming a more spindle cell configuration and mixed with lymphocytes. *(H&E)*

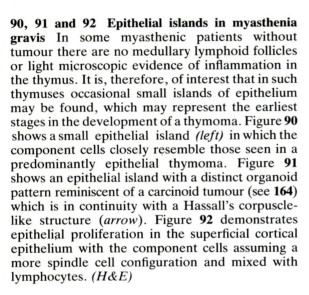

**93 Thymus in rheumatic heart disease** Thymuses from patients with rheumatic heart disease may show the presence of lymphoid follicles with germinal centres and, as in this example, an increase in the epithelial population with formation of numerous Hassall's corpuscles and abundant mucin production – stained red. Other diseases where the thymus may show inflammatory changes (thymitis) with or without abnormalities of the epithelial component, are rheumatoid arthritis, Sjögren's disease, systemic lupus erythematosus, Addison's disease and thyrotoxicosis. The lymphoid follicles are not generally so numerous as those seen in myasthenia gravis. *(PAS)*

**93**

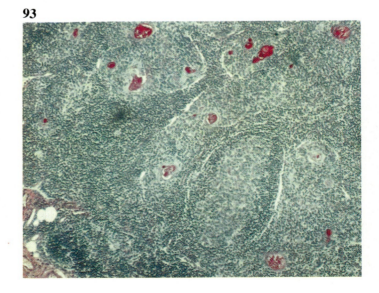

# Thymic tumours

Primary thymic tumours are not so rare as was thought. They are of particular interest in that approximately one third occur in patients who have evidence of other disease. Perhaps the best recognised association of thymic tumour with a disease is myasthenia gravis, which occurs in association with about 35 per cent of thymomas. Conversely, approximately 15 per cent of patients with myasthenia gravis have a primary tumour or thymoma of the thymus – *Thymomatous myasthenia gravis*. Whereas myasthenia gravis without tumour occurs predominantly in younger age groups and has a higher incidence in women, thymomatous myasthenia gravis occurs in older individuals and in some series is more common in men; it is also less likely to undergo remission following thymectomy and resection of the thymoma. The prognosis, however, so far as the thymoma is concerned is generally good, since the patients usually present with systemic symptoms before the tumours have grown to a large size and invaded neighbouring structures.

The association of thymomas with other disease processes is well documented (see **94**). For example, in acquired hypogammaglobulinaemia 12 per cent of patients have been found to have a thymic tumour, and in pure erythroid hypoplasia up to 5 per cent of patients have been found to have a thymoma. Thymomas also occur in a variety of diseases such as systemic lupus erythematosus, rheumatoid arthritis and Sjögren's syndrome, and in diseases with abnormalities of muscle such as myositis, myocarditis and dermatomyositis. All these thymic tumours are essentially a mixture of lymphocytes and epithelial cells and, therefore, are referred to conveniently as mixed epithelial/lymphocytic thymomas, though it is now generally considered that the epithelial cells represent the neoplastic population (see **104–111**). The entity known as a thymolipoma in which there is an overgrowth of fat and an absolute increase in the amount of thymic tissue of normal appearance should be considered separately. In recent years it has become recognised that another type of tumour occurs in the thymus; it is composed essentially of epithelial cells. This rare tumour, formerly referred to as a small cell carcinoma or adenoma often shows the features of a carcinoid tumour and is now increasingly designated as such. Not all these carcinoid-like tumours of the thymus appear to be associated with systemic symptoms (**94**), but it is important for the time being that they should be considered separately from the mixed epithelial/lymphocytic thymomas.

The majority of primary thymic tumours are not associated with any disease pattern and, usually, are picked up incidentally as a result of mass radiography or because the patient has presented with symptoms of mediastinal involvement. It is quite common for a thymic tumour to attain a large size before any symptoms are evident. The thymus may be involved also in a lymphomatous process. Hodgkin's disease, particularly of nodular sclerosing type (see **176-179**), quite commonly involves the anterior mediastinum and thymus and can result in a lesion which masquerades under the name of granulomatous thymoma. Diffuse lymphocytic lymphomas of well differentiated or poorly differentiated (lymphoblastic) type, including the recently defined convoluted cell lymphoma of T-cell origin (see **666–674**), may also involve the thymus as may some of the large (lymphoid) cell lymphomas (reticulum cell sarcoma). A third distinct type of malignancy which may involve the thymus includes all the variants of germ-cell tumours. Thus teratomas of the thymus are encountered, as well as a rather characteristic tumour occurring predominantly in young males – the seminoma or so-called seminomatous thymoma. Metastatic involvement of the thymus by carcinoma is rare. It is more common for mediastinal involvement to result from direct extension from a bronchial carcinoma. The thymus also may be the site of a leukaemic infiltrate.

## Categories of Thymic tumours

1 *Mixed epithelial/lymphocytic thymoma*
includes epithelial predominant, lymphocytic predominant and spindle cell thymomas
2 *Carcinoid tumour of the thymus*
with systemic effects
without systemic effects
3 *Lymphoma*
Hodgkin's disease
Lymphomas, other than Hodgkin's disease (including the mediastinal T-cell lymphoma – Sternberg's tumour)
4 *Germ cell tumours*
seminoma (germinoma)
teratoma and mixed germ cell tumours
5 *Myoid tumours and myosarcoma of thymus*
6 *(Thymolipoma)*
7 *Metastatic tumours*

**94**

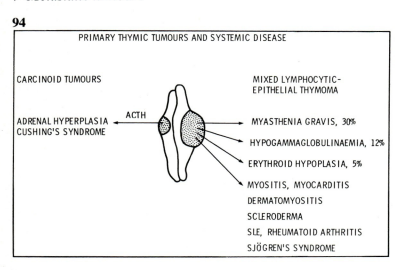

**95   Thymoma from a patient with myasthenia gravis**
This small thymoma, localised to one lobe, was an unexpected finding at thymectomy for severe acute-onset myasthenia gravis in a 43-year-old woman. Notice the circumscription of the tumour with the well-developed fibrous trabeculae and the surrounding residual fatty thymus (*arrow*).

**95**

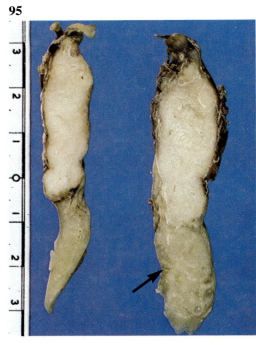

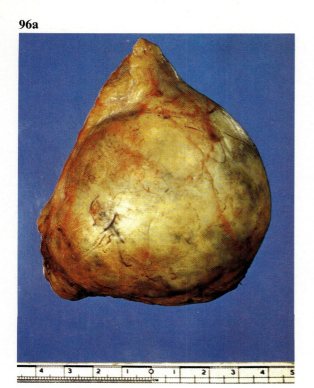

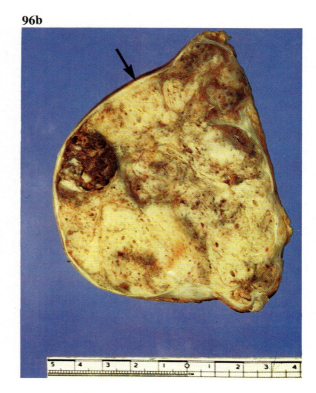

**96a and 96b  Thymoma from a patient without myasthenia gravis** Figure **96a** shows the tumour removed entirely with its thickened intact capsule. Figure **96b** shows the cut surface. The lobular appearance is characteristic and the thickened capsule with early calcification is clearly shown (*arrow*). The haemorrhagic areas and small cysts are other common findings. Even tumours of this size may remain localised to one lobe of the thymus without involvement of any neighbouring structures.

**97  Thymoma from a patient with myasthenia gravis** This thymic tumour was also localised to one lobe of the thymus. The cut surface shows extensive areas of cystic degeneration as a result of necrosis. The capsule is intact and shows no evidence of extension beyond its confines. The patient, a 38-year-old woman, also had an ectopic thymoma (see **155**), in the neck and a parathyroid adenoma.

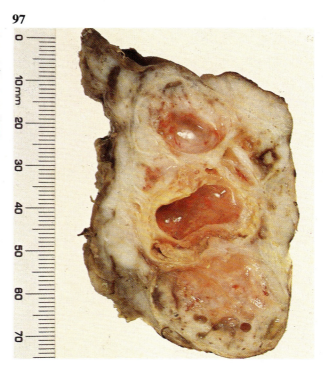

**98 Thymoma from a patient with hypo-gammaglobulinaemia** This thymoma was associated with severe hypogam-maglobulinaemia and, as in the majority of such cases, was of the spindle cell variety. Radiological evidence of a thymic tumour was equivocal, and it was not until a thoracotomy was performed for the purpose of a lung biopsy that the diagnosis of a thymoma was established. (See also **123–127**.)

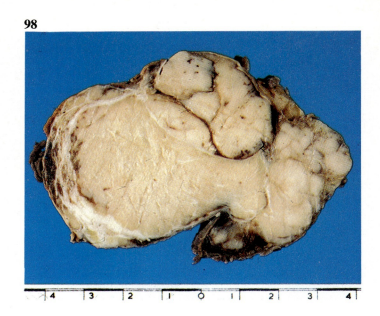

**99 Granulomatous response to endogenous lipid in thymomas** Not uncommonly, and particularly if there has been cystic degeneration in the tumour, a granulomatous response develops in the capsule in relation to inspissated fatty material – in this case, cholesterol as demonstrated by the needle-shaped spaces. This finding is also seen in the wall of some non-neoplastic thymic cysts. Necrosis with a granulomatous response accounts for some of the so-called granulomatous thymomas. *(H&E)*

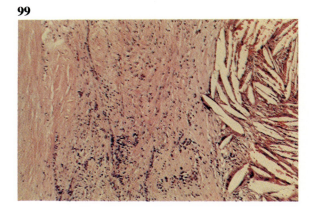

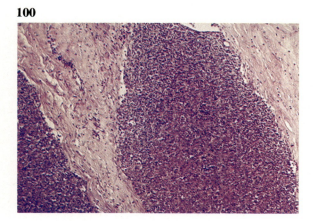

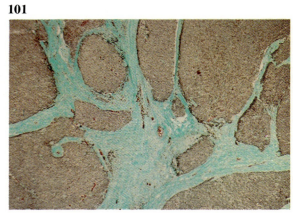

**100 and 101 Lobulation in thymomas** Thymomas characteristically show a lobular pattern due to intersecting bands or trabeculae of fibrous connective tissue. Figure **100** shows pink-staining connective tissue delineating the tumour lobules of a mixed epithelial/lymphocytic thymoma. Figure **101** shows broad bands of connective tissue – here stained green – enclosing variably-sized lobules of an epithelial predominant thymoma. (**100** *H&E;* **101** *Masson's trichrome)*

**102 Lobulation in thymomas** The coarse lobular pattern of thymomas is not always evident at low magnifications. Nevertheless, fibrous trabeculae are a characteristic feature of thymic tumours though, as here, they may be narrow and merge with the adjacent lobules of tumour. *(H&E)*

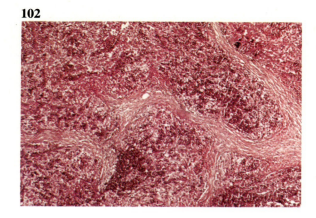

**103 Thymoma, reticulin content** The majority of mixed epithelial/lymphocytic thymomas are devoid of reticulin fibre except that associated with the vessels – seen here cut longitudinally (*arrow*) and transversely – and the fibrous trabeculae. This reticulin pattern is sometimes helpful in distinguishing thymomas from lymphomas. *(Gordon & Sweets)*

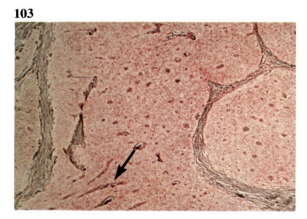

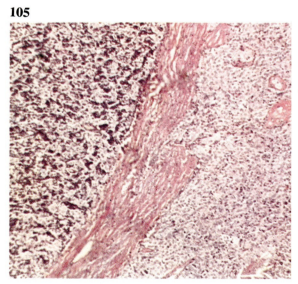

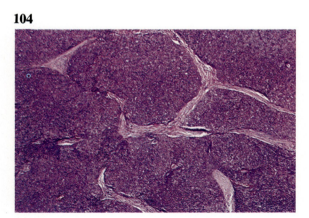

**104 and 105 Cellular composition of thymomas** Variation in the number of lymphocytes in different areas of a thymoma is very common. Figure **104** shows a predominantly epithelial appearance in what was essentially a mixed lymphocytic/epithelial thymoma. There may be, as shown in **105**, marked differences in the number of lymphocytes between one tumour lobule and another: one lobule contains mainly lymphocytes and is darkly stained, whereas the other consists predominantly of epithelial cells and is lightly stained. *(H&E)*

**106 Cellular composition of thymomas** At this magnification, it is possible to recognise the dual cell population in this mixed epithelial/lymphocytic thymoma (lymphoepithelioma) in a patient with myasthenia gravis. Approximately 50 per cent of the cells are small mature lymphocytes; the other half is composed of larger epithelial cells with open vesicular nuclei and abundant pale poorly-defined cytoplasm. Such epithelial cells are the type most frequently seen in thymomas associated with myasthenia gravis, as in this case, but are found also in thymic tumours from patients without myasthenia gravis. *(H&E)*

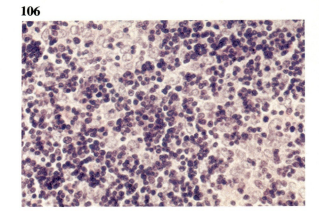

**107 Cellular composition of thymomas** In this field taken from a thymoma in a patient without myasthenia gravis most of the cells are epithelial. However there is a dual cell population due to a diffuse sprinkling of small lymphocytes, a feature which is extremely helpful in distinguishing a thymoma from a carcinoma involving the mediastinum. *(H&E)*

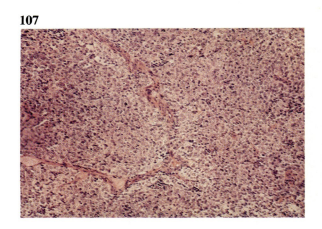

**108 Cellular composition of thymomas** Lymphocytes are very numerous in this tumour from a patient without myasthenia gravis and, because they tend to obscure the epithelial cells, such a thymoma is often misdiagnosed as a lymphoma. A feature which helps to differentiate a thymoma from a lymphoma is the presence of hyalinised strands of connective tissue originating from the perivascular spaces (*arrow*). *(H&E)*

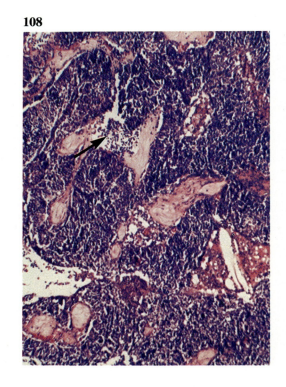

**109**

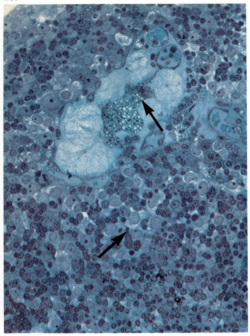
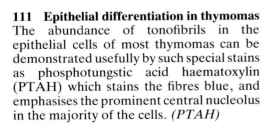

**109 Cellular composition of thymomas**
Difficulties in diagnosis of predominantly lymphocytic thymomas are resolved more easily by processing through epoxy resins. The superior fixation and thinner sections embodied in this technique clearly reveal the epithelial nature of the larger cells (*arrow*). Above is hyalinised perivascular connective tissue in which there are three vessels and fat-containing macrophages (*arrow*). *(Toluidine blue)*

**110**

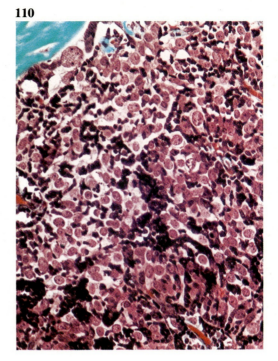

**110 Cellular composition of thymomas** A trichrome stain is also very helpful in distinguishing the finely dispersed stippled nuclear chromatin of the epithelial cells from the darker staining clumped chromatin of lymphocytes. It is the epithelial component which is considered to be neoplastic, the lymphocytes being viewed as reactive or residual. *(Masson's trichrome)*

**111 Epithelial differentiation in thymomas**
The abundance of tonofibrils in the epithelial cells of most thymomas can be demonstrated usefully by such special stains as phosphotungstic acid haematoxylin (PTAH) which stains the fibres blue, and emphasises the prominent central nucleolus in the majority of the cells. *(PTAH)*

**111**

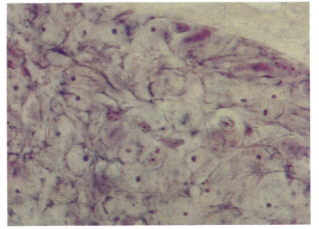

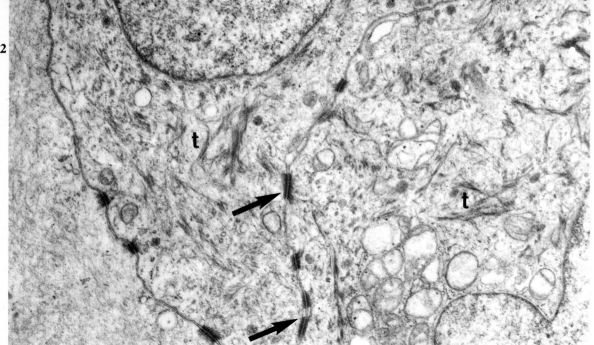

**112 Predominantly epithelial thymoma, ultrastructure** The ultrastructural features of the thymoma in **107** establishes the epithelial nature of the larger cells. Innumerable desmosomal attachments (*arrows*) are seen between the cytoplasm of three adjacent epithelial cells, and bundles of branching tonofilaments (t) are conspicuous in the cytoplasm of the nucleated cells. This thymoma is composed of plump, well-differentiated epidermoid cells, but the degree of epithelial differentiation and their shape can vary considerably in different thymomas. (× 18,000)

**113 Predominatly lymphocytic thymoma, ultrastructure** In this predominantly lymphocytic tumour the epithelial cells are less well differentiated. Their elongated processes show epidermoid characteristics with numerous bundles of tonofilaments (t), but lack the desmosomes seen in the better differentiated epithelial thymomas. The lymphocytic component (L) is composed mainly of small mature lymphocytes. (× 15,750)

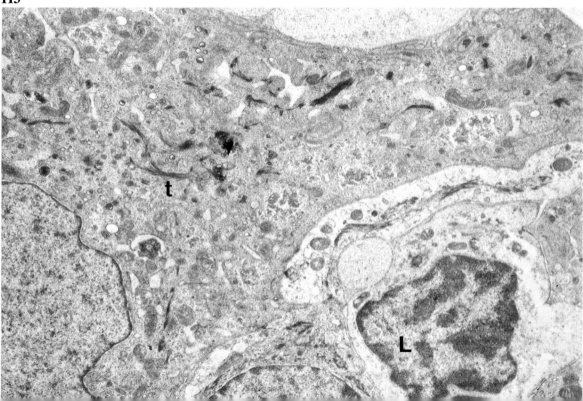

**114 'Cystic change' in thymomas** In this predominantly epithelial thymoma a cystic area is shown above. Such cystic change is common and is a feature helpful in the diagnosis of a thymoma since cystic change is not a characteristic of lymphomas or carcinomas. Most of these cysts are dilated perivascular spaces but occasionally there is such extensive tumour necrosis and resulting cyst formation that residual tumour may be overlooked and a diagnosis made of a thymic cyst or even of a mediastinal cyst. *(H&E)*

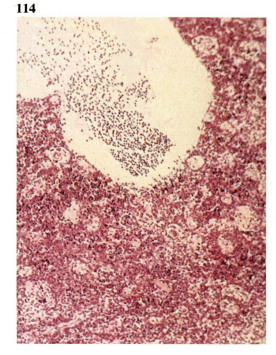

**115 and 116 'Cystic change' in thymomas** In the thymoma in **115** there are numerous small 'cystic' spaces resulting in a sieve-like pattern simulating the dilated lymphatic channels seen in a lymphangioma. The vast majority of these spaces, however, represent dilated perivascular spaces. In other thymomas, **116**, a somewhat similar lymphangiomatous pattern is seen between the islands of tumour cells but a derivation from the perivascular spaces cannot always be traced. The importance of this change in mediastinal tumours lies, on the one hand in not mistaking such an appearance for a lymphangioma and, on the other hand, as a helpful feature in distinguishing between thymomas and lymphomas. *(H&E)*

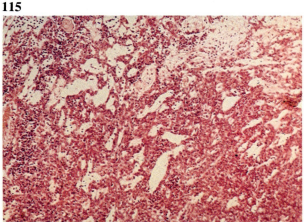

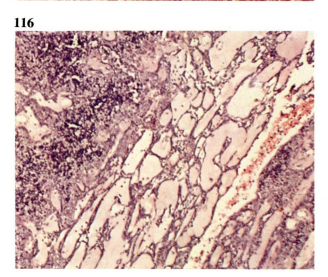

**117, 118 and 119  Perivascular spaces in thymoma mimicking cyst formation** Most 'microcysts' represent dilated perivascular spaces and show, as in **117** and **119**, the presence of a small vessel or vessels in addition to lymphoid cells. The 'microcyst' in **118** contains proteinaceous material admixed with lymphocytes, but no small vessel is identified. The epithelial cells lining the spaces are limited by a distinct basement membrane and exhibit a polar arrangement (see **133**). The plastic processed specimen, **119**, also shows that in addition to lymphocytes there are hairy macrophages (*arrow 1*) and epithelial tumour cells (*arrow 2*). (**117** *Giemsa;* **118** *H&E;* **119** *Toluidine blue*)

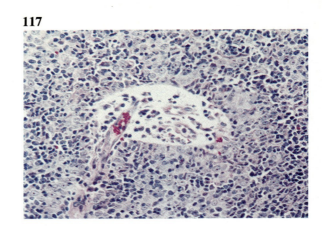

117

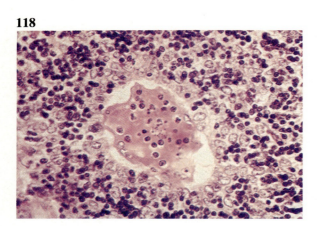

118

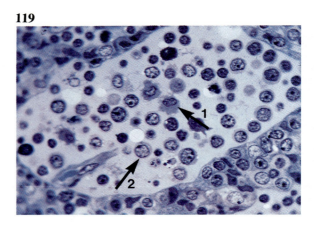

119

**120  Perivascular spaces in thymoma** Some thymomas, as here, show the presence of numerous greatly dilated perivascular spaces. Two of these seen here contain numerous red cells while the three others contain mainly lymphocytes and are becoming progressively hyalinised. The fibrosis starts in the walls of the vessels and gradually obliterates the space. Note that the vessels vary in size and appear to be of venous type. (*Masson's trichrome*)

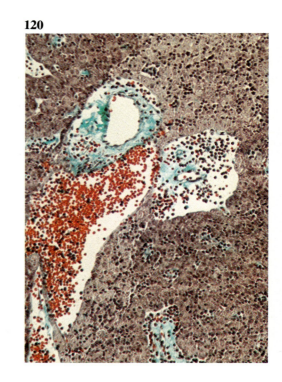

120

**121 Squamous differentiation in thymoma**
There are very few tumours which show
such extreme variation in appearance as
thymomas. This is due both to the dual
population of lymphocytes and epithelial
cells – with variable morphology and differing degrees of differentiation of the latter
cells – and to the different patterns resulting
from variations in the arrangement of the
epithelial component to the lymphocytes.
In this tumour from a patient without myasthenia gravis there is maturation towards a
keratinising tumour and to the left of the
field is a structure resembling quite closely a
Hassall's corpuscle. The presence of
perivascular spaces (*arrow*) and the
ubiquitous small lymphocytic component
helps in differentiating this thymoma from a
carcinoma. *(H&E)*

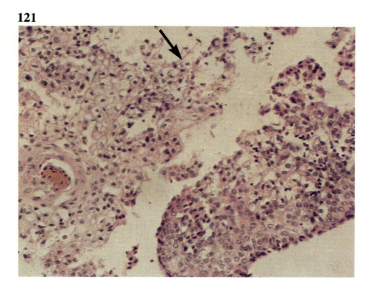

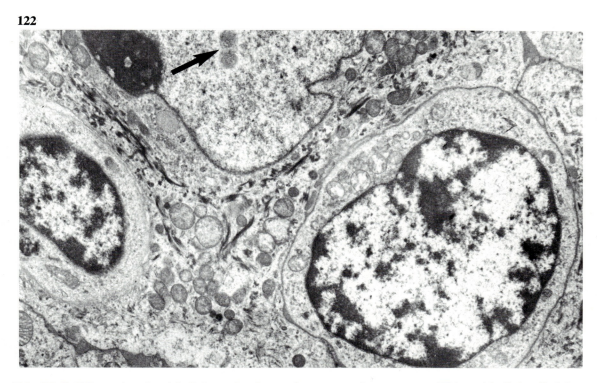

**122 Well-differentiated epithelial predominant thymoma, ultrastructure** This epithelial cell, lying
between two lymphocytes, shows numerous well-formed and dense bundles of tonofilaments. There is
a prominent nucleolus and a double nuclear body (*arrow*). The lymphocytes are mature and are
viewed as reactive. *(× 14,250)*

**123 Spindle cell thymoma** A common finding in thymic tumours are areas where the epithelial cells show a spindle cell morphology. A minority of thymomas, as this one, are entirely composed of spindle cells, when confusion with a mesenchymal tumour is likely to occur. It is when the cells are viewed in longitudinal section, as shown in the central part of this field, that the nuclear appearance so closely resembles that of fibroblasts. Note, however, the presence of scattered lymphocytes *(arrows)*. *(H&E)*

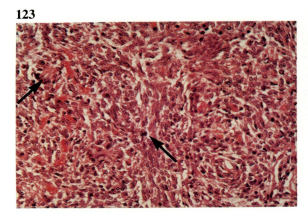

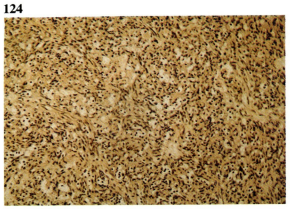

**124 Spindle cell thymoma** In this thymoma removed from a young man spindle cell change is extreme and, initially, a diagnosis of spindle cell sarcoma of the mediastinum had been made. Note, however, the sprinkling of small lymphocytes and the many scattered foamy macrophages. Spindle cell thymoma is uncommon in myasthenia gravis unless the patient has received radiotherapy prior to surgical resection – a procedure which in any case is to be deprecated. It is the commonest type of thymoma associated with hypogamma-globulinaemia – as in this patient – and red cell aplasia. *(Elastic Van Gieson (EVG))*

**125 and 126 Spindle cell thymoma** These are taken from the spindle cell thymoma in **123**. The patient, a 60-year-old man had severe hypogam-maglobulinaemia and later succumbed to an opportunistic cytomegalic virus infection. The spindle epithelial cells are seen well in the trichrome-stained sections, **125**, in which the vascular component and intercellular material also appear more conspicuous. The resin-embedded and toluidine-stained section, **126**, demonstrates the epithelial nature of the nuclei and also emphasises scattered lipid-containing cells. *(125 Masson's trichrome; 126 Toluidine blue)*

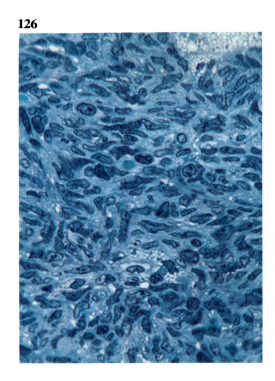

**125**

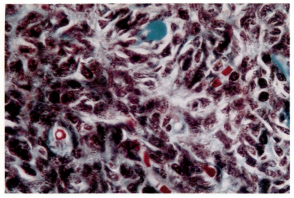

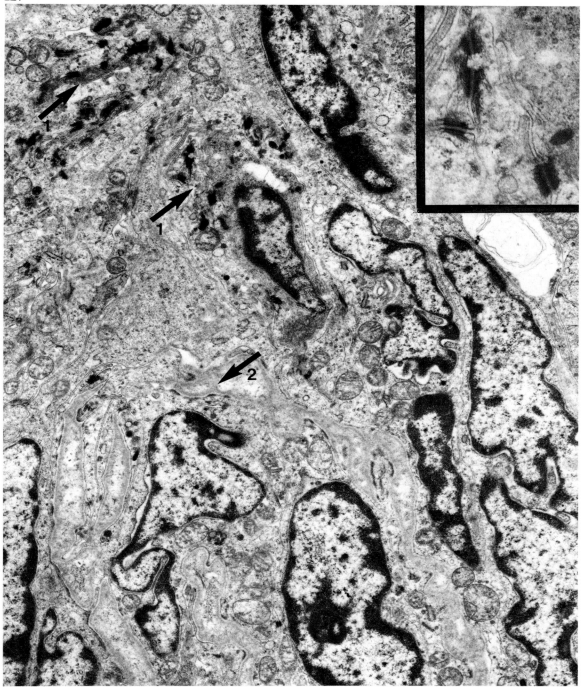

**127  Spindle cell thymoma, ultrastructure** In doubtful cases, electron microscopy is extremely useful in establishing the epithelial nature of the spindle cells. Although tonofilaments are inconspicuous, the elongated cytoplasmic processes show numerous desmosomal attachment sites (*arrow 1 and inset*) and basal laminae are more conspicuous (*arrow 2*) than in the 'ordinary' variety of epithelial thymoma. Conversely, not all spindle cell tumours of the thymus are epithelial; occasionally, true mesenchymal, for example smooth muscle tumours are encountered – and, again, electronmicroscopy is invaluable in establishing the correct diagnosis. *(× 11,000; inset × 31,000)*

**128 Poorly-differentiated epithelial predominant thymoma** Anaplastic or poorly-differentiated epithelial thymic tumours are likely to be confused with a diffuse lymphocytic malignant lymphoma of lymphoblastic or large cell type (reticulum cell sarcoma), and ultrastructure is invaluable where the diagnosis is in doubt. In this poorly-differentiated thymoma presenting in early pregnancy small lymphocytes, though present, are scanty, there is active mitosis and there are scattered macrophages giving a partial 'starry sky' effect. As with endocrine tumours, there is a poor correlation between the degree of differentiation of the epithelial cells and prognosis; neither is the mitotic activity a reliable index of behaviour. The most reliable single prognostic indicator is whether there is invasion of the capsule. *(PAS)*

**128**

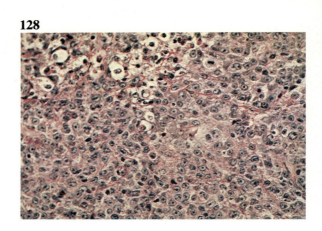

**129**

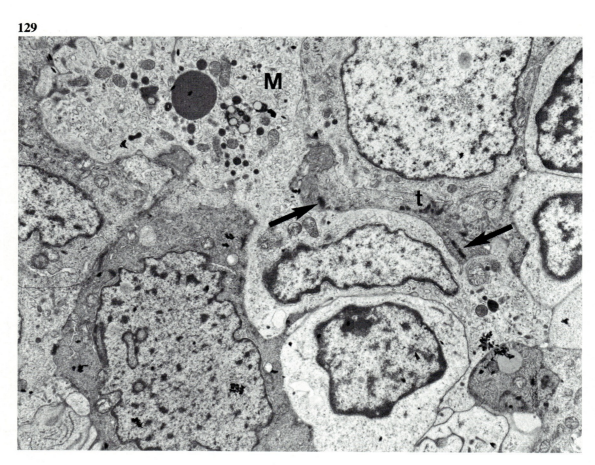

**129 Poorly-differentiated epithelial predominant thymoma, ultrastructure** Tonofilaments within the cytoplasm of these rounded epithelial cells are finely dispersed but show some aggregation into bundles (t). Desmosomes can be identified also (*arrows*). A macrophage (M) rich in lysosomes and phagocytosed material and small mature lymphocytes are seen in close association with the malignant epithelial component. *(× 5,350)*

**130 Thymoma with lymphocytic festooning** In addition to variations in appearance due to differing epithelial morphology, many differing patterns may be seen in thymomas as a result of the arrangement of the lymphocytic and epithelial components. In this mixed epithelial/lymphocytic thymoma a curious pattern has been produced by the festoons and clusters of lymphocytes. The epithelial cells are large and plump and show the vesicular nuclei and indistinct watery cytoplasm considered typical of myasthenia gravis. The patient did not have myasthenia gravis. *(H&E)*

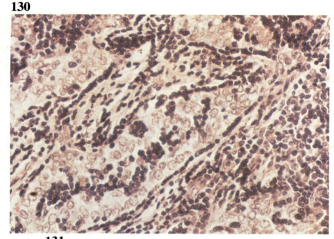

**131 Thymoma with lymphocytic vascular cuffing** In some thymomas, particularly those associated with myasthenia gravis, there is a very characteristic perivascular lymphocytic infiltrate, seen here around longitudinally sectioned vessels. This lymphocytic cuffing has been cited as supportive evidence for an auto-immune basis to the development of thymomas in patients with myasthenia gravis, since similar perivascular lymphocytic cuffing is seen in experimentally induced auto-immune disease. The numerous scattered microscopic 'spaces' represent vacuolated macrophages. *(H&E)*

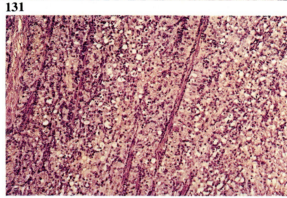

**132 Lymphocytic and epithelial segregation in thymoma** An uncommon separation of cellular constituents is shown in this thymoma, where the broad irregular islands of epithelial cells are quite separate from the intervening lymphocytic areas. Note the presence of a germinal centre within the lymphocytic area in the upper part of the field. *(H&E)*

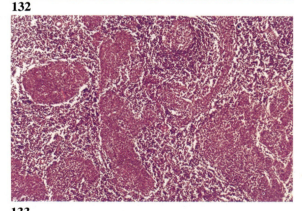

**133 Thymoma with epithelial palisading** The epithelial cells, where they abut on the perivascular spaces, sometimes assume a conspicuous palisade arrangement (*arrow*) and pseudoglandular appearance. Small mature lymphocytes are numerous within the perivascular compartment and throughout the epithelial component. *(H&E)*

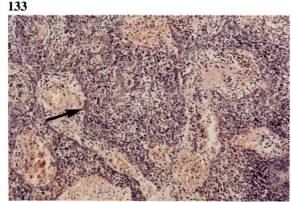

**134 Epithelial rosette formation in thymoma**
Some thymomas show the presence of rosette-like structures which may mimic the appearance of a neuro-epithelioma. The rosettes are formed by epithelial cells which are arranged around a fibrillar eosinophilic space. There is no true lumen as in rosettes seen in carcinoid tumours, and the fibrils in the space appear continuous with the cytoplasm of the epithelial cells. In these rosette-forming areas lymphocytes are not usually conspicuous. *(H&E)*

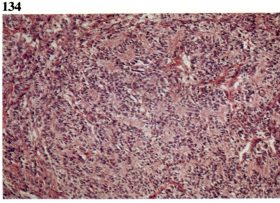

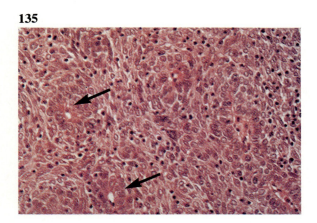

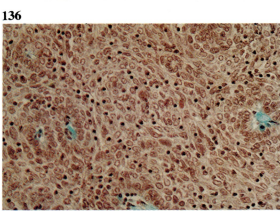

**135 and 136 Epithelial pseudorosettes in thymoma** In this epithelial predominant thymoma, **135**, there are several small 'rosettes' (*arrows*). These structures, however, have arisen by the polar arrangement of the epithelium around small perivascular spaces. This arrangement is visualised more easily in a trichrome stain of a similar field, **136**, where the connective tissue component around the vessels walls is stained green. *(135 H&E; 136 Masson's trichrome)*

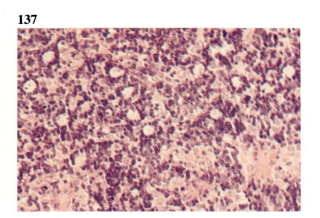

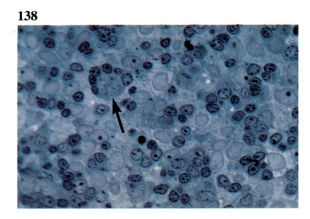

**137 and 138 Lymphocytic rosette formation in thymoma** Thymomas may contain reactive macrophages. In this thymoma, **137**, from a patient with myasthenia gravis, lymphocytes are ringed around macrophages to form rosettes. A true 'starry sky' effect is not achieved because of the conspicuous epithelial component. This close relationship of the lymphocytes to the macrophages is seen very clearly in semi-thin sections of plastic processed material, **138**, which shows the particulate matter within the macrophage (*arrow*) and emphasises the dispersed chromatin pattern of the epithelial nuclei and abundant cytoplasm. *(137 H&E; 138 Toluidine blue)*

**139  Inclusions of medulla in thymoma** Thymomas occasionally show the presence of scattered foci of thymic medullary tissue of normal appearance in which the usual components including Hassall's corpuscles can be identified. As in **139**, thymomas showing this feature are usually those composed of an even mixture of lymphocytes and epithelial cells or are predominantly lymphocytic. *(H&E)*

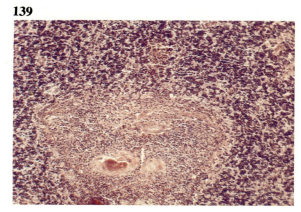

**140  Hassall's corpuscles in thymoma** Maturation of the epithelial component of a thymoma to form Hassall's corpuscles is uncommon but occasionally may be seen. This feature is to be differentiated from the Hassall's corpuscles found in the inclusions of normal medulla shown in **139**. *(H&E)*

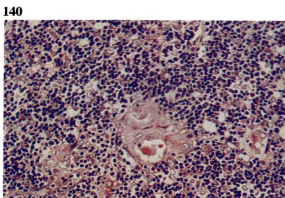

**141 and 142  Epithelial differentiation with Hassall's corpuscle, mucin and glycogen** In the low power view, **141**, of the thymoma shown in **140** there is Hassall's corpuscle formation in the epithelial predominant islands *(arrows)* as well as in the surrounding mixed epithelial/lymphocytic areas. Special stains here demonstrate the presence of mucin which is similar to that seen in normal and hyperplastic thymic tissue. The double staining technique has coloured the mucin reddish-purple. In addition to mucin production, there is accumulation of glycogen in both densely aggregated and finely particulate form, as shown in the high power view, **142**. Proof that the material is glycogen lies in its removal by digestion with diastase and by electron-microscopy. *(AB/PAS)*

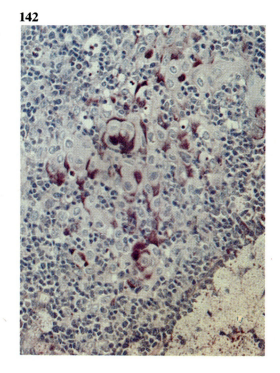

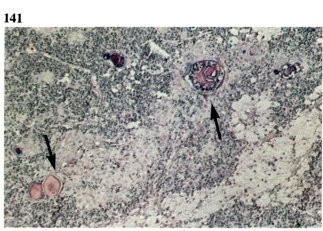

**143 and 144 Mucin secretion in thymoma** In this predominantly spindle cell thymoma, **143**, there are conspicuous small irregular spaces. These do not represent foci of microscopic degeneration but differentiation of the epithelium to secrete small pools of mucin. The mucus is coloured purple by a combined staining technique, **144**. No nuclear counterstain has been used. (**143** *H&E;* **144** *AB/PAS*)

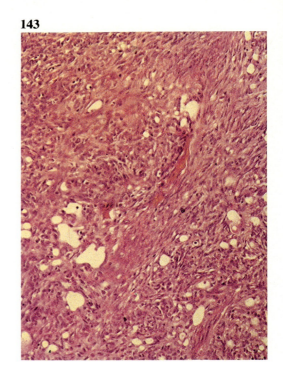

143

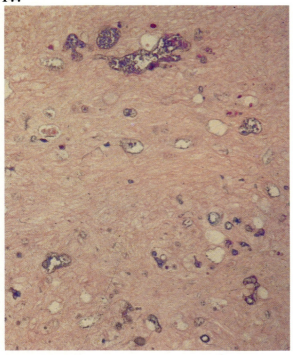

144

**145 Mucin secretion in thymoma** Mucin secretion can be demonstrated also in some lymphocyte predominant thymomas as shown here, and is a finding useful in differentiating such thymomas from lymphomas. Note that some of the mucin-filled glandular spaces – here lying alongside a fibrous trabeculum – are quite large (*arrows*) but are not associated with Hassall's corpuscles; nor do they resemble perivascular spaces. (*AB/PAS*)

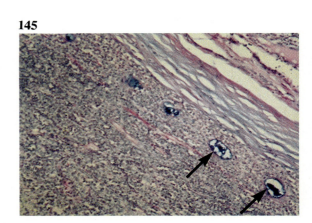

145

**146 Mucin secretion in thymoma, ultrastructure** In this mixed epithelial/lymphocytic thymoma, many of the epithelial cells contain mucin droplets at ultrastructural level. The cell shown here contains two vacuoles containing residual mucinous material and lined with stunted microvilli (*arrows*). Tonofilaments (t) and desmosome formation are also present. (× 7,800)

**146**

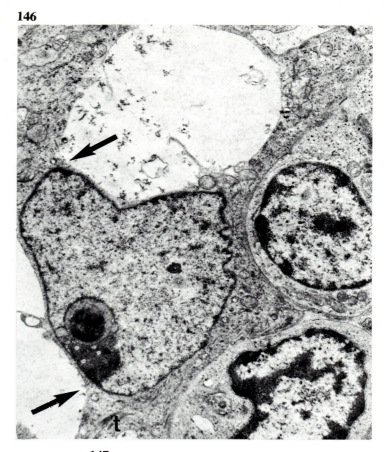

**147 and 148 Germinal centres in residual thymic tissue** Residual thymic medullary tissue in relation to thymomas commonly shows the presence of well-formed germinal centres which, as shown in **147**, in every way resemble those seen in lymph nodes and, as in non-thymomatous myasthenic thymuses, Hassall's corpuscles (*arrow*) and epithelial cells are ranged around them. In contrast to the lack of reticulin fibres characteristic of thymoma, seen on the right of **148**, subdivided by a fibrous band, the residual medullary tissue containing the germinal centre shows an increase in reticulin fibres (*arrow*) similar to that found in myasthenic thymitis. Such germinal centres are found in relation to thymomas of patients both *with* and *without* myasthenic gravis. (**147** *H&E;* **148** *Gordon & Sweets*)

**147**

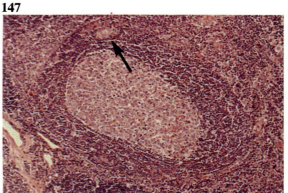

**148**

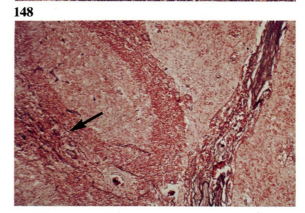

**149 Locally invasive malignant thymoma involving pleura** Distant metastases from a thymoma are exceedingly rare but recognised. It is on the basis of local invasion that thymomas are judged malignant. The incidence of invasiveness varies considerably in different series – averaging around 30 per cent. Although generally slowly growing, the thymoma, at first confined to one 'lobe', enlarges to involve the whole thymus and may then extend through the capsule to infiltrate pleura, interlobar fissures, pericardium, and the connective tissue around the great vessels of the neck, resulting in superior mediastinal obstruction. Tumour may grow also directly upwards into the neck, forwards through the sternum or downwards to involve the liver. The lungs are seldom directly invaded, but pleural infiltration may be so extensive that the lungs are encased in tumour, as shown here, simulating a mesothelioma. The structure at the top is the oesophagus. *(H&E)*

**149**

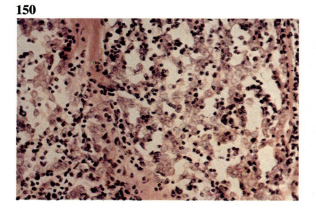

**150 Malignant thymoma with pleural involvement** There is, as previously illustrated, rather poor correlation between the histological appearance of thymomas and prognosis. This tumour is the same one as **149** and on the basis of mitotic activity there is little evidence of cellular proliferation. The epithelial cells are large with pale vesicular nuclei and ill-defined cytoplasm, similar to those usually associated with myasthenia gravis, and there is a lymphocytic component. The patient, however, was an elderly female without myasthenia gravis, who had had an inoperable thymic tumour diagnosed some years previously and, subsequently, had been treated with radiotherapy. *(H&E)*

**150**

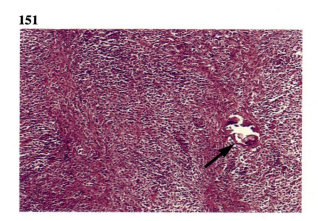

**151 Locally invasive (malignant) thymoma** This thymic tumour was removed from a young girl. The tumour was locally invasive and involved adjacent mediastinal structures including pleura. Not only are thymomas rare in young individuals and quite exceptional in children, but also the histopathological features of this tumour were somewhat atypical in that there was diffuse fibrosis but no well-formed fibrous trabeculae and, in many areas, the tumour cells lacked cohesion and assumed a rather 'histiocytic' appearance. Note the occasional degenerate and calcific Hassall's corpuscle *(arrow)*. *(H&E)*

**151**

**152 and 153  Malignant thymoma** In doubtful or atypical thymic tumours such as that in **151**, special techniques are necessary to enable a definitive diagnosis to be made. The PTAH-stained section, **152**, shows the presence of fine tonofilaments (*arrows*) and the toluidine blue-stained plastic section, **153**, enables the numerous desmosomal attachments to be visualised. Neither of these structures would be present in a histiocytic or any other type of lymphoma ( d-desmosomes). (**152** *PTAH;* **153** *Toluidine blue*)

**152**

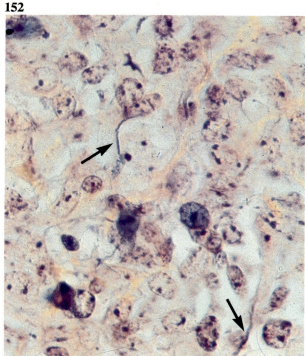

**153**

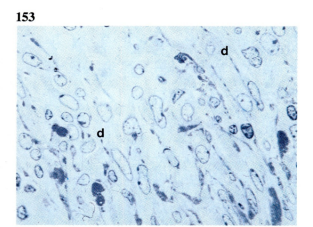

**154  Malignant thymoma with massive mediastinal lymph node involvement** This epithelial predominant thymoma presented with superior vena caval obstruction. The mediastinal nodes were replaced by tumour but can still be identified by the black residual carbon pigment. As judged by the cellular composition there is little to indicate such malignant (invasive) potential. It must be stressed that the single most important prognostic index is whether invasion through the tumour capsule has occurred. (*H&E*)

**154**

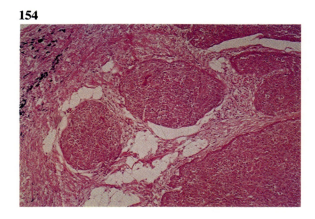

**155  Ectopic thymoma** Thymic tumours may arise in ectopic thymic tissue, usually in the neck, and are then a source of diagnostic confusion. Depending upon the number of lymphocytes in relation to the epithelial component, they are usually diagnosed as lymphomas or metastatic carcinomas such as nasopharyngeal carcinomas. This thymoma was an encapsulated lump in the lower neck with no continuity with the mediastinum. The microscopic features are those of a mixed epithelial/lymphocytic thymoma with a thick fibrous capsule and well-formed trabeculae. Focal areas of medullary tissue were also present. (*H&E*)

**155**

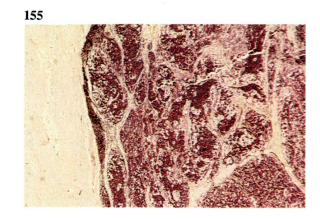

**156 Carcinoid tumour of the thymus** These rare tumours should be distinguished from the ordinary variety of thymoma since the cell of origin is considered to be a neuroendocrine cell, albeit one arising in the thymus. Some of these tumours are associated with Cushing's syndrome, as this one, and with multiple endocrine adenomatosis. The majority, however, are not associated with recognisable systemic effects; nor is there a consistent microscopic appearance. In this example, the tumour cells are arranged in solid islands lacking an organoid pattern and have shrunk away from the thick irregular fibrous trabeculae. There are no perivascular spaces and no lymphocytic component. *(H&E)*

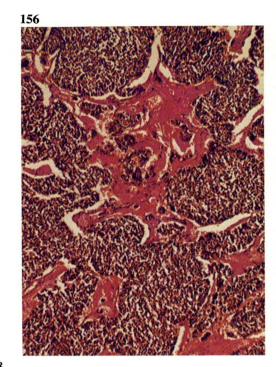

156

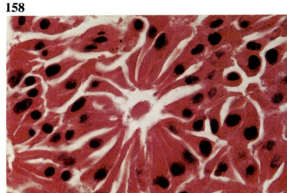

157

158

**157 and 158   Carcinoid tumour of the thymus** The connective tissue between the cords and lobules of tumour is variable in amount and may be quite extensive, as shown here. In **157**, it is possible to discern an ill-defined organoid pattern with the formation of rosette-like structures (*arrows*). One such rosette is shown in **158** and the granular eosinophilic cytoplasm of the radially arranged cells is striking. This patient presented with and died in status asthmaticus. *(H&E)*

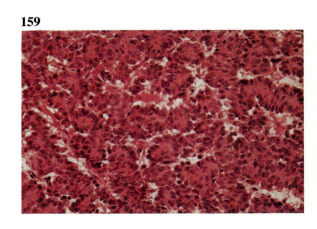

159

**159   Carcinoid tumour of the thymus** In this carcinoid tumour there is a prominent organoid pattern with 'rosettes', and winding ribbons of cells showing a palisade arrangement. There were, however, no recognised systemic symptoms. *(H&E)*

**160 Carcinoid tumour of the thymus** Some carcinoid tumours achieve a very large size as shown here. Delicate fibrous trabeculae separate the cords and column of cells, which exhibit the characteristic polar arrangement (*arrow*) associated with carcinoid tumour elsewhere. There were no associated systemic symptoms. (*H&E*)

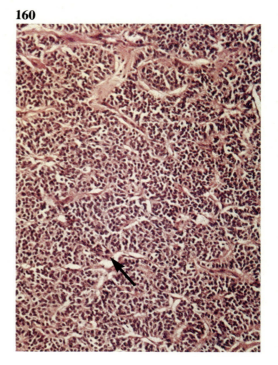

160

**161 Carcinoid tumour of the thymus** In this tumour which was associated with Cushing's syndrome, the cells are arranged in solid islands and show a very monomorphic appearance with round regular nuclei and no mitotic activity. The cells have shrunk away from the surrounding connective tissue, and the cytoplasmic vacuolation is also an artefact. Tumours showing this microscopic appearance were called originally thymic adenoma or small cell carcinoma of the thymus. (*H&E*)

161

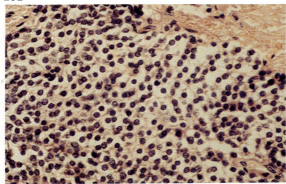

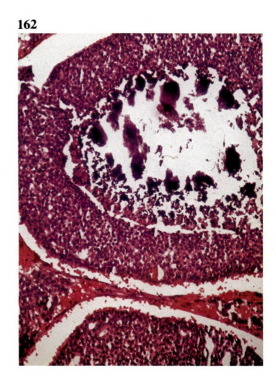

162

**162 Carcinoid tumour of the thymus** Some carcinoid tumours show a very distinctive feature of central necrosis with calcification within solid islands of tumour, as seen here. This finding, when present, is a useful aid to the recognition of the carcinoid nature of the thymic tumour, particularly one in which the cells are less well differentiated and lack an organoid component. (*H&E*)

**163**

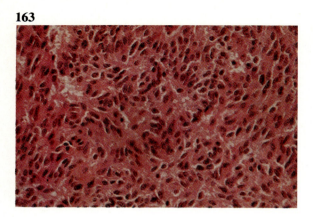

**163 Carcinoid tumour of the thymus** Rarely in carcinoid tumours, the cells assume a spindle shape as seen here. A vague organoid pattern can still be recognised, a feature helpful in distinguishing it from the more common spindle cell variant of the epithelial/lymphocytic thymoma. Note also the absence of lymphocytes. *(H&E)*

**164**

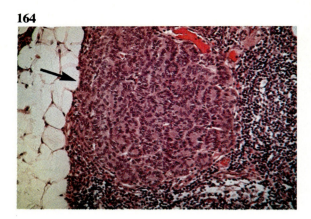

**164 Microcarcinoid of the thymus** Very occasionally, a microscopic focus of epithelial cells *(arrow)* with the morphological features of a carcinoid tumour is encountered in thymectomy specimens resected from patients with myasthenia gravis (see **91**). *(H&E)*

**165**

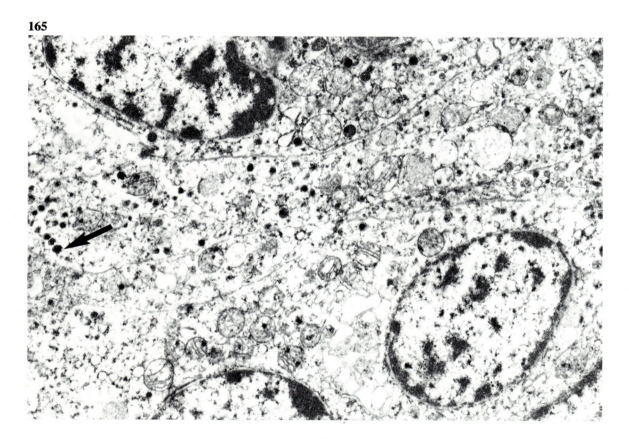

**165 Carcinoid tumour of the thymus, ultrastructure** In this electron micrograph of the formalin-fixed tumour cells illustrated in **160** the cytoplasm contains variable numbers of electron dense secretory granules *(arrow)*. Tonofilaments are absent and desmosomes are few in number. There were no overt systemic symptoms. *(× 11,250)*

**166** **Teratoma of the thymus** Part of a large cystic mediastinal teratoma arising in the thymus. Residual thymic tissue can be seen (*arrow*) outside the capsule which encloses a heterogenous collection of differentiated tissues such as skin (S), intestine (I), respiratory epithelium (R) and glands, cartilage (C), vascular and connective tissue and muscle (M). Most of these tumours are benign and are picked up on routine chest X-ray when their nature may be suspected sometimes by the presence of prominent calcification. (*H&E*)

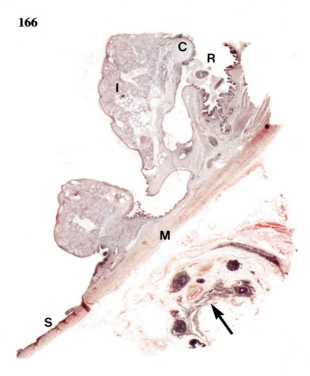

166

**167** **Teratoma of the thymus** A peculiar feature of mediastinal (thymic) teratomas is the frequency with which mature pancreatic tissue is found. In this example abundant pancreatic tissue was present containing numerous pale-staining Islets of Langerhan (*arrow*). In the bottom field there is glandular epithelium. (*H&E*)

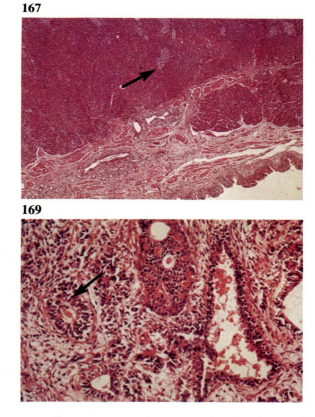

167

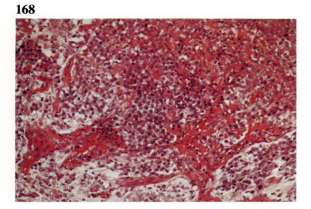

168

169

**168 and 169** **Mixed germ cell tumour of thymus** Two germ cell tumour areas from a mediastinal (thymic) teratoma with differentiated somatic constituents. Figure **168** shows embryonal carcinoma-like tissue; **169** shows irregular epithelial lined spaces occasionally containing vascular structures (*arrow*). It is probable that this tumour is an example of a mixed germ cell tumour incorporating both somatic and yolk sac elements. (*H&E*)

**170 Seminoma of the thymus** These tumours are histologically similar to gonadal seminomas and dysgerminomas and consist of cords of large cells with clear cytoplasm separated by fibrous septa infiltrated with mature lymphocytes. They occur in young male adults and children and following resection followed by radiation carry a good prognosis with a cure rate of 90 per cent. It is important, however, to exclude mediastinal metastases from a testicular seminoma. *(H&E)*

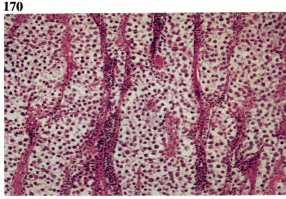

**171 Seminoma of thymus** As in gonadal seminomas and dysgerminomas, a granulomatous reaction consisting of epithelioid and giant cells is a common finding, and is helpful in distinguishing these germ cell tumours from mixed epithelial/lymphocytic thymomas. Occasionally, and particularly with biopsy specimens, the granulomatous response is so extensive that it may obscure the seminoma tumour cells, few of which could be distinguished with certainty in this specimen. *(H&E)*

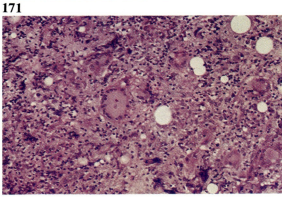

**172 Seminoma of the thymus** A second biopsy of the mediastinal tumour shown in **171** led to the correct diagnosis. A large mediastinal mass was subsequently resected and shows the familiar appearances of a seminoma with groups of tumour cells separated by slender fibrous trabeculae infiltrated with lymphoid cells. The tumour merged with the surrounding thymic tissue. The granulomatous response was very variable in different parts of the tumour and unrelated to the foci of necrosis. *(H&E)*

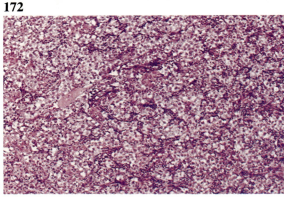

**173 Seminoma of the thymus** The large seminoma cells with clear cytoplasm contrasts strikingly in appearance with those of an epithelial thymoma, and this is very obvious in plastic processed material; tonofilaments and desmosomes are absent, glycogen accumulation is often conspicuous *(arrow)*, and the nucleoli also appear larger and less condensed. The thymic seminoma cells appear identical with those of testicular seminomas at both light and electron microscopical levels. Nevertheless, it cannot be stated dogmatically that mediastinal seminomas found within thymic tissue represent tumours of germ cells which have *migrated* into the thymus, and are thus unrelated to thymic cellular differentiation. In this context it should be remembered that although the thymus occupies a central anatomical position, it is in reality a paired organ. *(Toluidine blue)*

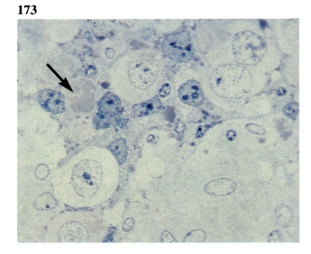

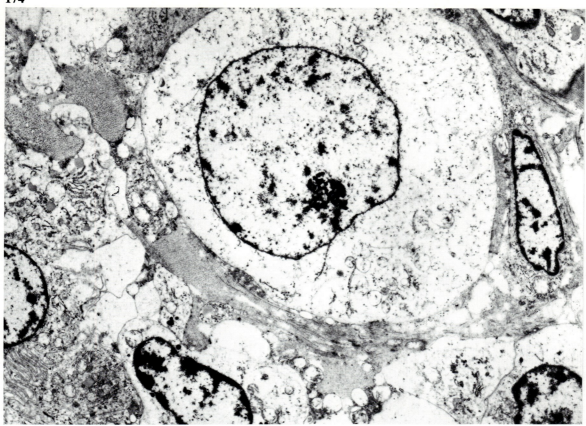

**174  Seminoma of thymus, ultrastructure** In this field there is one large seminoma cell surrounded by lymphocytes, and part of an epithelioid histiocytic cell. The nucleus of the seminoma cell shows a well-developed nucleolus with dispersed nucleonema, and the cytoplasm contains few organelles and no tonofilaments; there are neither desmosomes nor a basal lamina. *(× 6,000)*

**175  Foreign body granulomas in thymoma** In this epithelial predominant thymoma – part of which is seen on the right – there is a granulomatous response with large 'foreign body' type giant cells enclosing cholesterol clefts. Thymomas showing a prominent granulomatous response of this type have been designated previously as granulomatous thymomas. *(H&E)*

175

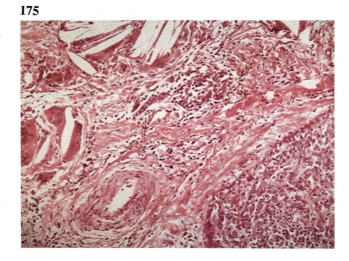

**176  Hodgkin's disease arising in the thymus** The most common type of malignant lymphoma arising in the mediastinum and involving the thymus is Hodgkin's disease, usually of the nodular sclerosing variety. As in lymph nodes, the nodules of neoplastic cells are surrounded by and demarcated by broad bands of birefringent collagen. However, the nodules of lympho-epithelioid tissue are of a different appearance from the lobular pattern seen in the majority of mixed epithelial/lymphocytic thymomas. At low magnification, not only is there often some retention of cortex and medulla, but the epithelial component can be seen to be disrupted and infiltrated by large cells (*arrows*). (*H&E*)

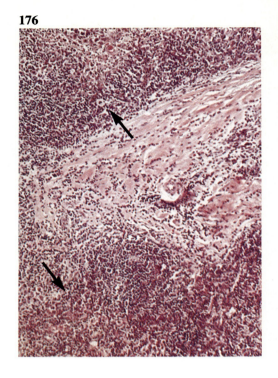

**176**

**177 and 178  Hodgkin's disease in the thymus** The microscopic appearance of Hodgkin's disease in the thymus can be confusing. The neoplastic lymphoid tissue frequently abuts on and merges with irregular but compact islands of epithelial cells (*arrow*), **177**, in which Hassall's corpuscles appear numerous and prominent. Only at high magnification can the distinction be made between the disrupted epithelial cells and the infiltrating lymphoid cells, **178**. Although lacunar cells can be identified, classical Reed-Sternberg cells are infrequent, and another source of confusion is the presence of multinucleate myoid cells. (*H&E*)

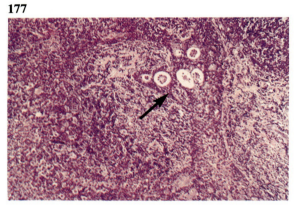

**177**

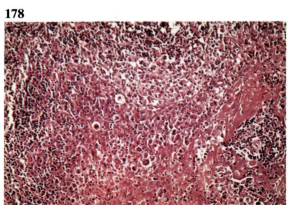

**178**

**179**

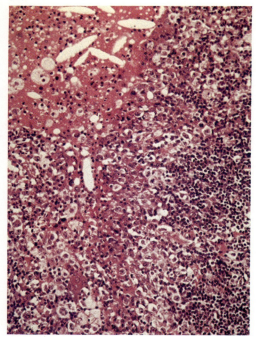

**179 Hodgkin's disease in the thymus**
Sometimes epithelial disruption and
necrosis is very marked: the degenerate
cells are mixed with cholesterol clefts producing a granulomatous appearance. The
majority of so-called granulomatous
thymomas are now considered to be
examples of Hodgkin's disease of nodular
sclerosing type involving the thymus.
*(H&E)*

**180**

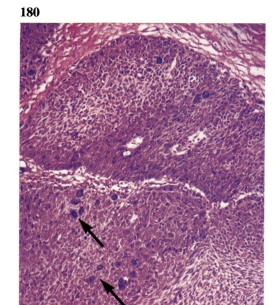

**180 Rhabdomyoepithelial cell tumours of
the thymus** Thymic myosarcomas are found
occasionally arising in the thymus and are
considered to derive from thymic myoid
cells. This tumour is composed predominantly of thymic epithelial cells but
scattered throughout are large granular
rhabdomyoblast-like cells (*arrows*) together
with some cells intermediate between
epithelial and myoid cells. *(PTAH)*

**181 Rhabdomyoepithelial cell tumour
of the thymus** This higher power view
shows rhabdomyoid cells (*arrow 1*) scattered among poorly differentiated
epithelial cells. To the left the epithelial
cells are better differentiated and show
a palisade arrangement in addition to
the presence of cytoplasmic tonofibrils
(*arrow 2*) The cytoplasm of the rhabdomyoid cells stains a granular blue due to
the content of myofibrils. *(PTAH)*

**181**

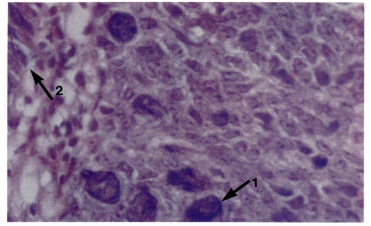

**182**

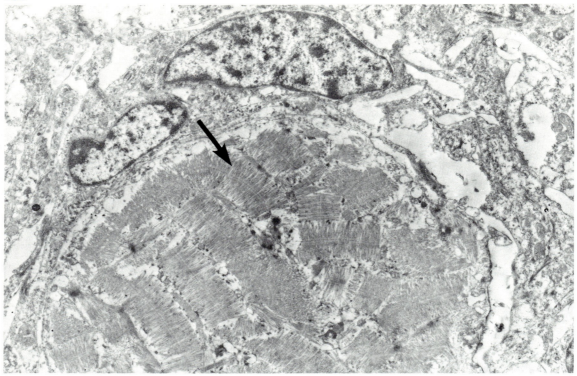

**182   Rhabdomyoepithelial cell tumour of thymus, ultrastructure** This shows part of a rhabdomyoid cell from the tumour in **180**, **181**. The abundant cytoplasm is filled with haphazardly arranged short sarcomeres (*arrow*) and has shrunk away from the surrounding epithelial cells due to poor fixation. (× 8,500)

**183**

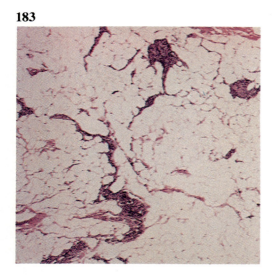

**184**

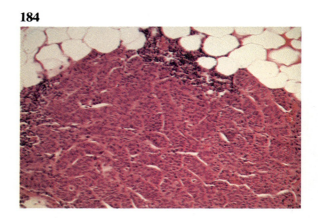

**183 and 184   Thymolipoma** A very rare questionable tumour is the so-called thymolipoma. These tumours may be huge and are composed of a mixture of mature fat and islands of normal-looking or involuted, **183**, thymic tissue such that the overall volume of thymic tissue is increased. Some of these masses have been associated with systemic effects and in one such thymolipoma from a patient with aplastic anaemia, **184**, there were several islands of thymic tissue containing microscopic carcinoid tumours. (*H&E*)

# Secondary (peripheral) lymphoreticular tissue

Lymph nodes form an important component of the peripheral or secondary lymphoreticular tissue, and are to be distinguished from the bone marrow and primary lymphoid organs such as thymus (see **0**). Other types of peripheral lymphoreticular tissues are spleen, bronchus- and gut-associated lymphoid tissue (BALT and GALT respectively) and other extra-nodal sites. In intimate communication and collaboration with the lymphoid cells are the cells of the mononuclear phagocytic system originating in bone marrow via the blood monocytes (see page 109). With age there is a progressive reduction in the amount of lymphoid tissue.

# Lymph Nodes

Lymph nodes are organised into different functional zones of which the most important are the lymphoid follicles with their germinal centres, the deep or paracortex, the medulla (medullary cords), the mononuclear phagocytic and sinusoidal systems, and the connective tissue framework.

## Lymphoid follicles and germinal centres

At birth the lymph nodes show a developed cortex but lack lymphoid follicles and germinal centres. These B-lymphocytic structures only develop following antigen challenge, and thus germinal centres (or follicle centres) are the morphological expression of an immunological response of B-lymphocytes to antigen. They will not develop in individuals reared in germ (pathogen)-free environments or in those with a defect of B-lymphocyte immunity. Normal reactive germinal centres contain a mixture of cells, of which lymphocytes predominate. The most characteristic lymphoid cell is the small follicle lymphocyte (small cleaved cell) which is not only larger than the small lymphocyte of the lymphocytic cuff (mantle zone) of the follicle but also shows a distinctive and characteristic nuclear irregularity. The small irregular follicle lymphocyte is at one end of a spectrum of irregularly nucleated lymphocytes; at the other end is the large irregularly nucleated lymphocyte. Regularly nucleated 'blast' cells and plasma cells form other constant lymphoid components of germinal centres (see **199**). The blast cells include the centroblast, plasmablast and the very large immunoblast or transformed lymphocyte. The small well differentiated 'mature' lymphocyte is rarely found. Of the non-lymphoid cells, the two most conspicuous are the tingeable-body macrophage belonging to the phagocytic system of cells, and the dendritic (antigen-trapping) cell (see **200**), the origin of which is debatable but which morphologically bears some resemblance to endothelial cells. The cytoplasm of centroblasts, plasmablasts, immunoblasts and plasma cells are intensely pyroninophilic on staining with methyl green-pyronin (MGP), by virtue of their content of ribonucleic acid (RNA) either free or bound as rough (granular) endoplasmic reticulum. The nucleoli, particularly those of immunoblasts, are also pyronin positive. The small and large irregularly nucleated lymphocytes, the dendritic cells and the macrophages show a negligible degree of pyroninophilia.

## Paracortex (deep or paracortical area)

The parenchyma of the lymph node between and deep to the lymphoid follicles is now known as the deep- or paracortex. In contrast to the B-dependent germinal centre, it is a T- or thymus-dependent area populated by T-lymphocytes. The prominence of the paracortex varies according to site, being particularly well-developed in cervical nodes, and relatively inconspicuous in abdominal nodes. The specialised vessels known as the postcapillary venules (PCV's), which are so important in the two-way lymphocyte traffic between blood and lymph, are to be found in the paracortex. In certain benign and neoplastic processes involving lymph nodes, these PCV's proliferate and may form a very conspicuous component of the reactive paracortex. Also present in the paracortex are the so-called interdigitating reticulum cells which we view as macrophage precursors (see **758**).

## Medulla

The medulla is that area of a node deep to the paracortex. The parenchyma consists of the medullary 'cords', and the sinuses between these cords are more conspicuous in the medulla than in other parts of the node. The medulla also varies considerably in prominence according to anatomical site and is usually most highly developed in abdominal lymph nodes. The medullary cords are viewed as B-cell areas and contain, in addition to lymphocytes, plasma cells in varying number. Maturation of the plasma cells series is defective in the immune deficiency states involving the B-lymphocytes.

## The mononuclear-phagocytic and sinusoidal systems

Throughout the node is a system of sinuses. These are in communication with the afferent lymphatics via the subcapsular sinuses on the one hand, and the efferent lymphatics at the hilum on the other. Lining the sinuses are the elongated sinus-lining cells which are believed to represent fixed macrophages, and which take their support from the fibre-forming cells. Scattered throughout the rest of the node are free cells of the mononuclear phagocytic system ultimately derived from monocytes and loosely called histiocytes. It is only when these mononuclear cells are actively phagocytic that they are recognised as macrophages. Macrophages tend to be most conspicuous in sinus histiocytosis and in active germinal centres where they are known as tingeable-body macrophages. Epithelioid cells, Langhans giant cells and foreign-body giant cells are also derived from mononuclear phagocytic cells, and it is our belief that so are the paracortical interdigitating reticulum cells.

## Connective tissue

The reticular or fibre-forming cells supply the connective tissue framework of the lymph node and support for the lymphatic sinusoidal system. Fibre-forming cells are inconspicuous at light microscopical level in most physiologically active nodes, though their presence may be recognised by the reticulin (argyrophilic) network present throughout the node. They are more active in some of the chronic reactive and infective processes and in certain neoplastic conditions.

Fibre-forming cells other than those associated with the blood vessels are absent from germinal centres. At ultrastructural level fibre-forming cells show the morphological features of fibroblasts and myofibroblasts and, because they too are engaged in the production of a fibrous protein, the cells may be strongly pyroninophilic by virtue of their RNA content.

# Spleen

The spleen normally weighs up to 250 gm and is an encapsulated organ which, in contrast to lymph nodes, lacks any pericapsular fatty tissue. Fibrous trabeculae pass down into the splenic substance which traditionally is divided into red and white pulp. The white pulp is composed of lymphoid tissue closely associated with the vessels passing out of the splenic trabeculae: on the basis of experimental studies, it can be divided into well-defined zones populated by either T- or B-dependent lymphocytes. The structures known as Malpighian bodies, in which well-defined germinal centres are normally seen in young individuals, are B-dependent areas, whereas the T-lymphocytes are grouped around the follicular arteries – the periarterial lymphocytic sheath or PALS.

The red pulp is made up of the sinusoidal system lined by endothelial (littoral) cells between which are the so-called Billroth cords containing a variable population of lymphoid cells, macrophages and polymorphs in transit. In the normal spleen the sinusoids are not well visualised but are readily seen in congested spleens when they are distended by red cells, and in reticulin preparations. With age the major change seen in the spleen is the progressive diminution in the amount of lymphoid tissue, particularly within the Malpighian bodies, and an absence of germinal centres. Splenic atrophy is also recognised in association with certain diseases such as coeliac disease.

# Gut-associated lymphoid tissue (GALT)

Throughout the absorptive alimentary tract, extending from Waldeyer's oropharyngeal ring down to and including the anal canal, is abundant lymphoid tissue either aggregated in non-encapsulated form or dispersed throughout the mucosal connective tissue (lamina propria). Waldeyer's ring is the lymphoid tissue made up of the tonsils (see **208**), adenoids and lingual tonsils, characteristically arranged in non-encapsulated lymphoid masses in intimate contact with the overlying epithelium. Hyperplastic follicles are common in young individuals and the active germinal centres are an important source of plasma cell production. The lamina propria of the intestinal tract contains numerous lymphocytes and plasma cells, the majority of which are engaged in the synthesis of IgA. From the stomach onwards non-encapsulated nodules of lymphoid tissue lying below the absorptive epithelium occur with increasing frequency, and towards the terminal part of the small intestine are very prominent. When these solitary nodules in the ileum coalesce they form the larger aggregates known as Peyer's patches, measuring up to 2 cm in their long axis. In the appendix also, particularly in children and young adults, large lymphoid follicles with prominent and active germinal centres are often found. Large masses of hyperplastic lymphoid tissue may also form in the rectum and anus, the so-called anal-tonsils. Mononuclear phagocytic cells are another normal component of the gastrointestinal tract, as are vessels very similar in structure to postcapillary venules. The hallmark of the gut-associated lymphoid tissue, or GALT, is the fact that it is non-encapsulated and lies beneath the epithelial surface. At one time it was considered that GALT functioned as the equivalent of the avian bursa of Fabricius, and the B of the B-lymphocyte stood for Bursa. There is now evidence that bone marrow itself subserves a bursal activity, hence B now stands equally for bone marrow.

**Component cells of peripheral lymphoreticular and mononuclear phagocytic system (LRMPS)**

On the basis of ultrastructural studies the indigenous cells of this system can be sub-divided into five categories:
1 Lymphoid cells, T- and B-lymphocytes, including plasma cells.
2 Mononuclear phagocytic cells, free and fixed.
3 Follicular dendritic (reticular) cells.
4 Endothelial cells.
5 Fibre-forming cells, fibroblasts and myofibroblasts.

# Lymph node biopsy

The pathologist should receive from the surgeon the fresh unfixed lymph node which has been carefully dissected to avoid any trauma, particularly crushing. It is then the pathologist's responsibility to ensure that adequate and representative material is processed for routine histopathology. It is convenient and often essential to process at the same time material for electron microscopy, and for histochemical and immunological studies. Ideally, the lymph node should be cut in the longitudinal (sagittal) plane. Samples for electron microscopy should be taken immediately from the cortex and medulla and either cut into 1 mm cubes or into larger (but only 1 mm thick) slices and placed in 3 per cent cacodylate buffered glutaraldehyde. One half of the node should then be placed in neutral buffered formol saline or formol calcium for conventional paraffin processing. In the event of immunocytological and histochemical investigations, additional samples from the unfixed half should be taken for snap freezing and storage, and for fixation in formol calcium. If imprints are needed these can be prepared by gently pressing clean glass slides on to a cut unfixed surface. It is desirable also, and particularly if a lymphoproliferative disorder is suspected, that some unfixed tissue should be made available for cell marker studies (and possibly also for cell culture) and transported without delay in tissue culture media.

**185**

**185 Lymph node biopsy** Shown here is a perfectly dissected lymph node sent fresh, unfixed and intact to the pathologist.

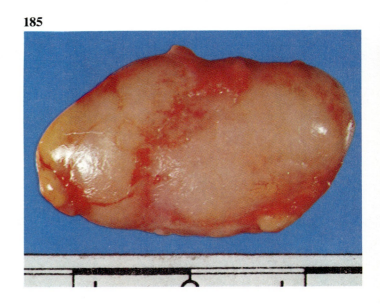

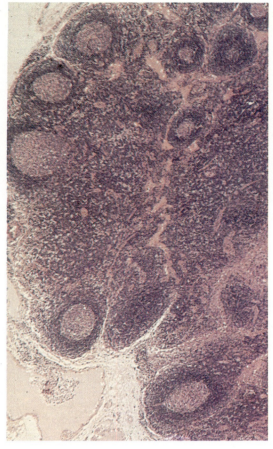

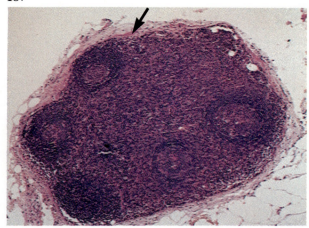

**186 and 187   Normal lymph node, anatomy** It is only by sectioning a lymph node in the sagittal plane that the normal anatomical relationships can be appreciated fully. In a typical cervical lymph node, **186**, the capsule encloses the circular sinus beneath which is the cortex containing the lymphoid follicles with germinal centres. Between and deep to these lymphoid follicles is the area called the deep – or paracortex – in which the characteristic postcapillary venules are to be found, and which merge with the medulla. The germinal centres and medullary cords are known to be the B-lymphocyte dependent areas containing a mobile population of B-lymphocytes – including plasma cells in contrast to the deep or paracortex through which T-lymphocytes circulate and which comprises the thymus dependent area. (The B was applied originally to lymphocytes considered to originate from, and depend upon the mammalian equivalent of the bursa of Fabricius, but now generally is understood to stand for the B of bone marrow). The relative prominence of these different areas within lymph nodes varies considerably according to site, and to the age and immunological activity of the individual. It also varies according to the plane of section, so that in the small abdominal node sectioned transversely through the cortex, **187**, no medulla is visible and the paracortex appears disproportionately large. That the plane of section is incorrect is apparent by the manner in which the nodal parenchyma is enclosed completely by the capsule and subcapsular sinus (*arrow*). *(H&E)*

**188**

**188   Abdominal lymph node, at birth** This abdominal lymph node from a full-term stillborn infant shows the development of cortex and medulla, but the cortex (*arrow*) consists almost entirely of closely packed small lymphocytes and lacks germinal centres. Lymphoid follicles with germinal centres develop only after immunological challenge and, thus, are not seen at birth; nor will they develop if the individual is reared in a germ-free environment. The medulla is well-formed and consists of sinuses lying between the medullary cords (*arrows*). *(H&E)*

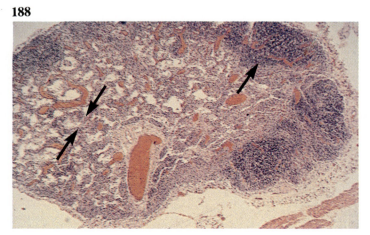

**189 Abdominal lymph node** In contrast to cervical lymph nodes, the cortex of abdominal nodes is usually rather small compared with the medulla. In this example the subcapsular sinus is well seen as are the dilated medullary sinuses. Another feature which is sometimes seen in abdominal nodes is a 'pseudofollicular' appearance (*arrow*) due to the packing and expansion of medullary cords by small lymphocytes. (*H&E*)

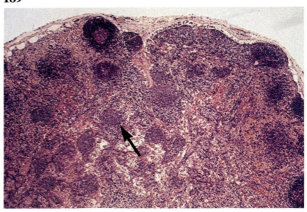

**190 Axillary lymph node** Fatty replacement of lymph node parenchyma with increasing age is particularly prominent in axillary and, to a lesser degree, femoral lymph nodes and can be seen even in relatively young individuals. In this axillary node the parenchyma forms only a very small crescentic area of the cut surface most of which consists of mature adipose tissue. Note, however, that the general configuration of the node is preserved. (*H&E*)

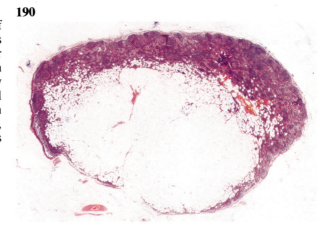

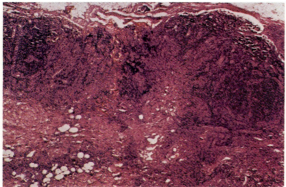

**191 Femoral lymph node** In this femoral lymph node from a young adult there is already advanced fibrosis in the hilar region. This fibrosis reflects the vulnerability of this group of lymph nodes to the effects of drainage from repeated trauma and minor infections of the lower extremities. Note also the fatty infiltration. (*H&E*)

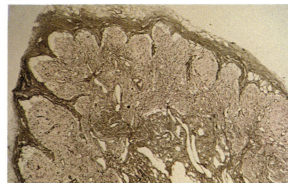

**192 Femoral lymph node** This reticulin stain emphasises the capsular thickening and the fibrotic process in the hilum extending up into the medullary area. Because of the common finding of a chronic lymphadenitis with fibrosis, groin glands are the least suitable to excise for diagnostic purposes where a choice exists between these and another group of nodes. (*Gordon & Sweets*)

**193  Normal activated lymph node** Subjacent to a
dilated and easily seen subcapsular or circular
sinus are two lymphoid follicles containing round
and clearly delineated germinal centres (follicle
centres, Fleming's centres). The scattered pale
cells giving a miniature starry sky appearance are
the tingeable-body macrophages. In between and
deep to the follicular structures are the closely
packed small lymphocytes of the paracortex
among which are the postcapillary venules
(*arrow*). *(H&E)*

**193**

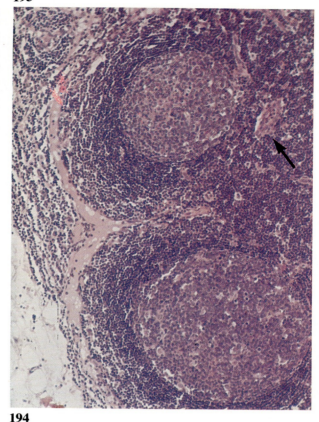

**194  Activated lymph node, normal fibre content**
Adjacent to the collagen of the capsule is the
subcapsular sinus. A rich reticulin network is
present throughout the node (cf. the pattern of
thymus, **6**) but fibres are relatively sparse in the
germinal centre (*arrow* ) where they tend to be
seen mainly in association with the small vessels.
The postcapillary venules are seen easily by this
technique. The reticulin is the product of the fibre-
forming cells. *(Gordon & Sweets)*

**194**

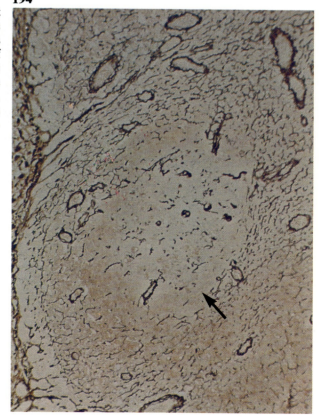

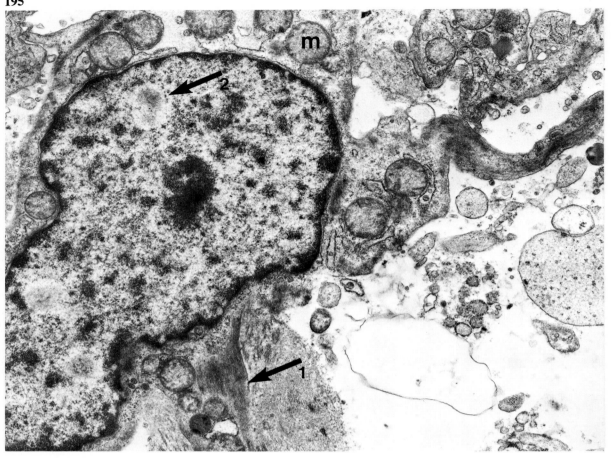

**195 Fibre-forming cells, ultrastructure** The cells responsible for the production of fibre resemble quite closely fibroblasts and myofibroblasts. The cytoplasm contains dilated rough endoplasmic reticulum (rer) and the elongated processes characteristically show dense fibrillary material abutting on the cytoplasmic borders (*arrow 1*). In an active cell of this type, as seen here, the nucleus is large with an irregularly dispersed chromatin arrangement, a fairly prominent nucleolus and often prominent nuclear bodies (*arrow 2*). m = mitochondria. (× *10,500*)

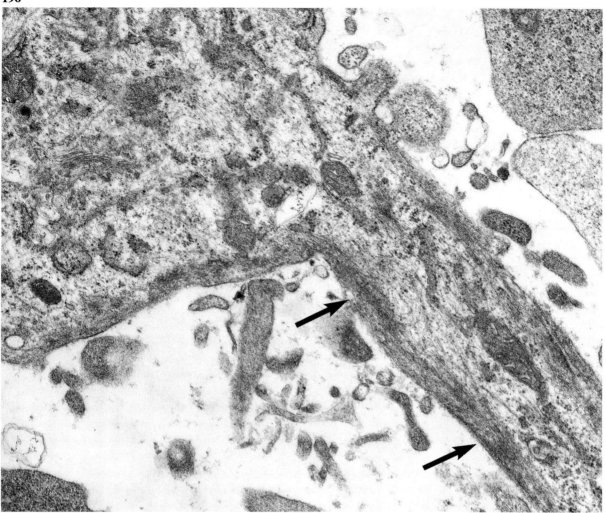

**196  Fibre-forming cells, myofibroblast, ultrastructure** Nodal myofibroblasts are indistinguishable from the myofibroblasts occurring at other sites of the body and in wound-healing. The cytoplasm which is abundant and drawn out into long processes contains a variety of organelles including rough endoplasmic reticulum: however, the characteristic feature is the fibrillary material (myofilaments – *arrow*) present along the cytoplasmic border which is similar to the myofilaments of smoth muscle. (× *25,200)*

**197 Active germinal centre** The component cells – *see page 75* – of parts of a germinal centre are here seen under the oil immersion lens in conventional paraffin-processed material. The nuclear irregularity of the majority of the lymphoid cells is in marked contrast to the nuclear uniformity of the small lymphocytes in the mantle zone (*arrow 1*). The follicle centre irregularly nucleated (cleaved) lymphocytes consist of small and large cells. Other larger lymphoid cells with regular nuclei are present also and range from immature lymphocytes or blasts (centroblasts) to large transformed lymphocytes or immunoblasts. Two cells are seen in mitosis. The elongated and vesicular nuclei (*arrow 2*) belong to the cytoplasm-rich dendritic cells. *(H&E)*

**198 Active germinal centre** The Masson's trichrome stain is excellent for demonstrating nuclear detail. In this active germinal centre most of the cells in this field are small irregularly nucleated follicle centre lymphocytes. Centroblasts with several peripherally arranged nucleoli (*arrow*) are seen easily and tingeable-body macrophages are prominent. *(Masson's trichrome)*

**199 Germinal centre cells** Staining with the methyl green and pyronin dyes (MGP) is invaluable in the interpretation of both normal and abnormal lymph node histology. In this active germinal centre several different types of pyroninophylic (MGP positive) cells can be seen. The large cell (*arrow 1*) is an immunoblast with a strongly MGP positive nucleolus and cytoplasm. The smaller MGP positive lymphoid cells are either immature lymphocytes (centroblasts) – cells which characteristically show the presence of up to four peripheral nucleoli in association with the nuclear membrane (*arrow 2*) – or plasma cells (*arrow 3*). Plasma cells – not readily apparent in routine H&E stained sections – are an invariable component of active germinal centres and may be very conspicuous in reactive nodes. Note that the cytoplasms of the irregularly nucleated (cleaved) lymphocytes (*arrow 4*) and dendritic cells (*arrow 5*) are only faintly stained (MGP negative) since they do not contain sufficient RNA, either as free cytoplasmic RNA or bound as rough endoplasmic reticulum, to combine with the red dye pyronin. *(MGP)*

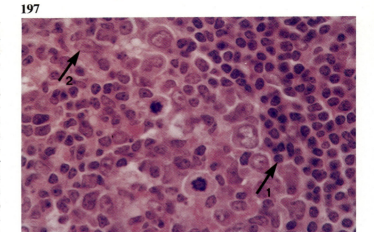

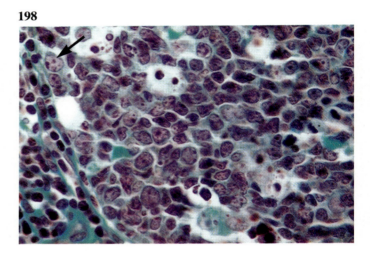

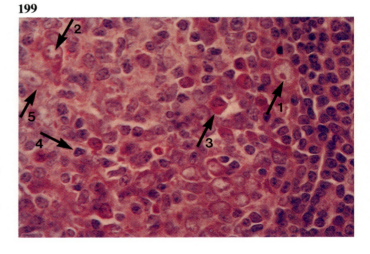

**200 Germinal centre, semi-thin plastic section** With gluteraldehyde fixation followed by plastic (epoxy resin) embedding there is minimal distortion of cellular morphology and the different features of immunoblasts (*arrow 1*), centroblasts (*arrow 2*) and the irregularly nucleated follicle lymphocytes are easily appreciated. Note that some small irregularly nucleated follicle lymphocytes are present within the surrounding mantle or cuff. The dendritic cell nuclei (*arrow 3*) resemble those of endothelial cells and macrophages but the limits of their extensive cytoplasm are poorly discerned. (*Toluidine blue*)

**200**

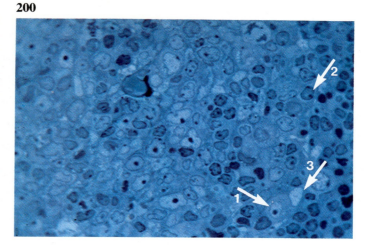

**201**

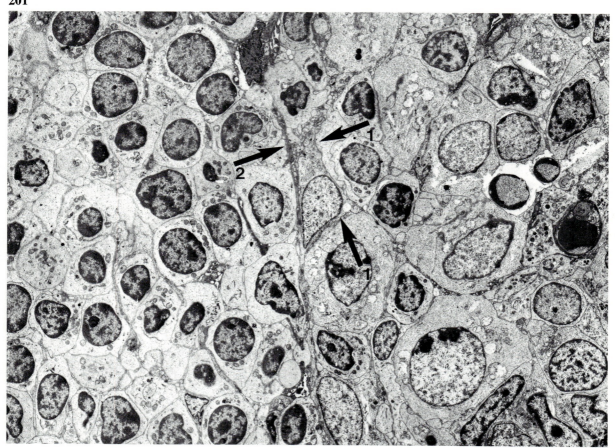

**201 Germinal centre, ultrastructure** The junctional zone between a germinal centre and its surrounding cuff of small lymphocytes shows that the elongated processes separating these two zones are derived both from dendritic 'reticular' cells (*arrow 1*) and from fibre-forming cells or fibroblasts (*arrow 2*). The nuclei of the dendritic cells are elongated with finely dispersed chromatin in contrast to the fibroblast nucleus which contains more electron dense heterochromatin. The immunoblast nuclei are rounded and regular and show a finely dispersed chromatin pattern. The large prominent nucleoli tend to be central or to lie in continuity with the nuclear margin. Their cytoplasm appears granular due to the presence of free ribonucleic acid (RNA). (× 2,770)

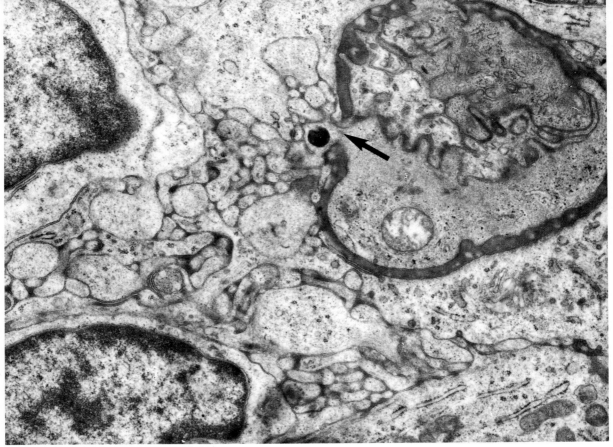

**202  Germinal centre, dendritic cells, ultrastructure** Shown here is the labyrinth formed by the ramifying processes of the dendritic cells which appear to be in direct continuity with the cytoplasm of a capillary endothelial cell (*arrow*). Electron dense fibrillar material between the dendritic cell processes is a common finding. The cells in the left-hand side of the field are lymphocytes. Note the close contact between the cytoplasmic processes of dendritic and lymphoid cells. *(× 12,000)*

**203**

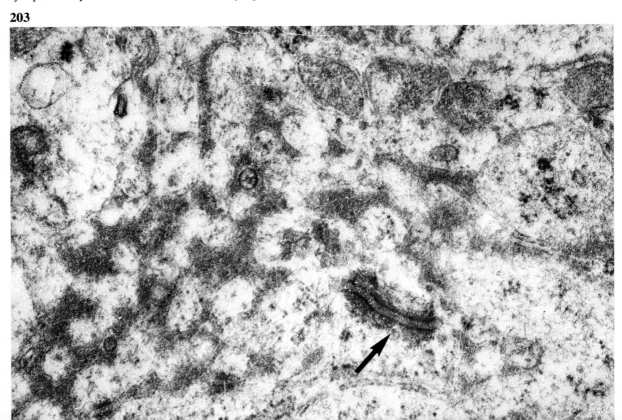

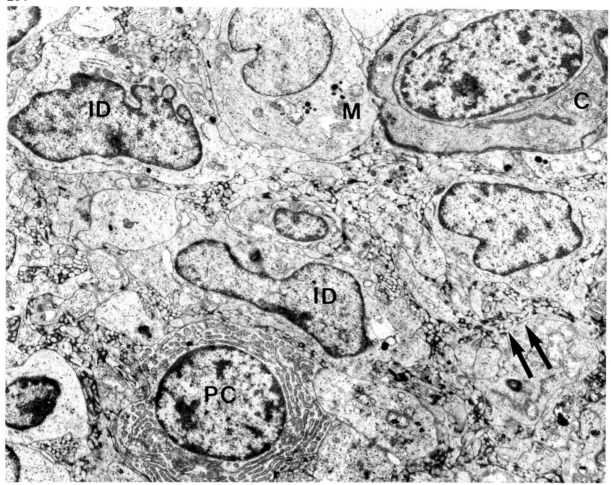

**204 Germinal centre, lymphoid cells, ultrastructure** The two lymphoid cells (ID) are typical follicle centre lymphocytes showing an irregular nuclear contour with clefts and nuclear protrusions or pockets *(left)*. The cytoplasm is more abundant than in the mature small lymphocytes of the mantle zone. The round cell at the bottom (PC) is a plasma cell with a cytoplasm containing stacks of rough endoplasmic reticulum. Interestingly, the nuclei of plasma cells found within germinal centres often exhibit irregularity, a feature which is present but rarely recognised at light microscopical level (see **199**). In between the lymphoid cells are numerous dendritic cell processes enclosing electron-dense proteinaceous material *(double arrow)*. Part of a capillary (C) and a macrophage (M) are included. *(× 6,800)*

◄**203 Germinal centre, dendritic cells, ultrastructure** In addition to possessing long cytoplasmic extensions, dendritic cells show the presence of desmosomal attachments *(arrow)* between one cell and another. This morphological feature is a useful marker at EM level in the identification of dendritic cells but it must be noted that in lymphoreticular tissue desmosomes are formed also by endothelial cells, by fibre-forming reticular cells or fibroblasts, and by sinus-lining cells in the form of autosomes (see **218**). *(× 48,000)*

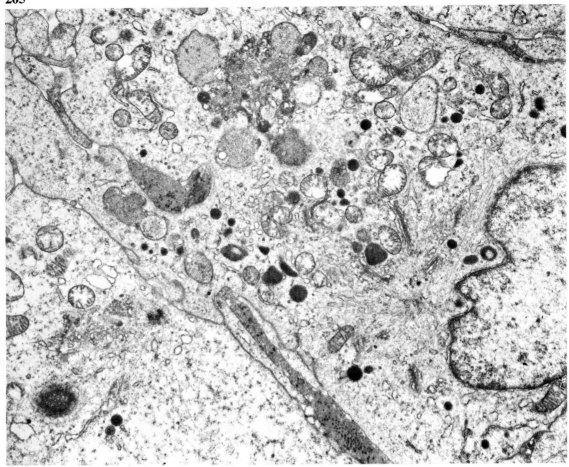

**205 Germinal centre, tingeable-body macrophage, ultrastructure** The macrophages within the germinal centres avidly phagocytose cell debris derived from dying cells and are known as tingeable-body macrophages. In contrast to the fixed sinus-lining cells, the abundant cytoplasm contains numerous electron-dense lysosomal bodies incorporating lysosomal enzymes and phagocytosed material. Both free and fixed macrophages are believed to derive initially from monocytes and form part of the mononuclear phagocytic system of cells. *(× 9,250)*

**206**

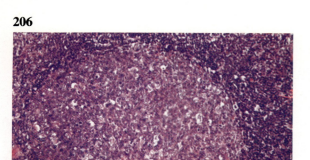

**207**

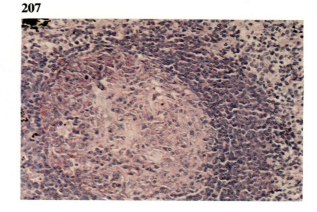

**208**

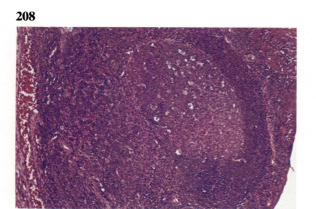

**209**

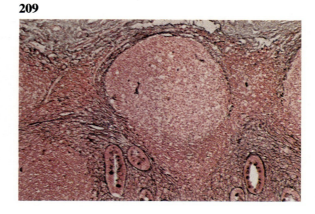

**210**

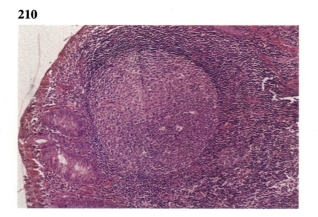

**206, 207, 208, 209 and 210  Polarity of germinal centres** Lymph node germinal centres, **206**, often show a definite biphasic staining pattern due to the different cellular composition at either pole; the dark-staining pole consisting mainly of lymphocytes, and the pale-staining pole containing numerous cytoplasm – rich dendritic cells. Evident polarity is largely dependent on the plane of section and is seen also in spleen, **207**; tonsil, **208**; appendix, **209**; intestine, **210** and wherever there is a formation of follicles with germinal centres. In all sites the pale-staining zone is nearer the source of antigen which in lymph nodes and spleen is the sinusoidal system and in gut the lumen. Note the small blood vessel at the pale pole in **206**. Polarity is absent in follicular lymphomas and, therefore, is of prime importance in separating reactive follicular hyperplasia from follicular lymphomas. (**206** *H&E;* **207** *MGP;* **208** *H&E;* **209** *Gordon & Sweets;* **210** *H&E*)

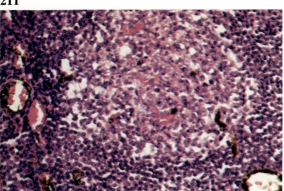
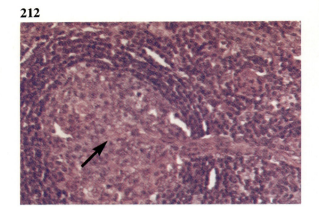

**211 and 212   Vascularity of lymphoid follicles** In the injected specimen, **211**, the venous vessels surrounding a lymphoid follicle have been filled with Colorpaque and some of the smaller capillaries within the germinal centre have also been filled with contrast media. This technique serves to emphasise the essential vascularity of germinal centres, a characteristic which is not generally appreciated. In favourable sections through lymphoid follicles, it is sometimes possible to visualise an apparent continuity between the branching small vessels of the germinal centre, **212**, and the cytoplasm of the dendritic cells (*arrow*) (see **202**). *(H&E)*

**213   Vascularity of lymphoid follicles** A good routine method for studying the vasculature of lymphoid follicles and lymph nodes in general is the Gordon & Sweets technique for reticulin. This method, as used here, demonstrates the reticulin fibre in association with vessels. *(Gordon & Sweets)*

**213**

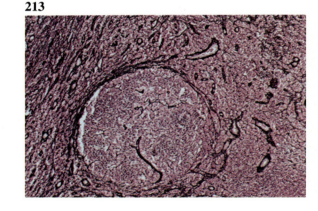

**214   Paracortex, semi-thin plastic section** The lymphocytes found in the paracortex are generally composed of small regularly nucleated lymphocytes. In plastic processed material, however, a few irregularly contoured lymphoid cells are invariably present. A few histiocytes or macrophages and larger lymphoid cells or immunoblasts are found also, but vary in number according to the reactivity of the node. The rounded structures are cross-sections of postcapillary venules and are characterised by tall endothelial cells, very narrow lumina and the presence of lymphocytes apparently within their walls (*arrows*). Well shown is the surrounding collar of adventitial cells. Postcapillary venules are an important site in the traffic of lymphocytes and enable these cells to pass from the blood into the lymphatic compartment and vice versa. *(Toluidine blue)*

**214**

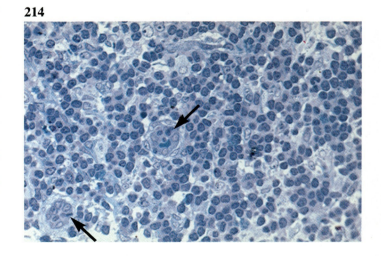

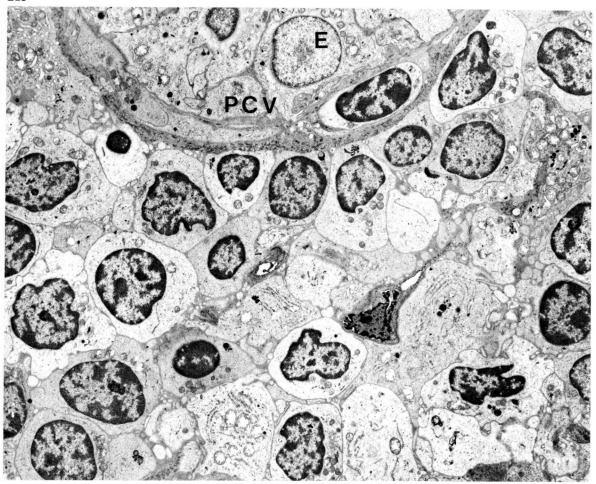

**215 Paracortex, ultrastructure** Part of a postcapillary venule (PCV) is shown above in cross-section. The lumen is considerably narrowed due to the large bulky endothelial cells (E) and there is a well-developed basal lamina which, in active lymph nodes, is often split into several layers and which may stain intensely with the periodic acid-Schiff (PAS) technique (see **278**). A migrating lymphocyte is present between endothelium and basal lamina. The generally rounded contour of the paracortical lymphocyte nuclei in contrast to those of the germinal centres is emphasised. *(× 4,800)*

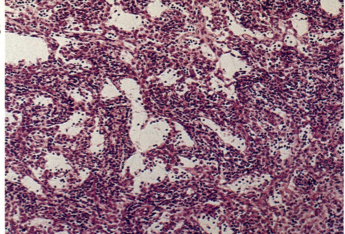

**216 Medulla, sinusoidal system** Between
the medullary cords are irregular dilated
lymphatic channels or sinuses lined by the
'fixed' sinus lining cells. Some of the sinuses
contain a few lymphocytes but in this
example little proteinaceous fluid is
evident. Such mild sinus catarrh is a
common finding in abdominal nodes. The
medullary sinuses are in continuity with the
subcapsular sinus and provide a system
whereby lymph-containing antigenic and/or
particulate material enters via the afferent
lymphatics, percolates through the
substance of the node, and then drains out
via the efferent lymphatics at the hilum.
*(H&E)*

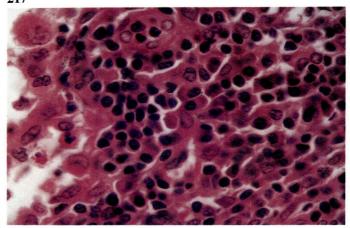

**217 Medulla, plasma cells** The so-called
medullary cords in addition to lymphocytes
contain plasma cells in variable numbers. In
some reactive nodes, as seen here, these
medullary cords are populated almost
entirely with plasma cells. Plasma cells and
their immediate precursor, the plasmablast, are specialised B-lymphocytes
committed to the synthesis of immunoglobulin. Note the very different
morphology of the sinus-lining cells present
on the left. *(H&E)*

**218 Medulla, sinus-lining cell,
ultrastructure** The sinus-lining
cells show a somewhat irregular
cytoplasmic contour characteristically enclosing bundles of collagen
fibres. A distinctive feature is the
presence of autosomes (desmosomal attachments between the
cytoplasm of the same cell –
*arrow*). These sinusoidal cells have
some features in common with the
mononuclear phagocytic cells from
which they are believed to derive.
Lysosomes, however, are inconspicuous in this resting cell. Note
the prominent network of fine filaments in the cytoplasm. *(× 21,150)*

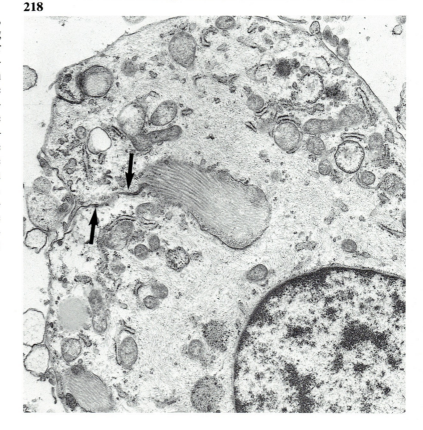

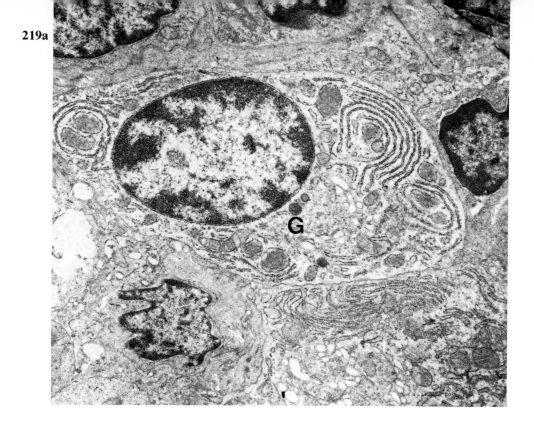

**219a**

G

**219a and 219b  Plasma cells, ultrastructure** A mature plasma cell is shown in **219a** with cytoplasm containing abundant rough endoplasmic reticulum with electron-dense secretory products (immuno-globulin). Adjacent to the eccentric nucleus is a large Golgi apparatus (G), the structure which is responsible for the perinuclear halo, or hof, seen at light microscopical level. In **219b**, a mature plasma cell, and the immediate precursor cell, the plasmablast are both intensely MGP positive due to their high cytoplasmic RNA content. In contrast to the immunoblast there is more abundant rough endoplasmic reticulum (rer) and nuclear chromatin in the plasmablast. *(219a × 9,000; 219b × 11,150)*

**219b**

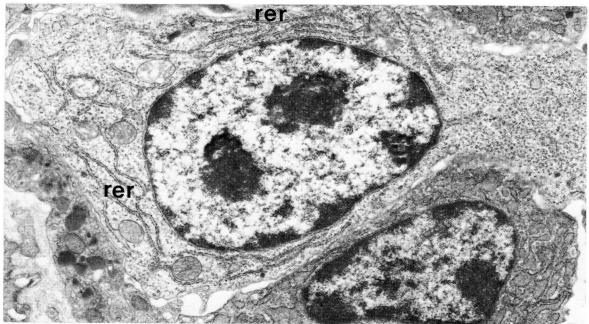

rer

rer

# Reactive processes affecting the peripheral lymphoreticular tissue

## Non-specific reactive changes

Any of the cells normally present in peripheral lymphoreticular tissue may proliferate in response to a variety of different antigens/infections. In practice, the areas or structures most frequently involved are (1) the B-dependent lymphoid follicles and germinal centres; (2) the paracortical T-cell areas which include the postcapillary venules; (3) the sinuses and mononuclear phagocytic system of free and 'fixed' macrophages; (4) the medullary cords.

**220**

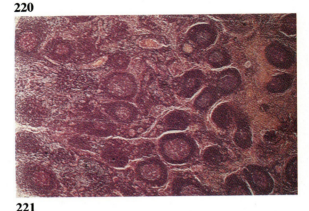

**220 Follicular hyperplasia** A common finding in enlarged lymph nodes is the presence of numerous lymphoid follicles with prominent and active germinal centres. Follicular hyperplasia may be confined to the cortical areas or may involve the entire substance of the node. This type of response is non-specific and is seen following a number of different stimuli ranging from infective processes to drainage of various substances including tumour products. *(H&E)*

**221**

**221 Follicular hyperplasia** The lymphoid follicles contain germinal centres which are often very large and irregular. The population of cells within the germinal centres is that normally found but shows increased cellular proliferation, with prominent mitotic activity and cell breakdown and, consequently, increased numbers of tingeable-body macrophages. Germinal centres which contain numerous mitotic figures and tingeable-body macrophages, and show a well-developed mantle, are unlikely to be neoplastic. *(H&E)*

**222 Follicular hyperplasia in rheumatoid arthritis** One disease sometimes associated with a striking degree of follicular hyperplasia is rheumatoid arthritis, as in this trichrome-stained section. The lymphoid proliferation may result in generalised lymphadenopathy and even splenomegaly. The lymphoid follicles vary considerably in size and may show variation in the shape of the germinal centres. This condition is confused sometimes with follicular lymphoma. Note the very sharp outline of the germinal centres and the well-defined mantles. *(Masson's trichrome)*

**223 Follicular hyperplasia in rheumatoid arthritis** At higher magnification and with methyl green-pyronin staining of the node in **222**, the germinal centres are seen to contain numerous variable-sized pyroninophilic cells, many of which are immunoblasts *(arrow)*. Some of the smaller pyroninophilic cells are plasma cells and plasmoblasts and these may be found also in large numbers in the paracortex. *(MGP)*

**222**

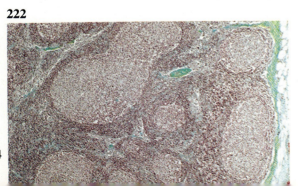

**223**

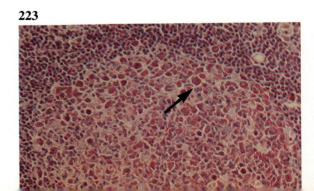

**224 Follicular hyperplasia** Marked follicular hyperplasia is a feature of many infectious processes and is a common finding in the early stages of toxoplasmosis, glandular fever, and the primary and secondary stages of syphilis. Coalescence and some necrosis of the germinal centres, producing a bizarre and irregular pattern, is particularly common in children. In this example, the follicles and germinal centres are very large as well as being of irregular contour – an appearance sometimes referred to as giant follicular hyperplasia. An infectious aetiology cannot be established always and the importance of the condition lies in its ready confusion with a follicular lymphoma. Note, however, the preservation of the lymphocytic mantles.

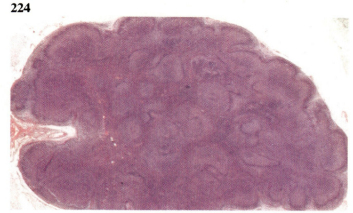

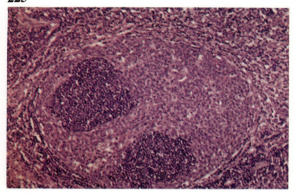

**225 Follicular hyperplasia** In some reactive nodes the plane of section through the large and irregular follicles results in an unusual appearance of small lymphocytes apparently contained within the germinal centre. These lymphoid clusters are, however, part of and continuous with the mantle zone. *(H&E)*

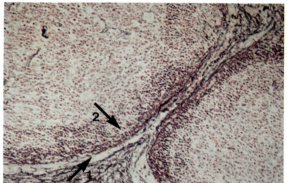

**226 Follicular hyperplasia, reticulin pattern** Reticulin preparations, particularly in a typical follicular hyperplasia are usually quite helpful in demonstrating the basic normality of nodal architecture. This example shows preservation of the subcapsular sinus (*arrow 1*) and a scant amount of reticulin within the germinal centres. Note the virtual absence of reticulin within the mantle zone (*arrow 2*). *(Gordon & Sweets)*

**227 Follicular hyperplasia, germinal centres** The appearance of the germinal centres in some examples of follicular hyperplasia may be extremely worrying particularly if there are large numbers of centroblasts as illustrated here, and immunoblasts. However, there are numerous tingeable-body macrophages containing much nuclear debris, (*arrows*) which favours a reactive rather than a neoplastic process. *(H&E)*

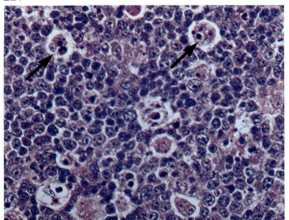

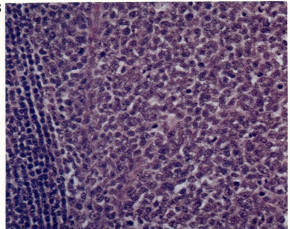

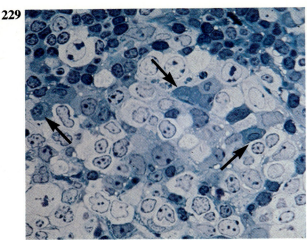

**228 Follicular hyperplasia, germinal centre** In this unusual type of follicular hyperplasia the germinal centres contain a relatively mono-morphous population of small follicle centre (cleaved) lymphocytes showing high mitotic activity but a relative absence of tingeable-body macrophages. This atypical appearance may be confused with a follicular lymphoma. However, the mantle of small mature lymphocytes is well developed, a feature which tends to be absent in neoplastic follicles. *(H&E)*

**229 Follicular hyperplasia, semi-thin plastic sections** The cellular components of this atypical reactive germinal centre in a patient with tonsillar lymphoid hyperplasia are particularly well visualised in plastic-processed material. Although there is a preponderance of large lymphoid forms, the small follicular centre cells are now seen easily, and there are several *(arrows)* plasma cells. The upper area shows the preservation of the mantle zone of small mature lymphocytes. *(Toluidine blue)*

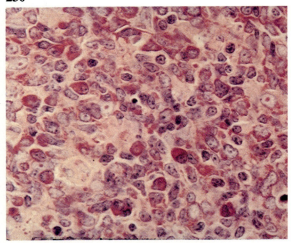

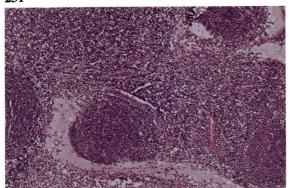

**230 Follicular hyperplasia, germinal centre** In follicular hyperplasia, plasma cells may be extremely numerous in the active germinal centres, a feature which usually escapes recognition in routine H&E preparations. In methyl green-pyronin stained sections the plasma cell component is clearly evident as demonstrated by the intense cytoplasmic pyroninophilia and the delineation of the perinuclear hofs. *(MGP)*

**231 Follicular hyperplasia** In abdominal nodes, in addition to sinus catarrh the formation of rounded lymphoid aggregates lacking germinal centres is quite a common finding. When the change is prominent it may lead to confusion with a follicular lymphoma. *(H&E)*

**232 Follicular hyperplasia** Germinal centres may form within the follicular structures and, when surrounded by concentric rings of lymphocytes as shown here, simulate the appearances of some forms of angio-follicular lymph node hyperplasia. The finding of polarity in the germinal centre is very useful in resolving the difficulty, since polarity is not seen in either angiofollicular lymph node hyperplasia, or in neoplastic follicles. *(H&E)*

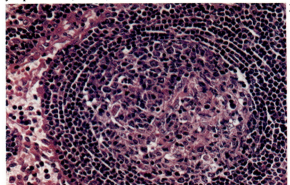

**233**

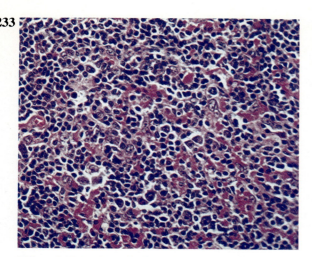

**234**

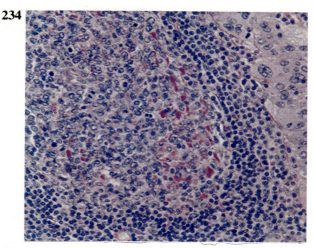

**233 and 234  Germinal centres, post-reactive change** Following the formation of active germinal centres a number of changes may occur. One of the most common is the presence of eosinophilic (pink) proteinaceous material, **233**, between the cells which later becomes organised and undergoes fibrosis. This feature is also seen in some follicular lymphomas (see **593**). The proteinaceous material is often PAS positive, **234**, as shown in this germinal centre from a lymph node with secondary carcinoma and emphasises that the intercellular material is predominantly within the dendritic cap. *(233 H&E; 234 PAS)*

**235**

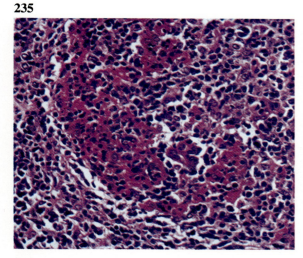

**235  Germinal centres, post-reactive change** In some instances, as seen here, the intercellular pink material appears to derive mainly from the seepage or haemorrhage of red cells from the small capillaries present within germinal centres. What determines this process is not fully understood, but may be due to an underlying inflammatory reaction. *(H&E)*

**237  Germinal centres, post-reactive change** In this high power view of **236**, the eosinophilic cells can be identified as secretory cells with globules of immunoglobulin (Russell bodies) distending their cytoplasm. The nuclei also are distorted and eccentric and not identified readily as plasma cell nuclei. *(arrows) (H&E)*

**236**

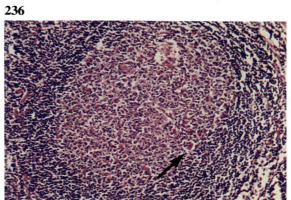

**236  Germinal centres, post-reactive change** Rarely, germinal centres may appear 'pink', because of the presence of cells with abundant pink-staining cytoplasm and not because of intercellular red cell deposition or acellular proteinaceous material *(arrow).(H&E)*

**237**

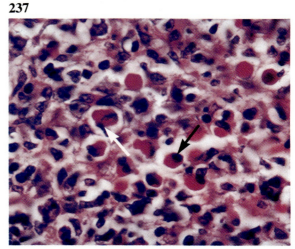

**238**

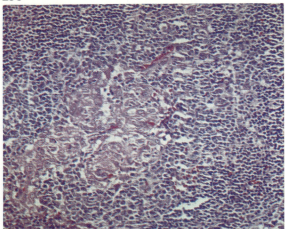

**238 Germinal centres, post-reactive changes** With continued activity, atrophic changes may occur within the 'exhausted' germinal centre consisting of prominent loosely aggregated dendritic cells and fewer lymphoid cells; mitotic figures and tingeable-body macrophages are generally absent. *(H&E)*

**240**

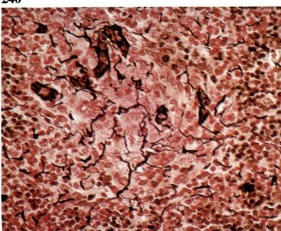

**241**

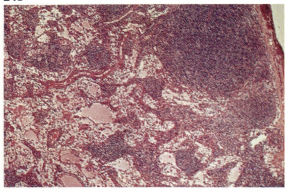

**241 Sinus histiocytosis (sinus catarrh)** This is a common and non-specific occurrence, particularly frequent in abdominal lymph nodes where the sinuses usually appear dilated and contain an abundance of proteinaceous fluid in addition to conspicuous sinus lining cells, free macrophages

98

**239**

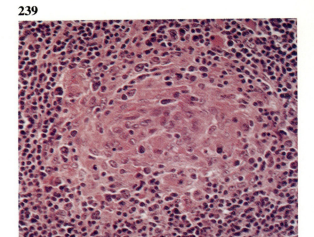

**239 Germinal centres, post-reactive changes** Occasionally, the histiocytic and dendritic cells in the involuted germinal centre assume an epithelioid appearance, and there are only a few lymphoid cells and an absence of a mantle zone of small lymphocytes. Note the resemblance of this atypical 'centre' to some of those seen in examples of angiofollicular lymph node hyperplasia. *(H&E)*

**240 Germinal centres, post-reactive changes** 'Epithelioid' centres may contain increased amounts of reticulin fibre, much of which is seen in relation to the walls of small vessels as well as to the intercellular ground substance. The vascularity and sclerosis of involuted centres is not readily apparent in H&E stained sections. *(Gordon & Sweets)*

**242**

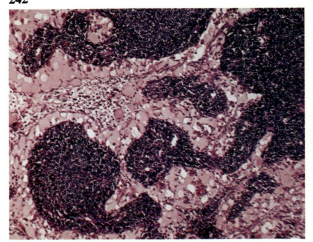

**242 Sinus histiocytosis (sinus catarrh)** In many otherwise normal abdominal lymph nodes the sinuses are extremely prominent and filled with protein-aceous fluid (lymph) but show little mononuclear – phagocytic activity. It is probable that such an appearance reflects normal physiological activity in this anatomical location. *(H&E)*

and lymphocytes. In this example there is relative inactivity of the cortex and an absence of germinal centres. *(H&E)*

**243**

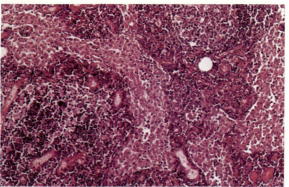

**244**

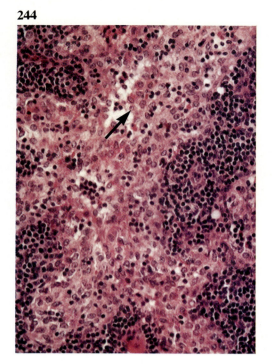

**243 Sinus histiocytosis** Except in abdominal nodes, sinuses are not normally well seen. In this cervical lymph node the sinuses are widely dilated, however, and filled with free phagocytic cells (histiocytes), admixed with a few lymphocytes. Such sinus histiocytosis is a response of the mononuclear phagocytic system of cells and can be quite independent of any immunological mechanism and merely reflect the innate filtering function of phagocytes. *(H&E)*

**245**

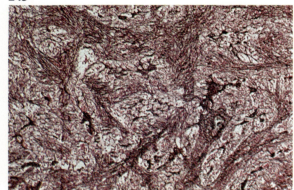

**244 Sinus histiocytosis** At this magnification, the proliferating histiocytes (mononuclear phagocytes) appear mature and reveal no atypical forms. Phagocytosis may be seen, including erythrophagocytosis (*arrow*) but is rarely so marked as in histiocytic medullary reticulosis or in histiocytic lymphomas. *(H&E)*

**245 Sinus histiocytosis** Reticulin preparations emphasise the dilated sinuses between the framework of the medullary cords. Reticulin fibre is also present within the sinuses. This example is slightly unusual in the very rich reticulin content of both parenchyma and sinuses. *(Gordon & Sweets)*

**246 Sinus histiocytosis** In some cases, the proliferation of histiocytes within the sinuses may simulate an appearance of a neoplastic proliferation of histiocytes. In other cases, as seen here in this poorly fixed preparation, the histiocytic proliferation may suggest sinus involvement by secondary carcinoma. *(H&E)*

**246**

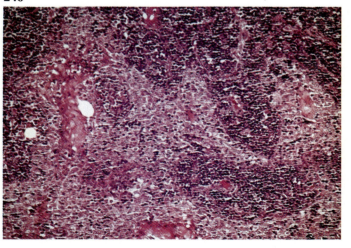

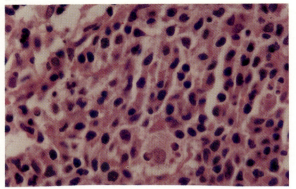

**247 Sinus histiocytosis** Sometimes, the mono-nuclear cells filling the sinuses in reactive nodes appear smaller, less mature and possess darkly staining nuclei – so-called unripe sinus histio-cytosis. There is some debate as to whether these cells are lymphocytic or histiocytic in origin. They are particularly common in toxoplasmosis. This example is from a node draining a breast carcinoma. *(H&E)*

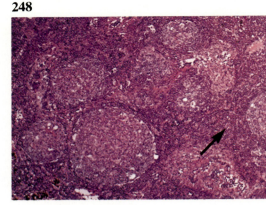

**248 Generalised hyperplasia of lymph nodes** Re-active lymph nodes are frequently encountered in which there is follicular hyperplasia and sinus histiocytosis combined, as in this mediastinal node with paracortical hyperactivity as shown by in-creased numbers of PCV's *(arrow)*. *(H&E)*

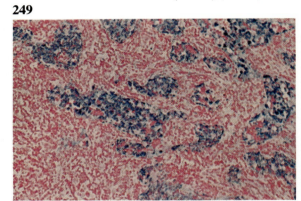

**249 Sinus histiocytosis** One of the most common of the many causes of sinus histiocytosis is the response to particulate matter. In this lymph node from a patient with advanced haemosiderosis re-sulting from multiple blood transfusions, the sinusoidal system is mapped out by the abundance of blue-staining iron within the proliferating sinus-oidal macrophages. *(Perls)*

**250 Sinus histiocytosis** In this mediastinal lymph node carbon pigment is seen within the proliferating histiocytes. This finding is useful since its presence will help to dis-tinguish macrophages from metastatic carcinoma cells with which sometimes they may be confused. At this magnifica-tion, however, the morphological features of reactive histiocytes (phagocytes) with their pale vesicular nuclei and abundant cytoplasm containing black pigment are readily identified. *(H&E)*

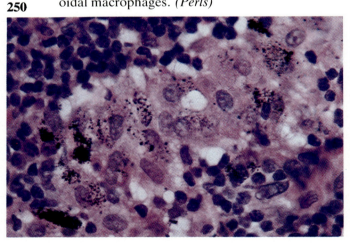

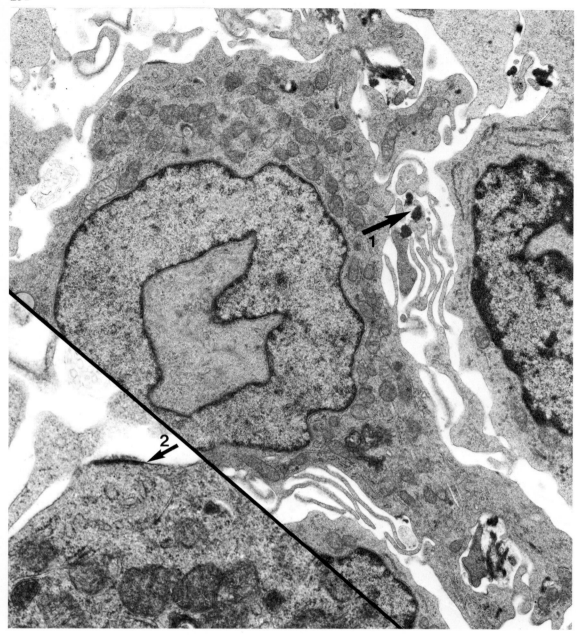

**251 Lymph node, free sinusoidal macrophage (histiocyte), ultrastructure** The cytoplasmic contour is irregular due to innumerable cytoplasmic projections varying from filiform to rather larger broader processes engulfing electron-dense material (*arrow 1*). The nucleus shows a rather characteristic finely dispersed chromatin pattern with condensation at the nuclear membrane. The apparent cytoplasmic nuclear inclusion seen in the centre is due to the plane of section through an indented or reniform nucleus. The cytoplasm contains an abundance of mitochondria but, in this particular view, lysosomes are few. The presence of focal areas of density along the cytoplasmic membrane (*arrow 2*), which superficially resemble hemidesmosomes is another characteristic feature of the histiocytic series. The inset shows these linear densities to include a superficial fuzzy coat and an absence of converging filaments. (× 9,500; inset ×28,500)

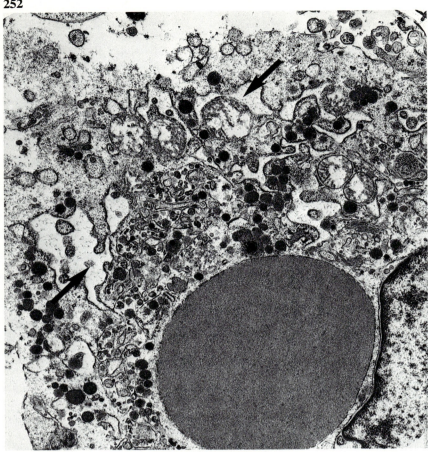

**252  Lymph node – a free macrophage (histiocyte), ultrastructure** Part of
the nucleus of a free macrophage is seen at the lower right-hand side, and
immediately adjacent is an ingested red cell (RBC). The cytoplasmic
contour is extremely irregular due to innumerable flaps and folds and
results in the appearance of cytoplasmic vesicles. These 'vesicles', however, are continuous with the extra-cellular space  *(arrows)*. A typical
feature of this cell is the numerous electron-dense membrane-bound
granules – the secondary lysosomes. The number of lysosomes varies
considerably from one macrophage to the other depending upon its degree
of activity and maturity. *(× 15,150)*

**253**

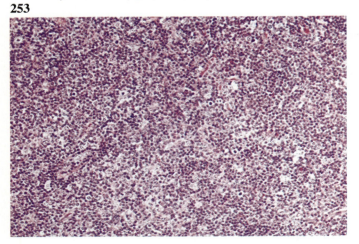

**253  Paracortical hyperplasia** The paracortical area of the lymph node frequently
enlarges in reactions to a variety of different stimuli and usually indicates a proliferation of the T-dependent lymphocytes.
It is most commonly seen in cervical
lymph nodes and occasionally may be so
marked that the expanded cortex results
in an apparent reduction of the lymphoid
follicles (see also **273**). *(H&E)*

**254**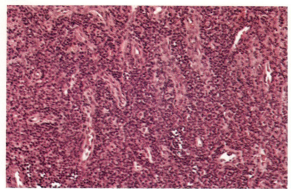

**255**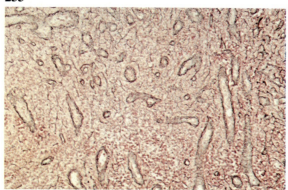

**254 Paracortical hyperplasia, postcapillary venules** A characteristic accompaniment of the proliferation of lymphoid cells within the paracortex is the presence of numerous and hyperplastic PCV's. In its extreme form this vascular proliferation is seen in angioimmunoblastic lymphadenopathy. Less marked examples are very common and are seen in a number of different conditions. This inguinal lymph node from a patient with chronic lymphadenitis also shows sclerosis of PCV's, which further adds to their prominence. (H&E)

**256 Paracortical hyperplasia, postcapillary venules** The proliferating vessels in this reactive node show extremely tall and plump endothelium between which migrating lymphocytes are seen in increased numbers. Sclerosis is not a feature and at low magnifications such hyperplastic vessels may be mistaken for epithelial inclusions. (H&E)

**257 Paracortical hyperplasia, post capillary venules** A feature occasionally seen in the actively proliferating vessels is mitosis (*arrow*) of the endothelial cells. Postcapillary venule proliferation in addition to more common non-specific reactive processes is seen as a fairly common accompaniment of lymph nodes which are the site of Hodgkin's disease and follicular lymphomas. (H&E)

**255 Paracortical hyperplasia, postcapillary venules** The lymph node shown in **254** has been stained for reticulin fibre. This method is a useful means of emphasising the marked vascular prominence in the paracortex. Another good technique for demonstrating PCV's is the periodic acid-Schiff technique (see **278**).
(*Gordon & Sweets*)

**256**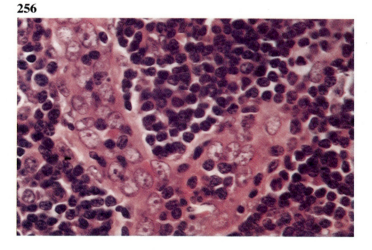

**257**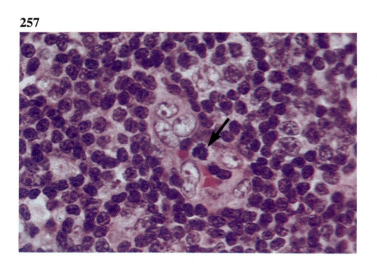

**258**

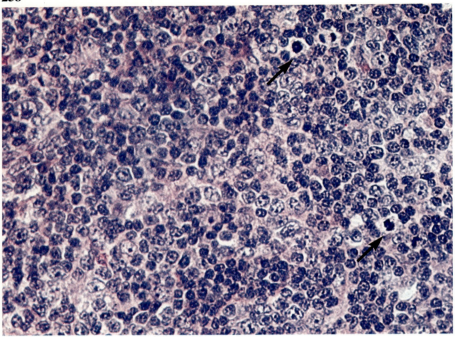

**258  Paracortical hyperplasia** The constituent cells in the hyperplastic paracortex will vary according to aetiology. Usually the predominant cell type is a small, relatively mature lymphocyte but among this population will be found larger imunoblast-like cells – many in mitosis (*arrows*) – and plasma cells. The histiocytic and interdigitating reticular components are very variable and in some conditions such as dermatopathic lymphadenopathy, are the most conspicuous cells present in the expanded paracortex. *(H&E)*

**259**

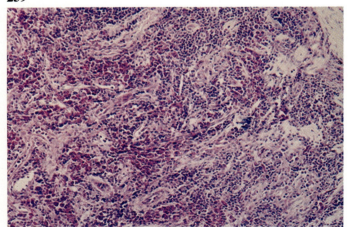

**259  Paracortical hyperplasia** In the paracortex from this patient with rheumatoid arthritis there are large numbers of relatively mature plasma cells. Lymph nodes showing increased numbers of immunoblasts in addition to plasma cells, a variable distortion of nodal architecture and striking postcapillary venule proliferation as shown here, are now generally included within the entity 'angioimmunoblastic lymphadenopathy'. *(MGP)*

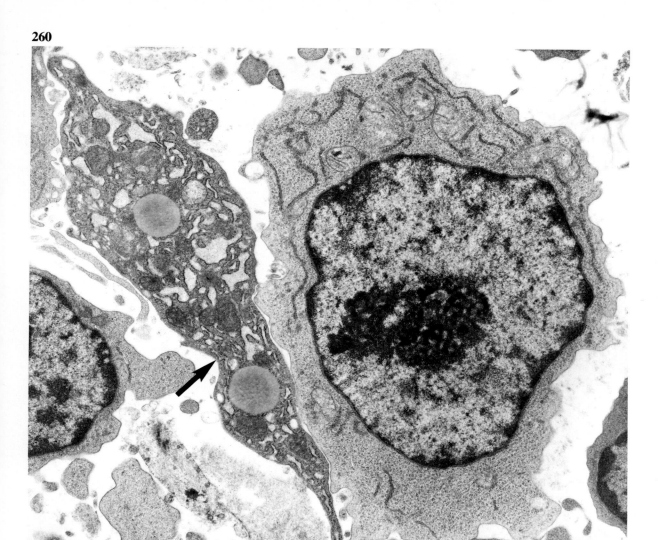

**260 Paracortical hyperplasia, immunoblast, ultrastructure** The immunoblasts in the paracortex in reactive conditions may be of both B- or T-lymphocyte origin. The ultrastructural appearances of both types of immunoblast are very similar. Adjacent to the immunoblast is part of the process of a fibre forming reticular cell or fibroblast (*arrow*). Both the immunoblast and the fibre forming cell will exhibit pyroninophilia due to the presence of free ribosomes in the former and an abundance of rough endoplasmic reticulum (rer) in the latter. Lipid droplets can be seen in the fibroblast, a not unusual finding (see **267**). (× *11,000*)

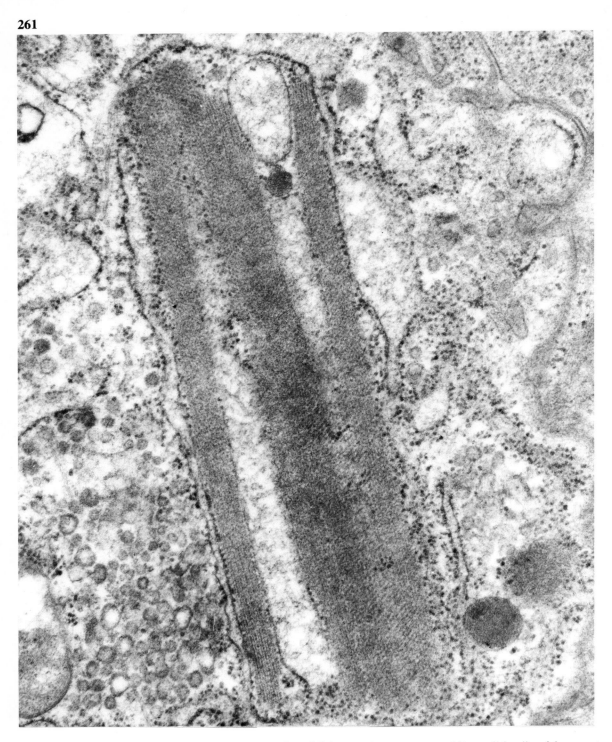

**261 Plasma cell differentiation, ultrastructure** In addition to the presence of Russell bodies (shown at EM level, **76** ) ultrastructure occasionally may demonstrate the presence of crystalline inclusion within the rough endoplasmic reticulum of reactive plasma cells. Crystalline products are however more common in the neoplastic proliferation of plasma cells. *(× 41,600)*

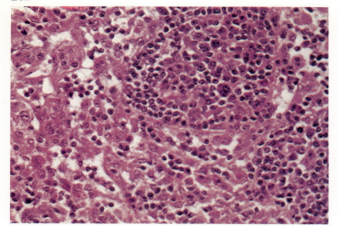

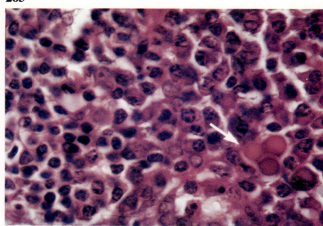

**262 Plasma cell proliferations** Plasma cell proliferation in the medullary cords is seen commonly in association with non-specific sinus histiocytosis as well as in some of the neoplastic histiocytic proliferations and is often accompanied by eosinophils, as in this example. Many plasma cells in the medullary cords of a node in combination with hyperplastic follicles favour the diagnosis of a reactive process. *(H&E)*

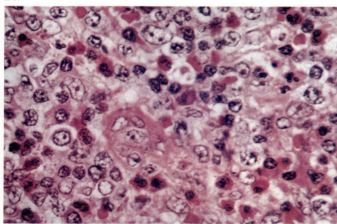

**263 Plasma cell proliferation** In some chronic reactive processes as shown here, there are increased numbers of plasma cells, some of which are distorted by (*arrow*) eosinophilic globules. These globules are Russell bodies and represent stored immunoglobulin. If the immunoglobulin is high in carbohydrate content such as IgA or IgM then the Russell bodies will stain red with the periodic acid-Schiff technique (see **282**). Atypical Russell bodies may also be seen in certain neoplastic plasma cell proliferations. *(H&E)*

**264 Eosinophilic lymphadenitis** Eosinophils are common in many reactive processes and sometimes are numerous in certain neoplastic conditions and in eosinophilic granuloma. Occasionally, as seen here, an isolated group of nodes show reactive changes accompanied by large numbers of eosinophils and increased numbers of large lymphoid cells and histiocytes; other parts of the nodes show focal necrosis. There was no known infectious cause nor evidence of an allergic disease, and the condition is probably an example of so-called eosinophilic suppurative lymphadenitis – a benign condition, albeit one of unknown aetiology. *(H&E)*

**265 Mast cells** Although the largest proportional increase in mast cells in lymph nodes is said to occur in the condition known as Waldenström's macroglobulinaemia, mast cells are found also in a number of chronic inflammatory processes and tend to be seen in association with plasma cells, as shown here. Mast cell granules stain a very distinctive orange (*arrow*) with the methyl green-pyronin stain in contrast to the rosy pink of the RNA rich cells such as plasma cells and immunoblasts; and assuming that the viewer is not red/green colour blind, pyronin is one of the best and most consistent stains with which to demonstrate mast cells. Another excellent method is Spicer's high iron diamine stain used in techniques for mucin demonstration. *(MGP)*

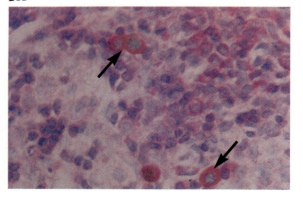

**266a**

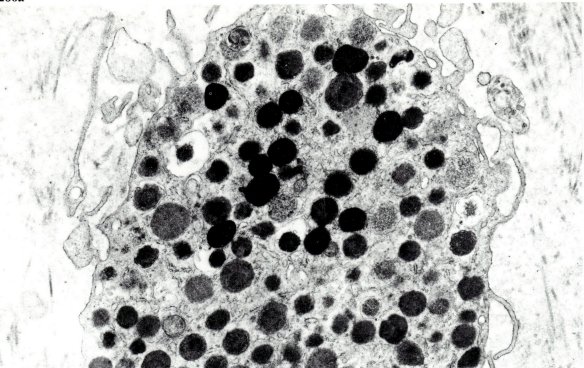

**266b**

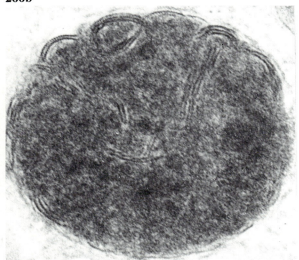

**267**

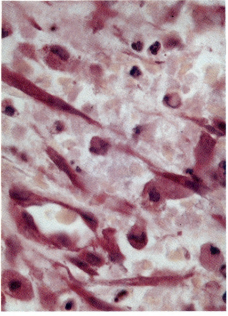

**266a and 266b  Mast cell, ultrastructure** Filling the cytoplasm, **266a**, are innumerable membrane bound lysosomal structures rich in glycoglucosamine, histamine and heparin and in certain species, but not man, serotonin, and which, **266b**, show a very characteristic scroll-like and whorled arrangement. Another feature of mast cells is the presence of delicate filiform cytoplasmic projections. (× 14,750; × 98,400)

**267  Fibroblast  proliferation** Fibroblastic proliferation is part of many reactive processes and is recognised most readily in lymph nodes where there is capsular thickening or fibrosis accompanying chronic lymphadenitis. Proliferating fibroblasts are rich in rough endoplasmic reticulum and this rich RNA content explains their very striking degree of pyroninophilia. *(MGP)*

## Mononuclear Phagocyte System

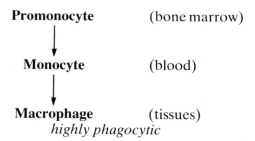

**Promonocyte**     (bone marrow)

**Monocyte**     (blood)

**Macrophage**     (tissues)
*highly phagocytic*

connective tissue (histiocyte)
liver (Kupffer cell)
lung (alveolar macrophage)
spleen (free and fixed macrophage, sinusoidal lining cell)
lymph node (free and fixed macrophage)
bone marrow (macrophages, sinusoidal lining cell)
serous cavity (peritoneal macrophage)
bone tissue (osteoclast)
nervous system (microglia)

# Reactive processes with characteristic nodal features

This descriptive phrase is used to cover a number of different conditions in which the pathology, although not absolutely specific, is sufficiently well characterised to enable a definitive diagnosis to be made and, sometimes, to infer the specific aetiology of the reactive process. As with the non-specific reactive hyperplasias seen in lymph nodes, these more specific reactive changes may involve the follicles and germinal centres, the paracortex and postcapillary venules, or the sinusoids and the medullary cords; these changes may occur either singly or in combination. The conditions which will be illustrated are:

Dermatopathic lymphadenopathy
Angioimmunoblastic lymphadenopathy
Massive sinus histiocytosis
Cholegranulomatous lymphadenitis
Fatal granulomatous disease of childhood
Sinus histiocytosis with ceroid bodies
Iatrogenic lymphadenopathy
    Post-lymphangiogram lymphadenopathy
    Drug-induced lymphadenopathy
    Post-vaccinial lymphadenopathy
Angiofollicular lymph node hyperplasia

Post-vaccinial or drug-induced lymphadenopathy cannot be differentiated on morphological findings alone, either from each other or, in some cases, from some other reactive processes such as angioimmunoblastic lymphadenopathy. They are included here for the sake of convenience.

**268**

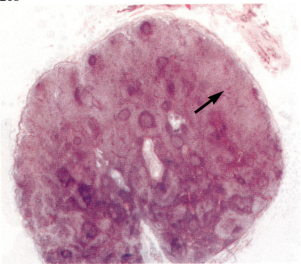

**268 Dermatopathic lymphadenopathy** Dermatopathic lymphadenopathy is a reactive condition in which enlargement of lymph nodes is found in association with a variety of chronic skin lesions – notably those characterised by pruritis, desquamation or hyperaemia. The cause of the enlargement, which is most common in the groin and axillary lymph nodes is thought to be a response to skin products draining into the regional nodes; the predominant area involved is the paracortex (*arrow*). In early or mild cases there is still retention of follicular structures, as seen here, but with further expansion of the paracortex these may be effaced. (*H&E*)

**269**

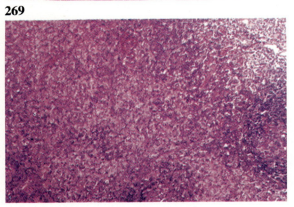

**269 Dermatopathic lymphadenopathy** Some of the most severe examples of dermatopathic lymphadenopathy are seen in generalised exfoliative dermatitis. The proliferating cells, predominantly the interdigitating reticular cells of mononuclear phagocytic origin, results in the expanded and rather palely staining paracortex. Note on the right a follicle with a rather indistinct centre. (*H&E*)

**270**

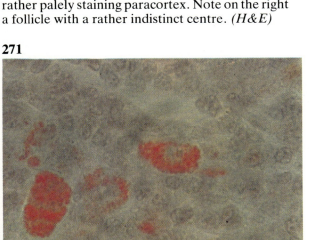

**270 Dermatopathic lymphadenopathy** Varying considerably in number are focal collections of macrophages containing brown pigment (*arrow*), which is predominantly melanin and ceroid pigment. Melanin pigment appears as finely divided brownish-black granules in contrast to the larger, more irregular lighter brown granules of iron pigment – which sometimes also may be present. (*H&E*)

**271**

**271 Dermatopathic lymphadenopathy** In addition to focal accumulations of melanin there is usually a significant amount of lipid within the macrophages which may result in a foamy appearance. The fatty material within the macrophages is more strikingly revealed in frozen sections stained with lipophilic dyes such as Oil red O·or Sudan black. The older term of lipomelanic reticulosis for this condition is deprecated since it provides a source of confusion with a lymphomatous process. (*Oil red O*)

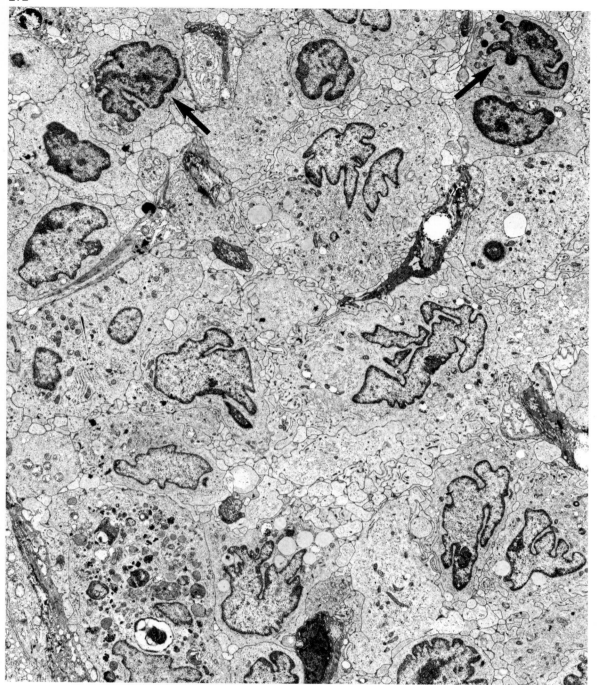

**272 Dermatopathic lymphadenopathy, ultrastructure** Electron microscopy confirms the essentially mononuclear phagocytic origin of the pale cells within the paracortical areas. They range from inter-digitating reticular cells to active macrophages whose cytoplasm varies considerably in amount and contains primary and secondary lysosomes, filled with ingested fat and pigment. Also seen in relation to the proliferating histiocytic cells are lymphocytes, some of which show the convoluted nuclei (*arrow*) characteristic of the Sézary/Lutzner T-lymphocytes. The patient, however, was a child with longstanding eczema. Dermatopathic lymphadenopathy is common in patients with the Sézary syndrome and mycosis fungoides; hence, sometimes it may be very difficult to decide whether increased number of T-cells in such patients' lymph nodes represents a non-specific proliferation of convoluted T-cells, or whether there is early involvement by neoplastic T-lymphocytes. (× 5,350)

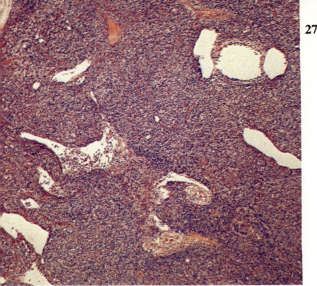

**273**

**273 Angioimmunoblastic lymphadenopathy (AILA)**
AILA or immunoblastic lymphadenopathy is a relatively
recently defined condition of unknown aetiology. The
patients are usually elderly, often present with bilateral
cervical lymphadenopathy of rapid onset following a
sometimes trivial upper respiratory tract infection, and
may suffer severe constitutional symptoms. Serological
and protein abnormalities are common and, in approximately one third of patients with dysproteinaemia, there
has been exposure to an allergen. The enlarged lymph
nodes may show either a partial or complete effacement
of architecture with loss of follicular and paracortical
demarcation, as shown here. *(H&E)*

**274**

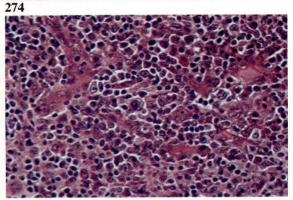

**275**

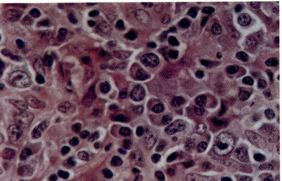

**274 AILA** The cause of the lymph node enlargement is a pleomorphic cellular proliferation which
involves the lymphoid cell series and the PCV's.
Thus, in addition to the presence of immunoblasts,
there is a constant though variable hyperplasia and
hypertrophy of the vascular component. Another
characteristic feature is the presence of amorphous
pink intercellular material. *(H&E)*

**276 AILA** Methyl green-pyronin staining
confirms, in addition to plasma cells, the many
large immunoblasts with pyroninophilic nucleoli
and thin rim of cytoplasm *(arrows)*. These
immunoblasts are consistent with a B-cell type,
since features which favour T-immunoblasts show
less cytoplasmic pyroninophilia, and in standard
preparations a rather clear cytoplasm. *(MGP)*

**275 AILA** The presence of many immunoblasts
and other cells including plasma cells may lead to a
diagnosis of a malignant lymphoma, particularly
Hodgkin's disease. It is important not to make this
error since it has been shown that the use of
chemotherapy in AILA results in fulminating and
fatal infections. Conversely, careful follow-up in
AILA is equally important since a significant
number develop a malignant lymphoma – usually
of non-Hodgkin's type. *(H&E)*

**277 AILA** The degree of accompanying vascular
proliferation is variable. In this example there is a
striking hyperplasia of PCV's. The endothelial
cells are tall and swollen and are seen in association
with migrating small lymphocytes. Although the
vascular changes are of great diagnostic value in
this condition, it should be borne in mind that
proliferation of PCV's is seen in some lymphomas,
such as Hodgkin's disease and follicular lymphoma,
as well as in other reactive processes. *(H&E)*

**276**

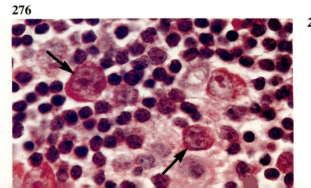

**277**

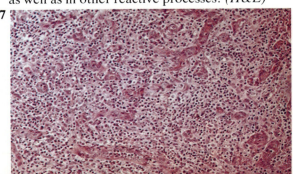

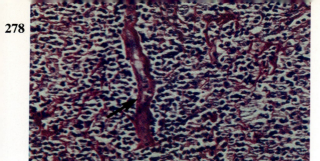

**278**

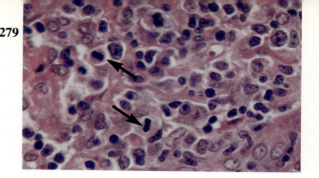

**279**

**278 Angioimmunoblastic lymphadenopathy** Delineating the proliferating vessels (*arrow*) is PAS positive proteinaceous material, which is seen also in an intercellular location. The vascular PAS positive material corresponds at ultrastructural level to basement membrane protein. A reticulin stain is a useful alternative to the PAS technique in outlining the arborizing vessels. *(PAS)*

**279 Angioimmunoblastic lymphadenopathy** The mitotic activity of the proliferating cells may be very intense. A helpful and characteristic feature is the way in which the cells in mitoses (*arrows*) are seen in close association with the postcapillary venules. Cells in mitosis may even be seen within the vessels when it is not always possible to indicate whether they are of lymphoid or endothelial origin (see **257**). Note the prominent intercellular pink proteinaceous material. *(H&E)*

**280 Angioimmunoblastic lymphadenopathy** In this case the diffuse proliferation of lymphocytes, immunoblasts and plasma cells, accompanied by numerous eosinophils, results in a pleomorphic appearance suggestive of Hodgkin's disease. Genuine Reed-Sternberg type cells are extremely rare – although there may be occasional very large mononucleated cells and even binucleate forms. *(H&E)*

**281 Angioimmunoblastic lymphadenopathy** In other examples, as shown here, there is a prominent mononuclear phagocytic cell proliferation leading to a histiocytic appearance. The histiocytes never appear atypical although sometimes they may assume epithelioid features. *(H&E)*

**282 Angioimmunoblastic lymphadenopathy** The focal collections of histiocytes may assume an epithelioid appearance and show the presence of cytoplasmic PAS positive material (*arrow*) as in other reactive histiocytic proliferations. The intensely PAS positive cell adjacent to a postcapillary venule is a plasma cell containing Russell bodies (immunoglobulin secretion). *(PAS)*

**280**

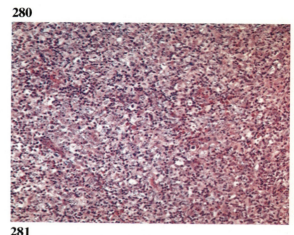

**281**

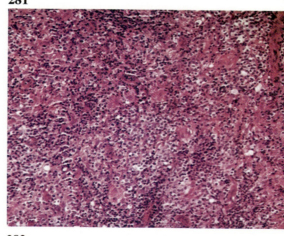

**282**

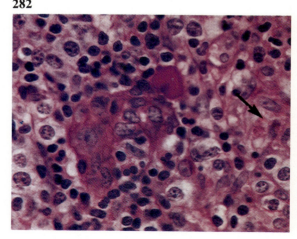

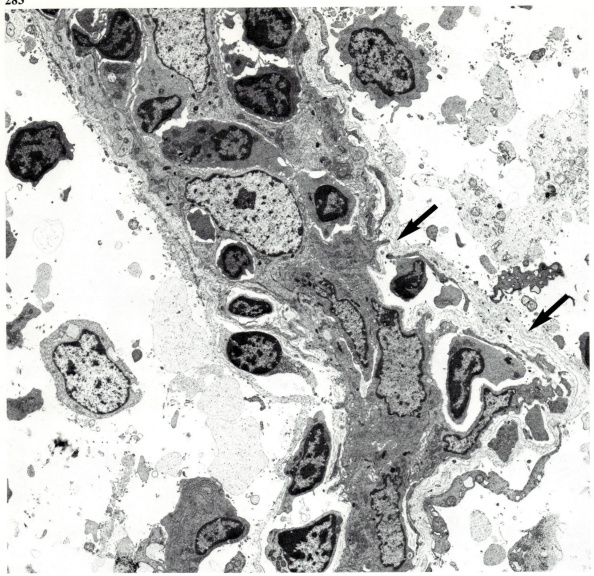

**283 Angioimmunoblastic lymphadenopathy, ultrastructure** This hyperplastic venule has been cut in longitudinal section. The lumen is markedly reduced in calibre, numerous lymphocytes are seen between the tall endothelial cells and there is prominent splitting (or reduplication) of the basal lamina (*arrow*). (× 4,800)

284

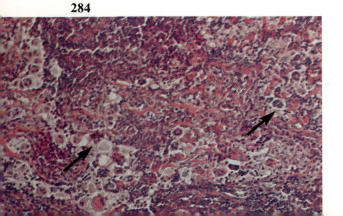

**284 Massive sinus histiocytosis** In this benign condition, also known as Dorfman's disease, the most striking clinical finding is massive enlargement, usually bilateral, of the cervical lymph nodes; hence the original term-sinus histiocytosis with massive lymphadenopathy. At low magnification, the enlargement of the lymph nodes is due mainly to greatly distended sinuses filled with large macrophages (*arrow*). The patients tend to be children or adolescents; the disease is rare after 20 years of age. There are very few constitutional symptoms and, after a variable time course, there is complete resolution of the lymphadenopathy. (*H&E*)

**285**

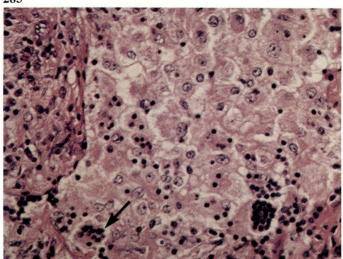

**285 Massive sinus histiocytosis** The appearance of the proliferating mononuclear phagocytic cells, or histiocytes, varies from one area to another. In their most characteristic form they are very large with abundant, pinkish granular cytoplasm enclosing variable numbers of lymphocytes (*arrow*), plasma cells and even occasionally polymorph neutrophils. Plasma cells are invariably seen in the adjacent medullary cords. *(H&E)*

**286**

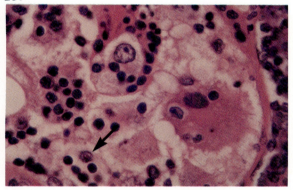

**286 Massive sinus histiocytosis** At high magnification, lymphocytes are identified readily within the cytoplasm of the macrophages and result in a highly characteristic and diagnostic appearance. Note also the occasional plasma cells (*arrow*). It has been suggested that these lymphoid cells have been phagocytosed; the authors believe that the lymphoid cells are actively travelling in and out of the macrophages – a process known as emperipolysis. *(H&E)*

**288 Massive sinus histiocytosis** With progressive resolution of the condition there is increasing fibrosis and loose textured connective tissue extends from the capsule and medullary cords into the sinuses. *(H&E)*

**287**

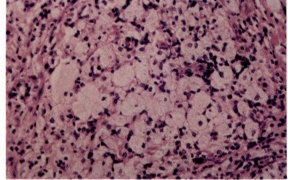

**287 Massive sinus histiocytosis** In other parts of the nodes the sinuses are filled with large, pale, foamy macrophages and emperipolysis is not obvious. These cells should not be confused with those present in the lipidoses. *(H&E)*

**289 Massive sinus histiocytosis** In this regressive phase fibrosis is advanced but it is still possible to identify the large macrophage cells with their characteristic lymphoid content . At no stage of the disease is it possible to identify infectious organisms, although an infectious aetiology seems the most likely cause. Interestingly, the disease appears to be more common in the black races. There is no sex difference. *(H&E)*

**288**

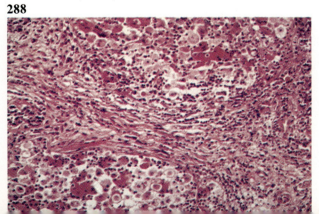

**289**

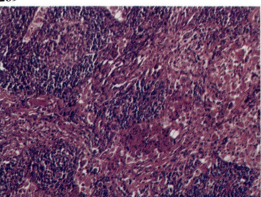

**290 Cholegranulomatous lymphadenitis** This condition occurs particularly in patients with cholecystitis and also may accompany obstructive jaundice. The nodes usually involved are the hepatic group and particularly the cystic node. The characteristic early lesions are collections of foamy macrophages within sinusoids in which vacuoles derived from fatty material are a prominent feature. Vacuoles are present also within the sub-capsular sinus. *(H&E)*

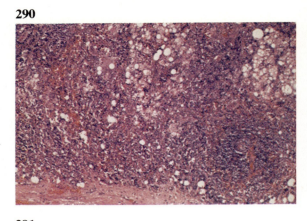

**291 Cholegranulomatous lymphadenitis** In addition to the foamy vacuolated macrophages, giant cells are a constant feature; typical sarcoid granulomas may be found. The identification of bile *(arrow)* in the macrophage epithelioid clusters distinguishes this lesion from other granulomatous lesions and, in particular, from Whipple's disease involving abdominal lymph nodes. *(H&E)*

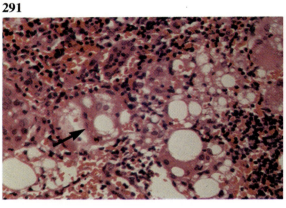

**292 Fatal granulomatous disease of childhood** Lymph node biopsy is useful in establishing the diagnosis of this condition, in which there is an inherited deficiency of bactericidal activity in the polymorph neutrophils. The key to the diagnosis is the presence of numerous large faintly pigmented macrophages which, superficially, resemble those of the lipidoses. *(H&E)*

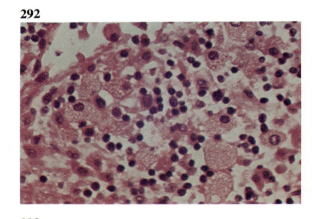

**293 Fatal granulomatous disease of childhood** The macrophages contain abundant granular cytoplasm due to the presence of sudanophilic material, which stains variably with the periodic acid-Schiff technique. The granular material is thought to be a lipochrome or ceroid and in some cases, fully formed ceroid or Hamazaki-Wesenberg bodies are present. Another property of this pigment is autofluorescence. *(PAS)*

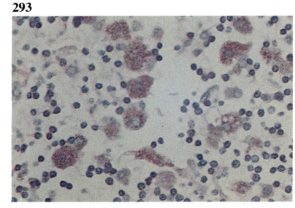

**294 Ceroid bodies (Hamazaki-Wesenberg bodies)**
In the macrophages of some reactive lymph nodes, usually those showing some degree of sinus histiocytosis, intracytoplasmic brown bodies can be observed (*arrows*). These Hamazaki-Wesenberg or ceroid bodies may be spindle-shaped, ovoid or round, and range in colour from yellow to dark brown or grey-brown. Because of their shape and sharp contour, and the simulation of a cell wall, they closely resemble fungal bodies with which they should not be confused. The are not stained by haematoxylin or eosin and in H&E stained sections the eosinophilia of cytoplasm may considerably mask their presence as shown here. *(H&E)*

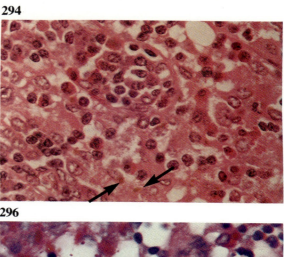

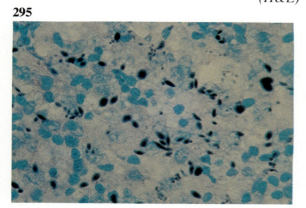

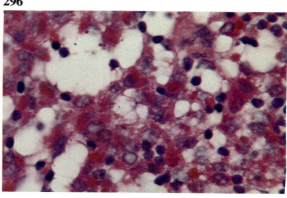

**295 and 296 Ceroid bodies (Hamazaki-Wesenberg bodies)** The two routine stains which most readily permit identification of these bodies are the Ziehl-Neelsen stain, **295**, which colours them an intense blue-black colour, and the periodic acid-Schiff technique, **296**, which stains them deep orange-pink. Sometimes the central area appears pale. Other stains which may be useful are Giemsa staining, which will impart a greenish colour to the bodies, and the Gram stain in which they are often quite strongly Gram positive. Methenamine silver techniques and stains for melanin pigment give variable results. *(295 ZN; 296 PAS)*

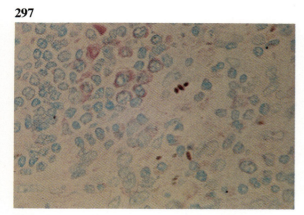

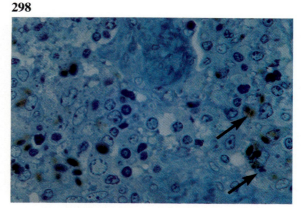

**297 Ceroid bodies (Hamazaki-Wesenberg bodies)**
Special stains which do not generally stain macrophage cytoplasm are also useful since the brown bodies will stand out in sharp relief within the unstained cytoplasm. Thus in methyl green-pyronin preparations, as shown here, and in stains for iron using the Perl's technique, these brown bodies are seen easily. *(MGP)*

**298 Ceroid bodies (Hamazaki-Wesenberg bodies)**
In plastic processed lymph nodes stained with toluidine blue, ceroid bodies are much more easily correctly identified. Although the darker outer zone surrounding a central paler area still further enhances their resemblance to organisms, it is now possible to appreciate their marked variation in size with many small particulate forms (*arrow*). *(Toluidine blue)*

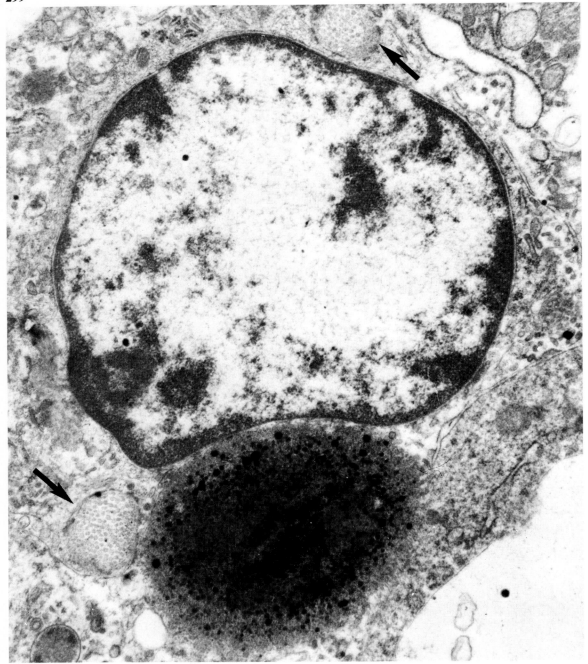

**299 Ceroid bodies (Hamazaki-Wesenberg bodies), ultrastructure** The debate as to whether these bodies represented organisms or collections of ceroid pigment was settled easily by ultrastructural examination, since the morphological features are not those of an organism. Note that the fatty osmophilic material tends to be most dense in the centre of the body. The cell containing the pigment is a fixed sinus-lining cell enclosing collagen bundles (*arrows*). (× 27,960)

300

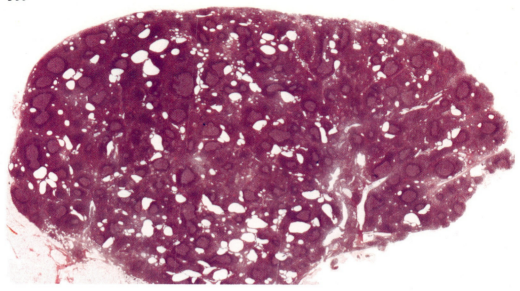

**300 Post-lymphangiogram lymphadenopathy** With the advent of lymphangiography and its increasing use, an oliogranulomatous response occurs in the draining lymph nodes in response to the oily base of the contrast medium. The appearance in lymph nodes is highly characteristic and likely to cause few diagnostic problems other than the consideration of Whipple's disease. However, the specimen is likely to be an abdominal lymph node removed during staging laparotomy. The sinusoidal system is prominent and contains numerous variable-sized vacuoles. The oily substance which was present cannot be seen, of course, in the paraffin-processed sections but may be demonstrated easily in frozen sections. *(H&E)*

**301 Post-lymphangiogram changes** The vacuoles are surrounded by phagocytic cells, including foreign-body giant cells (*arrow*). Characteristically, lymph nodes showing fully formed post-lymphangiogram changes are not those involved in a neoplastic process. Occasionally, however, with partial neoplastic involvement, one may see classical post-lymphangiogram changes adjacent to an area replaced by a lymphoma (see **537**). *(H&E)*

301

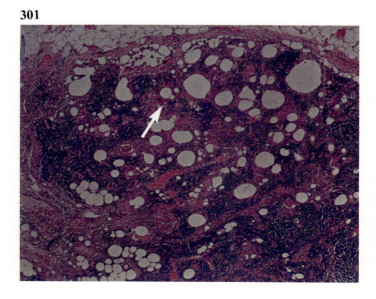

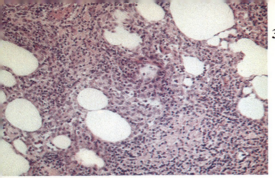

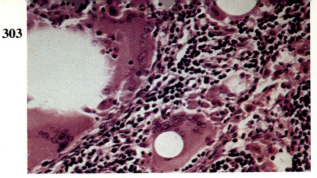

**302 and 303   Post-lymphangiogram lymphadenopathy** The appearances in different examples vary according to the date of the previous lymphangiogram. In early cases, **302**, while there is a considerable mononuclear phagocytic cell response and sinus histiocytosis, giant cells are absent. With time, **303**, there are numerous multinucleate giant cells of foreign body type. In contrast to Whipple's disease, the macrophages seen in both early and late lymphangiogram induced lymphadenopathy do not contain the characteristic PAS positive granules; nor do they tend to be aggregated into small epithelioid granulomas. *(H&E)*

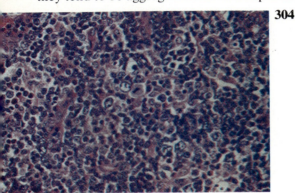
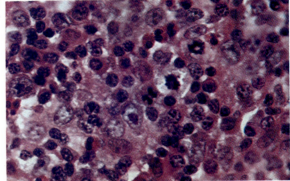

**304   Drug induced lymphadenopathy** Occasionally the administration of certain drugs, notably the hydantoin group, may be followed by lymphadenopathy. The most striking changes are seen in the paracortical areas, and may result in effacement of follicular structures. The large numbers of proliferating immunoblasts together with plasma cells and a few eosinophils and proliferation of the PCV's produce a picture, as shown here, very similar if not identical to that seen in AILA. This type of appearance has been described as Grade 2 hydantoin lymphadenopathy. *(H&E)*

**306   Post-vaccinial lymphadenopathy** In some patients following vaccination against smallpox, the regional lymph nodes (usually axillary) may enlarge progressively and, if biopsied show a very alarming appearance somewhat similar to that seen in drug induced lymphadenopathy. There may also be prominent PCV's. Here there is virtual obliteration of normal architecture and replacement by proliferating large lymphoid cells. Note the sprinkling of eosinophils. *(H&E)*

**305 Drug induced lymphadenopathy** The prominent mitotic activity, pleomorphic cellular content and large atypical mononuclear cells may suggest Hodgkin's disease. Even when the history of drug administration is known, diagnostic difficulty may remain since some cases of hydantoin lymphadenopathy progress to a malignant lymphoma. There is also evidence that lymphoma occurs with increased frequency in patients taking these drugs. *(H&E)*

**307   Post-vaccinial lymphadenopathy** At high magnification many of the proliferating cells are large lymphoid cells or immunoblasts and exhibit marked mitotic activity. A diagnosis of a large cell lymphoma (immunoblastic sarcoma) may be considered and if there are many eosinophils and occasional large binucleate cells (*arrow*) an erroneous diagnosis of Hodgkin's disease may be made. *(H&E)*

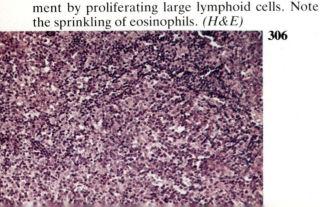
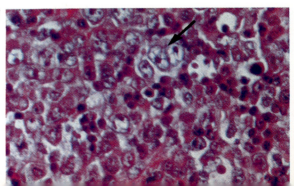

**308  Angiofollicular lymph node hyperplasia (giant lymphoid hamartoma)**
In our view this lesion is not a hamartoma but represents an unusual and abnormal response of peripheral lymphoid tissue, including lymphoid tissue in extra-nodal sites.

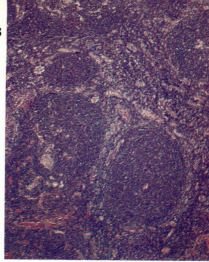

In the more common hyaline vascular variety, which presents usually in adults as mediastinal enlargement, the characteristic pathology is the presence of large follicular structures with absent, inconspicuous or poorly formed germinal centres, ( *right* ) and the presence of inter-follicular vessels with thickened walls. Some vessels are prominent and hyalinised *(left)* and superficially may resemble Hassall's corpuscles. It is this feature when seen in the abnormal mediastinal lymphoid tissue which has led to diagnostic confusion with a thymoma. *(H&E)*

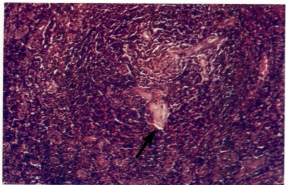

**309  Angiofollicular lymph node hyperplasia** Conspicuous hyalinised vessels (*arrow*) are seen frequently within the follicular structure and in this example one vessel is seen in continuity with an atrophic germinal centre. The combination of the atypical vessels and abnormal lymphoid follicles, together with the lack of identifiable sinuses, led some workers to consider that this condition represents a hamartoma, and one which involves *lymphoid tissue* rather than *lymph nodes*. In some series, however, normal nodal tissue has been identified. *(H&E)*

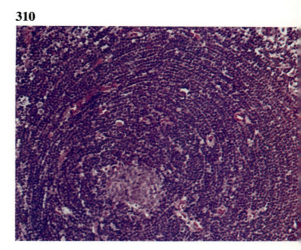

**310  Angiofollicular lymph node hyperplasia** In some of the follicular structures, the small lymphocytes are arranged in highly characteristic concentric festoons likened to 'strings of beads' around the small germinal centre. These follicular appearances are sometimes confused with those of a follicular lymphoma, particularly when found in sites outside the mediastinum, such as axilla and abdomen. *(H&E)*

**311 and 312  Angiofollicular lymph node hyperplasia** These are two atypical germinal centres at high magnification: **311** shows a mixture of cells, mitotic activity and a conspicuous feeder vessel ( *top* ) to which the centre appears related, **312** shows a structure which appears to consist almost entirely of endothelial and/or dendritic cells with abundant cytoplasm and vesicular nuclei, and scattered intercellular red cells (*arrow*). *(H&E)*

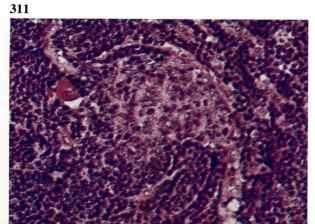

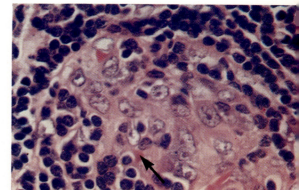

**313**

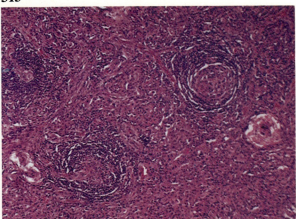

**314**

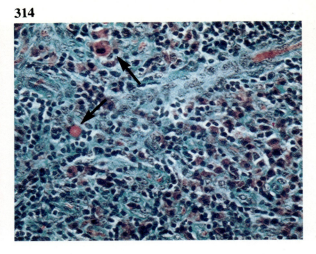

**313 and 314    Angiofollicular lymph node hyperplasia** In contrast to the more common hyaline vascular type in **311** and **312** which is not associated with systemic symptoms, there is an uncommon variant known as the plasma cell type. The characteristic morphology of this type are sheets of plasma cells, numerous vessels of postcapillary venular size in the interfollicular areas, **313**, and the presence of better-formed germinal centres. The plasma cells and secretory products (*arrows*) in between the small vessels, **314**, are particularly well seen in trichome-stained sections. In these patients symptoms include fever, fatigue, sweating and a raised ESR, and serological abnormalities such as hyperglobulinaemia – presumably the product of the proliferating plasma cells. Occasionally, mixed examples are encountered which combine the histopathological features of the hyaline vascular type with those of the plasma cell variant. (**313** *H&E;* **314** *Masson's trichrome*)

## Infective lymphadenitis

Lymph nodes are involved during the course of a number of infections. In many instances the changes found are non-specific and do not permit a definitive diagnosis to be made. In other infections while characteristic lesions such as granulomas develop they are not specific since they are shared by other infective and non-infectious processes. In this section only selected examples of infections which are commonly associated with lymph node involvement will be illustrated if they satisfy one or all of the following criteria: (1) the infectious disease is considered to be of prime importance in terms of morbidity and mortality; (2) the infectious lymphadenitis results in distinctive histopathological lesions; (3) the causal agent can be identified at microscopical level.

All three criteria are satisfied in some infections such as lepromatous leprosy. In other diseases such as toxoplasmosis and cat scratch disease, a presumptive diagnosis can usually be made on the histopathological appearances in the *absence* of identifiable organisms; while in the many infections characterised by granulomatous or tuberculoid lesions, a definitive diagnosis can be reached by the morphological identification of the infectious agent – as in tuberculosis, coccidiomycosis and histoplasmosis. Infections such as infectious mononucleosis and syphilis are included because although the diagnosis is usually made on the clinical and serological findings, in the rare event of lymph node biopsy being performed, the histopathological appearances may present diagnostic difficulties and even confusion with a lymphoproliferative process. These infectious lymphadenopathies, which may be of world-wide or geographically restricted distribution, common or rare in terms of incidence, are grouped in the following categories: bacterial, chlamydial, viral, protozoal, fungal and metazoal.

*Bacterial lymphadenitis*
Tuberculosis
Leprosy
Brucellosis
Yersinia enterocolitica
Syphilis
Typhoid
Whipple's disease

*Chlamydial infections*
Cat scratch disease
Lymphogranuloma venereum

*Viral lymphadenitis*
Measles
Infectious mononucleosis

*Protozoal lymphadenitis*
Toxoplasmosis
Visceral leishmaniasis
Malaria

*Fungal (deep) lymphadenitis*
Histoplasmosis
Coccidiomycosis

*Metazoal lymphadenitis*
Schistosomiasis
Onchocercosis
Filariasis (*Wucheria bancrofti*)

Diseases not illustrated but which have to be considered in the differential diagnosis are referred to in the text.

**315 Tuberculous lymphadenitis** Lymphadenopathy resulting from tuberculosis is almost always the result of primary infection by *Mycobacterium tuberculosis* of human or bovine type, or by atypical mycobacteria. In those countries in which there is an active campaign aimed at the eradication of tuberculosis, tuberculous lymphadenitis is becoming increasingly rare. The nodes most commonly involved are the cervical, mediastinal, abdominal and axillary lymph nodes. In this cervical node a number of tubercles varying in size, none of which show central caseation, are ranged around a lymphoid follicle with an active germinal centre. Note the occasional Langhans giant cell (*arrows*). *(H&E)*

**315**

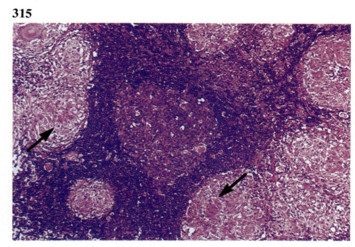

**316 Tuberculous lymphadenitis** In this classical tubercle there is commencing central necrosis (caseation). Giant cells are present in the surrounding zone of epithelioid cells (*arrow*) and lymphocytes form the outermost zone. *(H&E)*

**316**

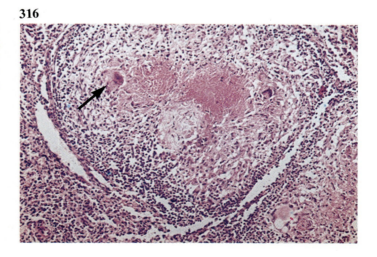

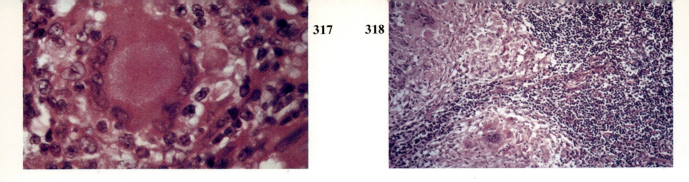

**317 and 318 Tuberculous lymphadenitis** Two types of giant cells are associated with tuberculosis. The classical type, **317**, is the Langhans giant cell, typified by peripherally arranged nuclei often in a horseshoe configuration, in contrast to foreign body giant cells in which the nuclei are centrally located, **318**. It should be emphasised that Langhans giant cells are not unique to tuberculosis and occur in other chronic granulomatous diseases as well as in lymph nodes which are the site of, or are draining malignant disease. *(H&E)*

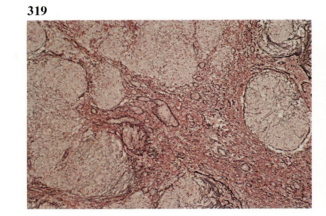

**319 Tuberculous lymphadenitis** Numerous coalescing tubercles are present in this field. Stains for reticulin demonstrate a relative paucity of fibre within the granulomas – most of which are often poorly demarcated by reticulin – a feature sometimes helpful in distinguishing tuberculous non-caseating granulomas from those of sarcoidosis. *(Gordon & Sweets)*

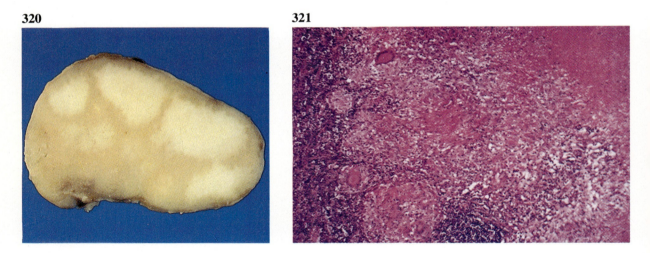

**320 and 321 Tuberculous lymphadenitis** With established tuberculous lymphadenitis necrosis may be extremely widespread and involve a major part of a node. Tuberculous necrosis is known as caseation since its macroscopic appearance, **320**, resembles that of a soft full fat cheese - like ripe Camembert. Caseation is a particular form of coagulation necrosis and occurs in other diseases. Histopathologically, **321**, caseation is characterised by its relative acellularity, eosinophilia and absence of reticulin fibre. The latter feature is helpful in distinguishing the necrotic process of tuberculosis from that found in syphilis and in rheumatoid nodules since in these conditions reticulin fibre is generally preserved. *(H&E)*

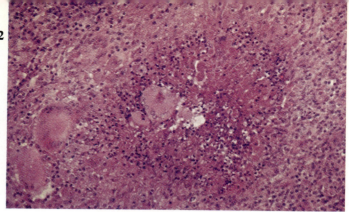

**322 Tuberculous lymphadenitis** This shows an atypical tubercle in that the central area of necrosis is cellular and the Langhans giant cells are scattered irregularly through the histiocytic zone. Such an appearance although atypical of tuberculosis should always initiate a search for acid fast bacilli which, in this case, were identified. *(H&E)*

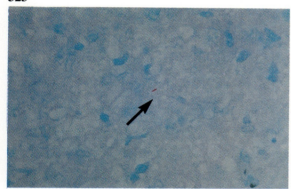

**323 Tuberculous lymphadenitis** In this Ziehl-Neelsen preparation of the lymph node in **322**, a solitary acid fast bacillus *(arrow)* is seen. Acid fast bacilli may be extremely sparse and the most rewarding technique in identifying these occasional organisms is systematically to scan, field by field, using the high × 40 dry lens. When present in lymph nodes, they are usually single and are found either in giant cells or the epithelioid cells. Rarely are they found in the caseous areas. *(ZN)*

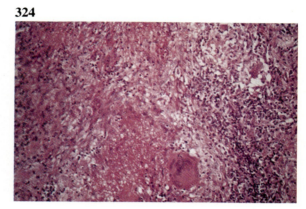

**324 Tuberculous lymphadenitis** In other examples of tuberculous lymphadenitis the appearances are even more atypical. Instead of caseating tubercles there is a diffuse inflammation with areas of cellular necrosis and, sometimes, these necrotic areas are bounded by a well defined histiocytic zone resulting in a close resemblance to the lesion seen in cat scratch disease. These uncommon histological appearances can be due to either an atypical host response to infection, or infection with an atypical mycobacterium. *(H&E)*

**325 Tuberculous lymphadenitis** This is an example of tuberculosis involving a mesenteric lymph node, most commonly the result of a gastro-intestinal infection with *Mycobacterium bovis*. Abdominal lymph nodes may be extensively involved and result in the condition known historically as *tabes mesenterica*. The natural history of such nodes is to undergo calcification, in which case they are usually accidentally discovered during the course of abdominal X-ray. *(H&E)*

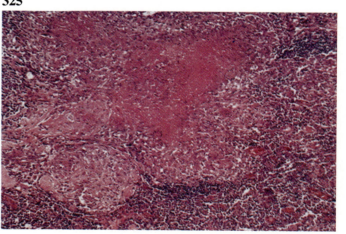

**326**

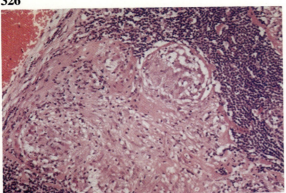

**327**

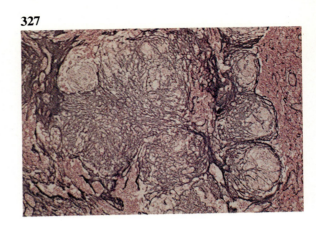

**326 and 327   Tuberculous lymphadenitis** In some patients the tubercles undergo a more extensive fibrosis and, when this feature is seen together with an absence of caseation and no identifiable acid fast bacilli, it may be difficult to make a distinction between tuberculosis and sarcoidosis. In such cases the Mantoux and Kveim tests can be very helpful. Fibrotic tubercles are shown here **326**, *H&E;* **327** *Gordon & Sweets.*

**328   Tuberculoid leprosy** Leprosy is caused by an acid fast bacillus and, with the exception of Northern Europe, has a world-wide distribution, being most common in the Tropics. Clinically and histopatho-logically there are two distinct types but with indeterminate and borderline variants. The tuberculoid form of leprosy shown here may involve superficial lymph nodes and reflects a high degree of immunity. The granulomas closely resemble sarcoidosis in that they are discrete epithelial giant cell systems without necrosis which may under-go progressive fibrosis. The diagnosis will not be made unless leprosy is considered in the differential diagnosis of non-caseating granulomas. Since acid fast bacilli are rarely demonstrated in the tuberculoid form, the lepromin test is necessary to confirm the diagnosis. *(H&E)*

**328**

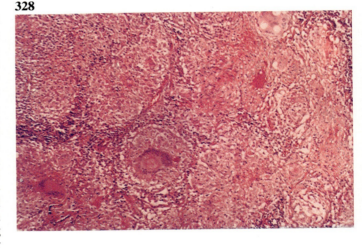

**329   Lepromatous leprosy** The lepromatous form of leprosy commonly involves lympho-reticular tissue and occurs in individuals with low immunity to the disease. It has a worse prognosis than tuberculoid leprosy even following treatment. Involved lymph nodes show sinus histiocytosis and collections of large foamy or vacuolated macrophages. There is no necrosis and lymph node architecture is preserved. In this example the 'globi' associated with well developed lesions are not evident within the vacuolated macrophages and such collections of macrophages may resemble closely a reactive response to the drainage of various substances, particularly silicone. *(H&E)*

**329**

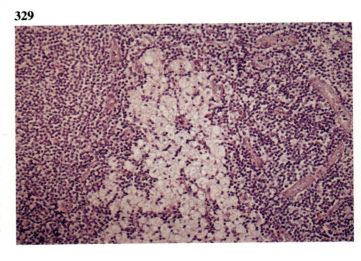

**330**

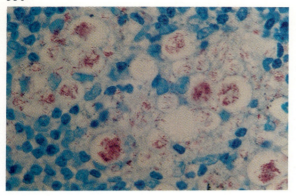

**331**

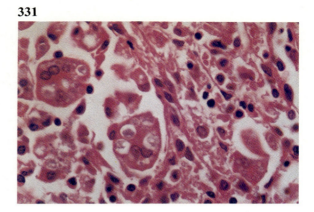

**330 Lepromatous leprosy** On staining with the Wade-Fite technique the apparently empty vacuoles are seen to contain surprisingly numerous acid fast bacilli. These bacilli – first described by Hanson – have not been successfully cultured yet on artificial media although they can cause the disease if transmitted to certain animals. *(Wade-Fite)*

**331 Lepromatous leprosy** In well developed disease, either in lymph nodes or spleen, there are large and frequent multinucleated mononuclear phagocytic cells containing prominent vacuoles. Within these vacuoles bluish-grey bodies known as globi are visible and consist of clumps of leprosy bacilli. *(H&E)*

**332**

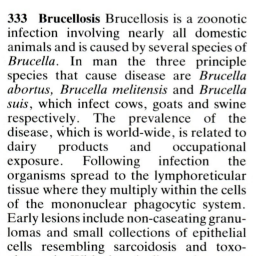

**332 Lepromatous leprosy** Confirmation that the intravacuolar structures are globi can be obtained easily by the Wade-Fite stain which demonstrates the clumps of acid fast bacilli. Cells containing leprosy bacilli, whether they are the apparently empty foamy vacuolated cells or those containing the tingeable globi are known as Lepra cells. *(Wade-Fite)*

**333**

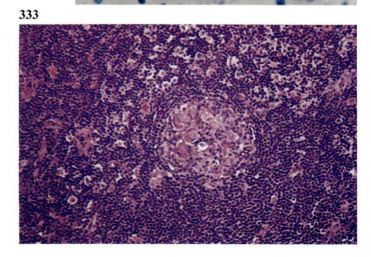

**333 Brucellosis** Brucellosis is a zoonotic infection involving nearly all domestic animals and is caused by several species of *Brucella*. In man the three principle species that cause disease are *Brucella abortus, Brucella melitensis* and *Brucella suis*, which infect cows, goats and swine respectively. The prevalence of the disease, which is world-wide, is related to dairy products and occupational exposure. Following infection the organisms spread to the lymphoreticular tissue where they multiply within the cells of the mononuclear phagocytic system. Early lesions include non-caseating granulomas and small collections of epithelial cells resembling sarcoidosis and toxoplasmosis. With chronic disease larger caseous granulomas may develop – particularly in *B. suis*. The differentiation from tuberculosis or some deep seated fungal infection can be made only by laboratory procedures. *(H&E)*

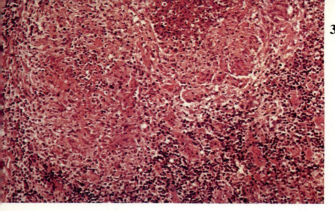

**334 Yersinial lymphadenitis** This enteric infection is caused by an invasive gram-negative zoonotic bacterium called *Yersinia enterocolitica*. The condition usually presents with diarrhoea or with abdominal symptoms suggestive of an acute appendix. Patients thus frequently undergo laparotomy when the mesenteric lymph nodes are found to be enlarged. The terminal ileum and colon are frequently affected and the appendix, which may look normal macroscopically, is often found to be involved. The pathological changes in nodes and intestinal tract are either those of a non-specific reactive process or a highly characteristic but not pathognomonic lesion as seen here, consisting of central areas of necrosis and polymorph neutrophils surrounded by a zone of histiocytes. *(H&E)*

**335**

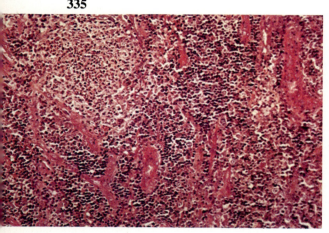

**335 Yersinial lymphadenitis** *Yersinia enterocolitica* has world-wide distribution and is now recognised with increasing frequency. The disease probably includes most of the cases previously diagnosed as pseudotuberculous mesenteric lymphadenitis (Masshoff's disease – thought to be due to infection with *Pasteurella pseudotuberculosis*) and many of the cases labelled as non-specific mesenteric lymphadenitis. In addition to the presence of microabscesses in various stages of development, reactive features in affected nodes often include a striking proliferation of the postcapillary venules as shown here. Occasionally vessels may show necrosis. *(H&E)*

**336**

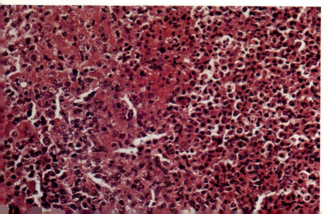

**336 Yersinial lymphadenitis** In the well developed lesion the histiocytes surrounding the central area of necrosis assume a palisade arrangement. In many cases the lesion may simulate closely the changes found in early lymphogranuloma venereum and cat scratch disease and in the lymphadenitis due to infection with *Listeria monocytogenes*. Giant cells are seen rarely. The gram stain may demonstrate the presence of gram negative bacilli but usually is not helpful. In doubtful cases the diagnosis is confirmed by culture of the organism and serological examination. *(H&E)*

**337**

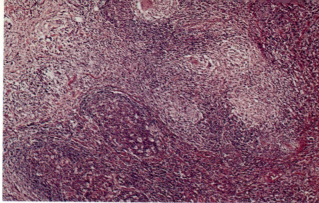

**337 Syphilitic lymphadenitis** Lymph node enlargement is a common manifestation of both primary and secondary syphilis and is characterised by a regional distribution in the primary stage and a generalised lymphadenopathy in the secondary stage. The histopathological features of the lymphadenitis are not diagnostic. They include variable degrees of follicular hyperplasia, large numbers of plasma cells, vascular changes, and granulomatous lesions. The changes seen in both the primary and secondary stages of the disease are essentially similar, except that they tend to be more marked or advanced in secondary syphilis. The granulomatous response varies from small clusters of epithelioid cells to larger defined epithelioid granulomas. In this field there are several non-caseating granulomas, one of which contains a Langhans giant cell. The lymphoid follicles contain large active germinal centres and there is a marked capsulitis. *(H&E)*

**338**

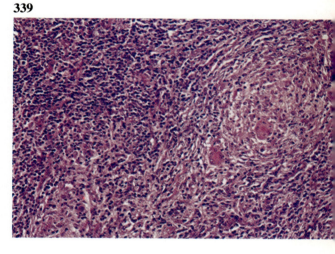

**338 Syphilitic lymphadenitis** *Treponema pallidum* are more abundant and easily demonstrated by appropriate silver impregnation techniques in the primary stage. Treponemes are particularly numerous in the acute necrotizing lymphadenitis which occasionally may compli-cate the primary stage. In such cases, many of the usual histopathological features are masked by extensive necrosis and infiltration of the necrotic tissue by polymorph neutrophils and histiocytes. In this example an occasional Langhans giant cell (*arrow*) is present adjacent to an area of necrosis. While it is important to consider syphilis in the differential diagnosis when faced with a biopsy of an acute necrotizing lymphadenitis, it is equally important to exclude a superimposed infection such as gonococcal lymphadenitis in those patients diagnosed as having acute syphilitic necrotizing lymphadenitis. *(H&E)*

**339**

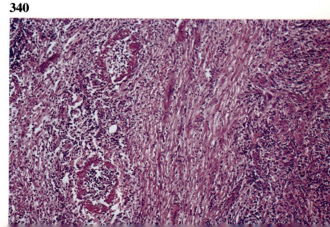

**339 Syphilitic lymphadenitis** Giant cells are very variable in number in the granulomatous lesions of both primary and secondary syphilis and congenital syphilis. In tertiary syphilis lymph node involvement is now rarely seen – par-ticularly the massive form of gummatous lymphadenitis, though the *miliary* form of gummatous lymphadenitis is slightly more common. Both forms of gummatous lympha-denitis are still occasionally seen in congenital syphilitics. In this example of secondary syphilitic lymphadenitis there are loosely aggregated epithelioid granulomas and two large Langhans giant cells, surrounded by numerous plasma cells and small vessels. Should central necrosis occur – a rare event – the appearances may resemble yersinial or chlamydial necrotizing granulomatous lymphadenitis. *(H&E)*

**340**

**340 Syphilitic lymphadenitis** Inflammation of capsule, trabeculae and the walls of both arteries and veins can usually be seen in syphilitic lymphadenitis and tends to be more prominent and associated with a greater degree of fibrosis in the secondary stage. In this field there is capsular thickening due to early fibrosis and inflammation which is extending into the perinodal tissue. The walls of two small veins show a cellular infiltrate and the PCVs in the under-lying parenchyma are prominent. With continuing disease the inflammatory process results in a fibrous endarteritis and considerable fibrosis of capsule and perinodal tissues. Treponemes may or may not be demonstrable. *(H&E)*

**341**

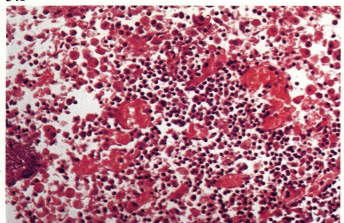

**341 Typhoid lymphadenitis** Salmonella infections always induce a mesenteric lymphadenitis which tends to be more severe in typhoid fever than in the paratyphoid infections. There may be generalised lymphadenopathy as a result of septicaemia. In this abdominal lymph node from a patient with typhoid, the enlarged node shows focal areas of necrosis and accumulation of large mononuclear cells. Note the clump of blue staining *Salmonella typhi* bacilli in relation to the necrosis. *(H&E)*

**342**

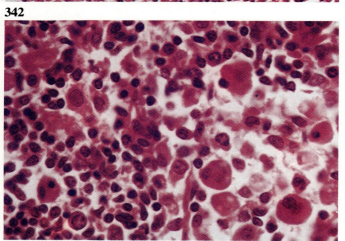

**342 Typhoid lymphadenitis** The characteristic and often predominant cell type is a large cell of mononuclear phagocytic origin with a single darker staining nucleus and abundant eosinophilic cytoplasm. These cells are seen in parenchyma as well as sinuses and are known as 'typhoid cells'. Occasionally they may be binucleate and their phagocytic nature is well demonstrated by the frequent finding of ingested red cells and lymphocytes within their cytoplasm. *(H&E)*

**343 Whipple's disease** Whipple's disease is a rare condition affecting chiefly middle-aged men. Because of its generalised nature it may present in a number of ways. The principal manifestations are related to the small intestinal pathology and include steatorrhoea and weight loss. The abdominal nodes are invariably involved (and occasionally superficial groups of nodes). One of the most striking features is a progressive accumulation of fatty material leading to enlargement and to a diffuse vacuolation similar to post-lymphangiogram lymphadenopathy as seen in this low power view. *(H&E)*

**343**

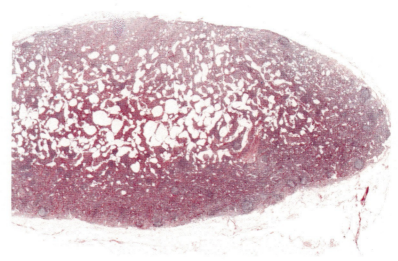

**344 Whipple's disease** The diffuse vacuolation due to fat deposition and the mononuclear phagocytic cell response including the presence of foreign body giant cells (*arrow*) result in an appearance again closely resembling post-lymphangiogram changes. When fatty change is present but mainly intracellular the lymph node appearances may be mistaken for cholegranulomatous lymphadenitis. At histopathological level the separation of the three entities depends upon the presence of distinctive intracytoplasmic PAS + ve granules in Whipple's disease. With progression of the disease the abdominal nodes may be almost entirely replaced by yellowish inspissated fatty material lacking a cellular response. *(H&E)*

**345 Whipple's disease** Originally this condition was considered to be a disorder of lipid metabolism as reflected by the alternative terms 'intestinal lipodystrophy' and 'lipophagic intestinal granulomatosis'. Electron microscopy subsequently showed the presence of small bacilli in relation to the lesions, and the condition is now considered to be essentially infective in nature. The bacilli excite little inflammation and accumulate within mononuclear cells in large numbers. The bacterial products are strongly PAS positive, and the finding of fatty spaces together with giant cell granulomas containing PAS positive granules, as shown here, is virtually diagnostic of Whipple's disease. *(PAS)*

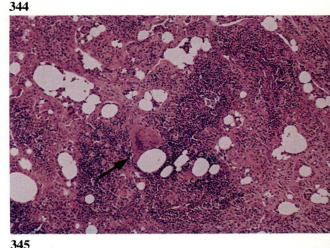

344

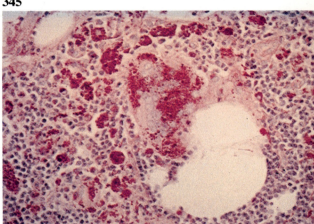

345

346

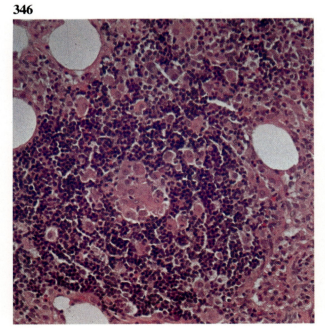

**346 and 347 Whipple's disease** The granulomas and fatty vacuoles are very variable in size and giant cells are not always present. Figure **346** shows a small accumulation of epithelioid cells within a lymphoid aggregate. On staining with PAS, **347**, the cytoplasm is seen to contain the characteristic diastase resistant PAS + ve granules. *(346 H&E; 347 PAS)*

347

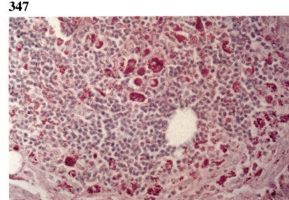

**348 Whipple's disease** Some patients, because of their abdominal symptoms, undergo a laparotomy and, when the abdominal lymph nodes are found to be enlarged and not obviously fatty, and the small intestine appears normal, a diagnosis of a lymphoproliferative disorder may be suspected. In this mesenteric lymph node from such a patient, the enlargement was due mainly to a marked sinusoidal histiocytic proliferation and increased numbers of plasma cells and eosinophils; there was little fatty accumulation or granuloma formation. Note, however, the bluish granularity of the cytoplasm of the mononuclear cells. *(H&E)*

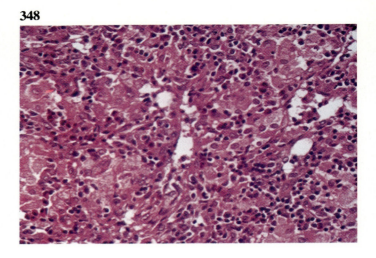

**349 Whipple's disease** The bluish colour of the cytoplasm in **348** is due to the presence of large quantities of bacteria and their products as revealed by the PAS technique. With fewer numbers of PAS positive cells or when the cells contain fewer PAS granules, and when fatty accumulation and granulomas are inconspicuous, caution should be exercised before making a diagnosis of Whipple's disease on the lymph node findings alone. *(H&E)*

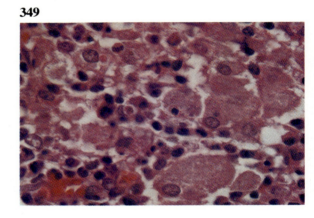

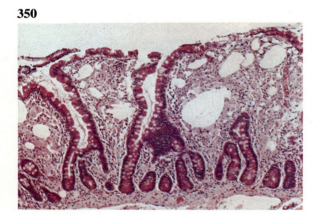

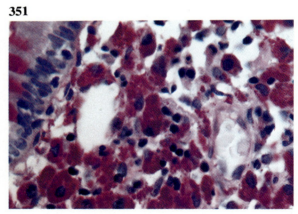

**350 and 351 Whipple's disease** A definitive diagnosis of Whipple's disease can always be made by peroral small intestinal (jejunal) biopsy when, in addition to changes in villous morphology, **350**, there are vacuoles of varying size and large numbers of macrophages within the lamina propria. The cytoplasm of these cells is strongly PAS + ve, and coarsely granular, **351**. *(350 H&E; 351 PAS)*

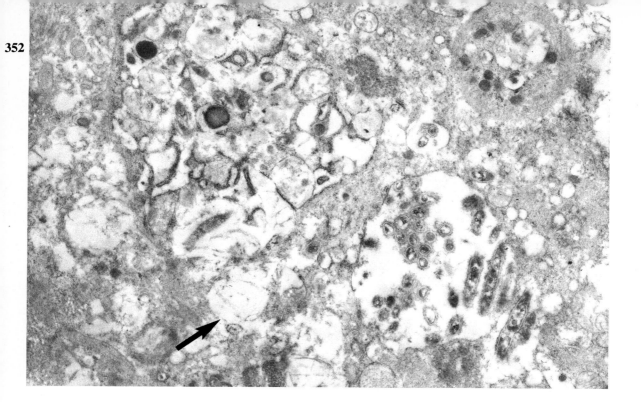

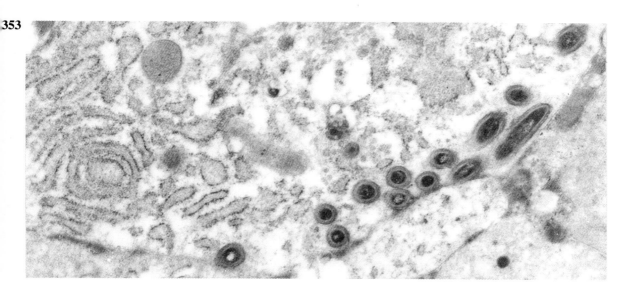

**352 and 353  Whipple's disease, ultrastructure** Ultrastructural study of the small intestine and lymph nodes in Whipple's disease shows the presence of many small bacilli in the intercellular tissues and in the cytoplasm of macrophages and plasma cells and in the epithelial cells of gut. The nature of the infectious agent has not been established. However, the most likely candidate to date is an L form of *Haemophilus influenzae*. Treatment with broad spectrum antibiotics results in cure, with a reversal to normal morphology and eradication of the bacilli. Figure **352** shows part of a macrophage with Whipple's organisms contained within vacuoles and showing early degradation (note the fatty vacuoles – *arrow*); in **353** part of a plasma cell with numerous organisms apparently lying free in the cytoplasm is seen. *(352 × 14,380; 353 × 19,820)*

**354**

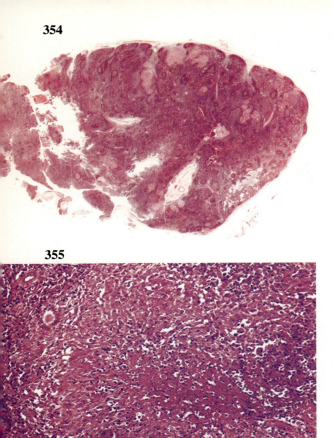

**354 Cat scratch disease** Cat scratch disease (cat scratch fever, non-bacterial regional lymphadenitis) is a relatively recently recognised condition of world-wide distribution. Although the causative organism has yet to be identified, the clinico-pathological findings together with the response to an intradermal inoculation prepared from affected lymph nodes, are so similar to those found in lymphogranuloma venereum that for the time being the putative organism is considered to be chlamydial. In the early stages of the disease there is follicular hyperplasia and sinus histiocytosis, together with epithelial aggregates resembling the findings in toxoplasmosis or brucellosis. In disease of longer duration in addition to the characteristic but not pathognomonic microabscesses, there is usually a periadenitis with capsular thickening. The microabscesses, as shown here, can often be seen to develop within the subcapsular cortical tissue. *(H&E)*

**355**

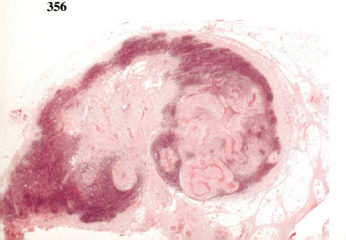

**355 Cat scratch disease** The source of infection in the majority of patients is the domestic cat and, frequently, there is a history of a cat scratch or even bite. A few weeks later the regional nodes enlarge and at presentation there is usually no trace of a skin lesion. In lymph nodes the microabscesses at first contain necrotic cellular debris and polymorph neutrophils, surrounded by a well developed histiocytic zone, as shown here. At this stage in addition to the similarity to lymphogranuloma venereum, the lesions resemble those of *Yersinia enterocolitica* except for the rarity of giant cells in the latter condition. Plasma cells are numerous in the zones between the abscesses and proliferation of postcapillary venules is often seen. *(H&E)*

**356 and 357 Cat scratch disease** Approximately one third of patients affected are children under ten years of age, and in adults females are more commonly infected than males. It is not unusual for the enlarged nodes to become adherent to surrounding structures including skin, to become fluctuant and to develop a draining sinus. At the late stage, **356**, there is considerable distortion of nodal architecture and replacement by variable sized and shaped abscesses including the classical stellate forms. The central contents of some abscesses undergo necrosis similar to caseation, and are acellular and eosinophilic. Often the caseous centres are surrounded by a prominent histiocytic zone, as in **357**. Tuberculosis, mycotic infections and tularaemia all have to be considered in the differential diagnosis. A presumptive diagnosis of cat scratch disease based on the clinico-pathological findings can be confirmed by a positive skin test to antigenic material prepared from a suppurative lymph node. *(H&E)*

**356**

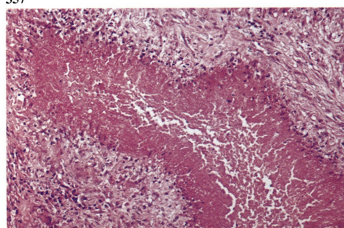

**357**

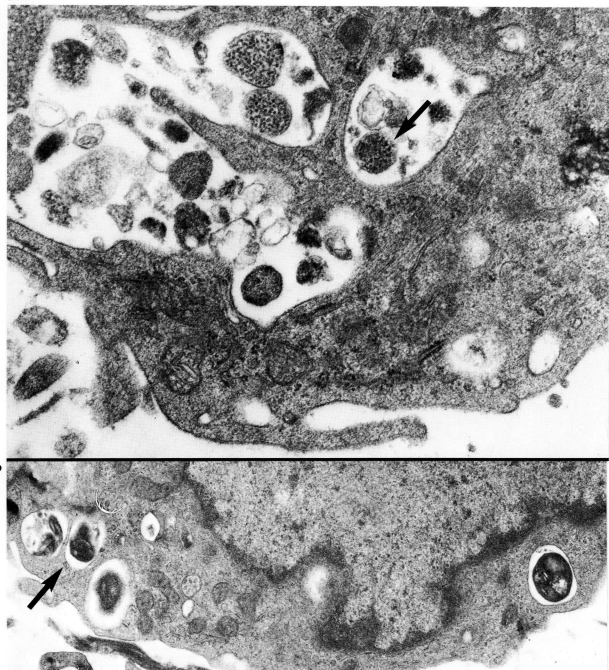

**358a and 358b   Cat scratch disease, ultrastructure** The peripheral parts of two macrophages are shown here, in the process of engulfing rounded Chlamydia-like organisms (*arrows*). The patient was a ten-year-old child presenting with an enlarged epitrochlear lymph node. (× *19,250*)

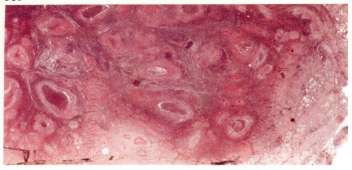

**359 Lymphogranuloma venereum**
Lymphogranuloma venereum (lymphogranuloma inguinale), sometimes referred to as the sixth venereal disease, is a chlamydial infection of world-wide distribution. The histopathological nodal findings are indistinguishable from those of cat scratch disease and some other cases of necrotizing granulomas and are seen in varying stages of evolution. In the early stages the lymph nodes may show only small aggregates of epithelial histiocytes closely resembling toxoplasmic lymphadenitis. Later, however, characteristic microabscesses develop which enlarge by a process of fusion and then collapse to produce the stellate abscesses with central necrosis as shown here. In addition there is very marked capsular thickening and periadenitis. *(H&E)*

**360 Lymphogranuloma venereum** The disease is usually transmitted by sexual intercourse, and the most commonly affected lymph nodes are the inguinal and pelvic nodes. However any group of nodes may be involved and occasionally there is generalised lymphadenopathy. The microabscesses develop first in the cortex and later in the medulla and characteristically show a central areas of cellular necrosis with numerous polymorph neutrophils. In some abscesses, instead of the more usual centres consisting of neutrophils and necrotic cell debris, the central zone contains numerous eosinophils. These may also be numerous in the areas surrounding the abscesses. Like cat scratch disease, the necrotic centres may assume a caseous appearance and when the surrounding histiocytic zone contains epitheloid cells and giant cells, tuberculosis and deep-seated fungal infections need to be considered. A definite diagnosis of lymphogranuloma venereum is made by a positive Frei test, complement fixation reactions, and the isolation of the chlamydial organism. *(H&E)*

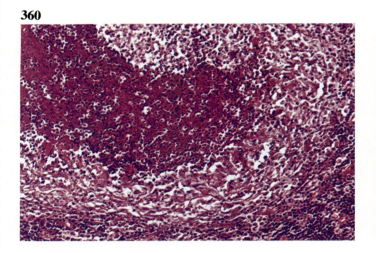

**361 Lymphogranuloma venereum** With progression of the disease, the abscesses enlarge and the necrotic centres lose their purulent character and become increasingly acellular and eosinophilic. At the same time the abscess walls may collapse to assume the characteristic stellate configuration. In other cases the 'acellular' necrotic zone containing the ghostly outline of the dead cells is surrounded by granulomatous and fibrous tissue and may simulate closely the appearance of a gumma – hence the term gummatous lymphogranuloma inguinale. In all cases and at all stages, plasma cells are regularly present and may be very numerous as shown here. *(MGP)*

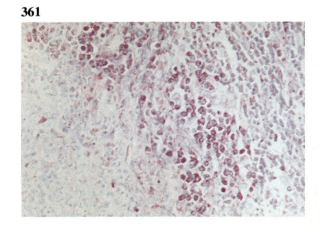

**362 Measles lymphadenitis** Measles (morbilli) is an exanthematous disease caused by a paramyxovirus. In the prodromal stages of the disease peculiar cells – to date seen only in relation to the measles virus – are regularly present in hyperplastic lymphoid tissue throughout the body, such as lymph nodes, spleen, GALT and thymus. These large multinucleate cells are called Warthin-Finkeldey cells (*arrow*) and are most commonly found within active germinal centres. They also occur in the lymphoid cuff and more rarely in the interfollicular areas. The identification of these cells enables the pathologist to make a definitive diagnosis of measles and, in patients known to be particularly vulnerable to infection, this early recognition may be of supreme importance. *(H&E)*

**363 Measles lymphadenitis** Before the onset of the morbilliform rash, if the mesenteric lymph nodes or appendiceal tissues are sufficiently hyperplastic, the resulting abdominal symptoms may suggest an acute appendicitis or mesenteric lymphadenitis. Laparotomy and biopsy of the enlarged nodes are then likely to follow. The Warthin-Finkeldey cells, four of which are shown here, are identified easily by their large size and the multiplicity of haemotaxyphil nuclei. These giant cells are of lymphoid origin and are not to be confused with the giant cells found in lung in measles pneumonia which are of epithelial origin. *(H&E)*

**364 Measles lymphadenitis** With the exception of abdominal lymph nodes, other lymphoid tissue showing the characteristic findings are likely to be seen in autopsy material either from patients dying of fulminating infection or in those dying from other causes in the prodromal stage of the disease. In this lymph node from an African child, Warthin-Finkeldey cells were very numerous and were present also in the interfollicular areas (*arrow*). Note the reactive changes and proliferation of postcapillary venules. *(H&E)*

**365 Measles lymphadenitis** A higher magnification of the previous figure reveals plasmocytic differentiation in the Warthin-Finkeldey cells outside the follicle, and is further evidence of the lymphocytic nature of these cells. It also indicates that the giant lymphoid cells are of B-cell type. *(H&E)*

**362**

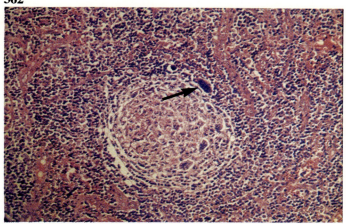

**363**

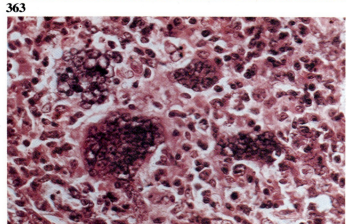

**364**

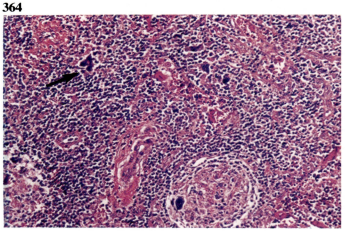

**365**

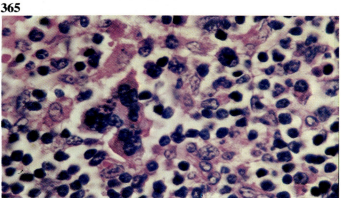

**366**

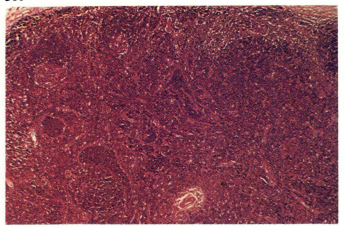

**366 Infectious mononucleosis** The usage of the term infectious mononucleosis should be reserved for an illness which is now known to be due to infection with the Epstein-Barr virus, and which is characterised by fever, lymphadenopathy, atypical mononuclear cells in the peripheral blood and, in the majority of patients, the presence of heterophile antibodies. The term glandular fever has been used in the past synonymously with infectious mononucleosis, but now should be restricted to the illness caused by *Toxoplasma gondii*, *Cytomegalovirus* and *Listeria monocytogenes*, all of which may cause a similar syndrome, but lack both the heterophile antibodies and antibodies to the E.B. virus.

Infectious mononucleosis so defined is a disease principally of the young. Diagnosis is usually made by serological means but occasionally an enlarged lymph node may be excised. In this example, lymphoid follicles with germinal centres are still present but there is obvious expansion and cellularity of the interfollicular areas, packing of the sinuses with lymphocytes and postcapillary venules are conspicuous. *(H&E)*

**367**

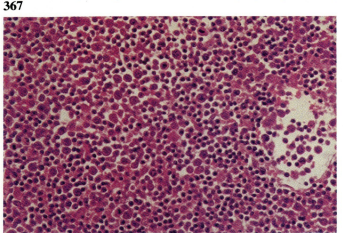

**367 Infectious mononucleosis** There are no consistent changes present in lymph nodes removed from patients with infectious mononucleosis. Some nodes as seen here show effacement of normal architecture due to the proliferation of lymphoid cells, which vary considerably in size and include both large and small forms. The importance of these changes is that without the benefit of clinical and serological data the lymphoproliferative process may be misinterpreted as a malignant lymphoma. A helpful finding is the presence of the atypical mononuclear cells within sinuses, including the subcapsular sinus, and their presence within the small vessels of the capsule. *(H&E)*

**368**

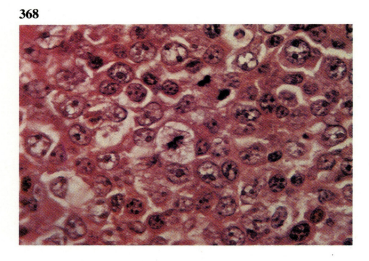

**368 Infectious mononucleosis** Occasionally there is a very marked degree of pleomorphism of the proliferating lymphoid cells. If in addition there are binucleate cells, the changes may superficially resemble Hodgkin's disease. In other cases mitotic activity among the large blast forms is very prominent and a non-Hodgkin's lymphoma of either lymphocytic poorly differentiated or large cell type may be considered, as in this example. The spleen is also involved and may be greatly enlarged. In those patients presenting with rupture of the spleen the histopathology can appear extremely worrying and suggest a lymphomatous or leukaemic infiltrate. The proliferation of lymphocytes is now known to represent a B-lymphocyte response to E.B. virus infection. *(H&E)*

**369 Toxoplasmic lymphadenitis** Either localised or generalised lymph node enlargement resulting from infection with the protozoal organism *Toxoplasma gondii* is common; the cervical – particularly the posterior cervical – nodes are the most commonly involved. The reservoir of infection is usually the domestic cat (kitten) and young children are especially at risk. Sometimes the infection presents as one type of 'glandular fever' but heterophile antibodies are absent and the Monospot and Paul-Bunnell tests are consequently negative. This cervical lymph node shows periadenitis with capsular thickening, lymphoid follicles with active germinal centres and small scattered cellular foci in the paracortex. Lymph node architecture, however, is preserved. *(H&E)*

**370 Toxoplasmic lymphadenitis** The affected nodes show a number of histopathological features which, although individually are non-specific, when seen in combination present a rather characteristic appearance such that a presumptive diagnosis of toxoplasmosis can be made. In this field there are numerous small aggregates of epithelioid cells surrounding an active germinal centre. Part of a sinus *(arrow)* is also included and this can be seen to be widened and cellular. The epithelioid aggregates seldom achieve the size or rounded neatness of those seen in sarcoidosis, for although the cellular clusters may run together to form larger aggregates they are very loosely combined. There is no fibrosis or necrosis – in particular caseous necrosis – and Langhans giant cells are rarely found. The proliferating sinusoidal histiocytes appear smaller than those seen in the ordinary variety of sinus histiocytosis. This change is sometimes referred to as unripe sinus histiocytosis or sinus histiocytosis of immature type. *(H&E)*

**371 Toxoplasmic lymphadenitis** Groups of epithelioid cells have formed within the highly active germinal centre. Sometimes as seen here, the cells making up the epithelioid clusters appear eosinophilic and possess a more abundant and vacuolated cytoplasm than the epithelioid cells seen in sarcoidosis or tuberculosis and, therefore, are not so easily defined. In the many other conditions where reactive epithelioid foci may be found – as in lymph nodes draining malignant disease – the germinal centres are generally spared. *(H&E)*

369

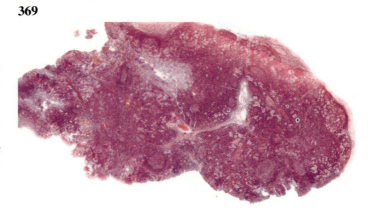

370

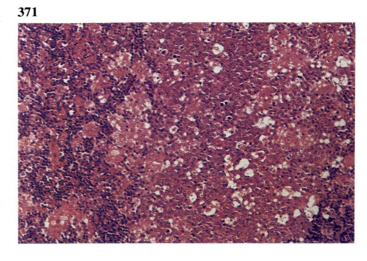

371

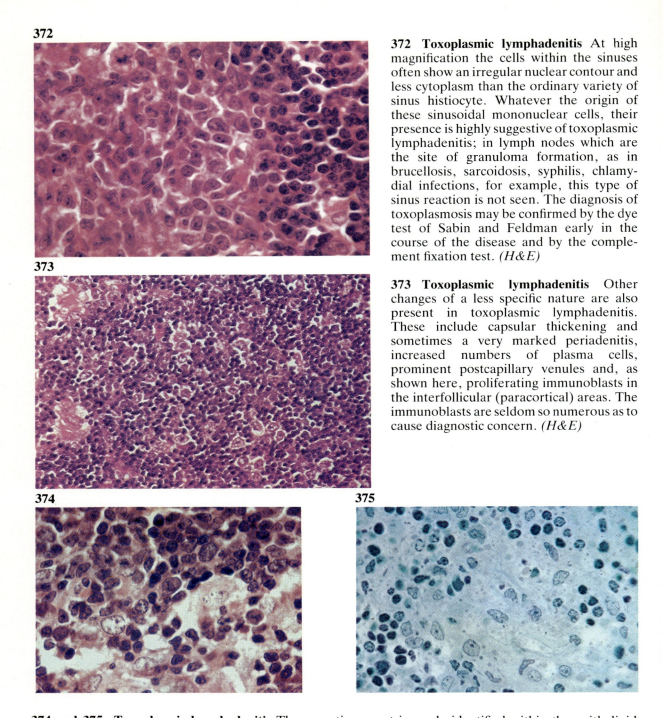

**372** Toxoplasmic lymphadenitis At high magnification the cells within the sinuses often show an irregular nuclear contour and less cytoplasm than the ordinary variety of sinus histiocyte. Whatever the origin of these sinusoidal mononuclear cells, their presence is highly suggestive of toxoplasmic lymphadenitis; in lymph nodes which are the site of granuloma formation, as in brucellosis, sarcoidosis, syphilis, chlamydial infections, for example, this type of sinus reaction is not seen. The diagnosis of toxoplasmosis may be confirmed by the dye test of Sabin and Feldman early in the course of the disease and by the complement fixation test. *(H&E)*

**373** Toxoplasmic lymphadenitis Other changes of a less specific nature are also present in toxoplasmic lymphadenitis. These include capsular thickening and sometimes a very marked periadenitis, increased numbers of plasma cells, prominent postcapillary venules and, as shown here, proliferating immunoblasts in the interfollicular (paracortical) areas. The immunoblasts are seldom so numerous as to cause diagnostic concern. *(H&E)*

**374 and 375** Toxoplasmic lymphadenitis The causative agent is rarely identified within the epithelioid granulomas and if toxoplasma cysts are present they are generally lying free in the tissue. When the epithelioid cells are viewed under the oil immersion lens, particulate material is seen within their cytoplasm but as in **374**, it is not possible to be certain whether such particulate material represents protozoal organisms or nuclear dust. Plastic processed material emphasises the particulate matter within the epithelioid cell cytoplasm, **375**, and is helpful in demonstrating that such matter does not represent the infectious agent. The paucity of organisms is in fact one of the few features helpful in distinguishing the epithelioid granulomas found in toxoplasmosis from those seen in leishmanial lymphadenitis, since in the latter condition the leishmanial organisms are numerous and readily identified within the epithelioid cells. *(374 H&E; 375 Toluidine blue)*

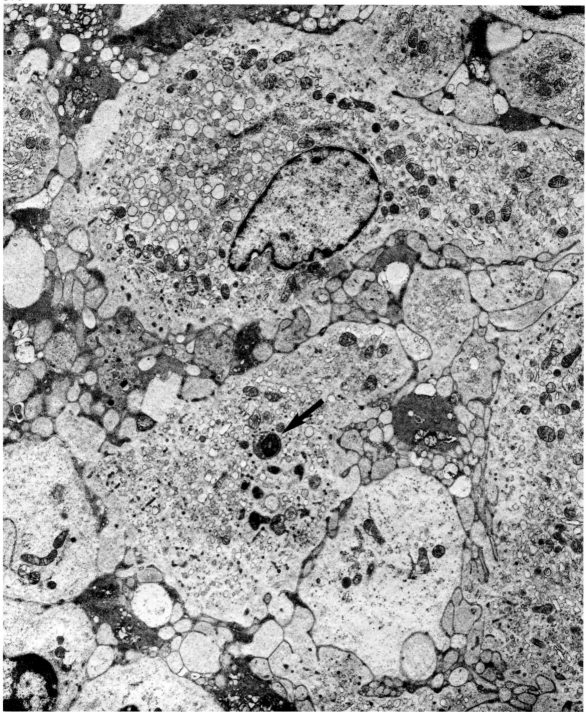

**376 Toxoplasmic lymphadenitis, ultrastructure** Part of an epithelioid cell cluster is seen here. The abundant cytoplasm shows dilated endoplasmic reticulum which partially accounts for the foamy appearance seen at light microscope level, numerous mitochondria, small secondary lysosomes and a few autophagic vesicles (*arrow*). No structures identifiable as protozoal organisms are seen. Note the complex cytoplasmic contour of the epithelioid cells and the interdigitation between one cell and another. (× *7,800*)

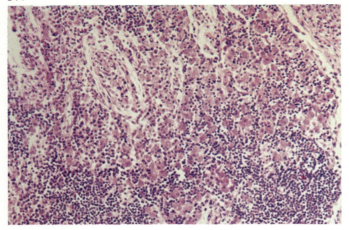

**377 Visceral leishmanial lymphadenitis**
Lymph node involvement is very rare in cutaneous leishmaniasis. Lymph nodal, splenic, hepatic and bone marrow involvement are usual, however, in the visceral form of the disease. The causative organism – the protozoa *Leishmania donovani* – is inoculated through the skin by the bites of infected sand flies. The disease has a wide geograpical distribution but is most common in South America, Africa, the Mediterranean basin and Asia. In this lymph node there are numerous large histiocytes filled with intracytoplasmic ingested leishmania, imparting a bluish granularity to the cytoplasm. *(H&E)*

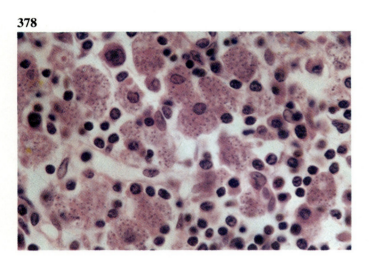

**378 Visceral leishmanial lymphadenitis**
Under the oil immersion lens the intracytoplasmic bodies of *Leishmania donovani* are seen easily. In contrast to *Toxoplasma gondii* where intracytoplasmic organisms are rare, they are numerous in leishmaniasis and are readily distinguishable from toxoplasma protozoa by their kinetoplasts· (best seen in Romanovsky stains). They may be differentiated from the fungus *Histoplasma capsulatum*, with which they are sometimes confused, by their smaller size and by special stains for fungi such as the PAS and Grocott techniques. *(H&E)*

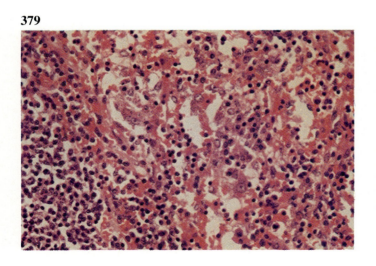

**379 Visceral splenic leishmaniasis** The infected spleen (and liver) may enlarge to enormous sizes, and weights of 1,000–3,000 gm are not uncommon, even in children. The substance of the spleen is firm and red and with long-standing infection there is capsular thickening and sometimes infarction. The enlargement is due to hyperplasia of the mononuclear phagocytic cells in the red pulp at the expense of the white pulp, which is atrophic. In this field histiocytes with granular cytoplasm are prominent in cords and sinuses and are mixed with mononuclear lymphoid cells. *(H&E)*

**380**

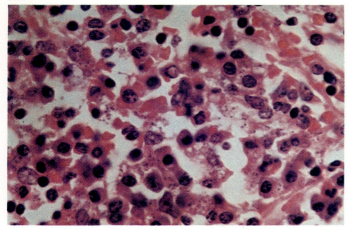

**380 Visceral splenic leishmaniasis** At this high magnification the *Leishmania donovani* bodies appear as bluish dots in the histiocyte cytoplasm. The lymphoid mononuclear cells consist mainly of plasma cells and it is this plasma cell proliferation in response to infection which accounts for the hypergammaglobulinaemia which may be a feature of the disease. *(H&E)*

**381**

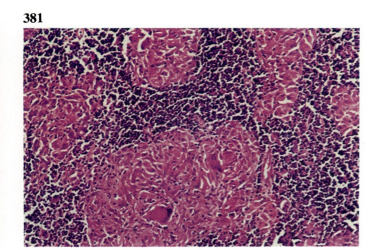

**381 Visceral leishmanial lymphadenopathy** Superficial lymphadenopathy may be the presenting feature in visceral leishmaniasis and is particularly common in the infantile and childhood forms of the disease acquired in the Mediterranean belt. In this cervical lymph node there is a granulomatous response. The epithelioid cell granulomas lacking any evidence of caseation, bear some resemblance to toxoplasmosis on the one hand and sarcoidosis on the other. *(H&E)*

**382**

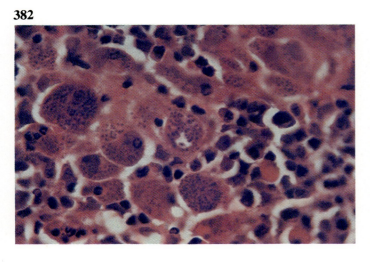

**382 Visceral leishmanial lymphadenopathy** At higher magnification and in contrast to toxoplasmosis and sarcoidosis, the epithelioid and giant cells (not shown) contain numerous and easily visualised *Leishmania donovani* bodies. It is the identification of these bodies that provides the most reliable means of diagnosis and, since their morphology is not always optimal in histopathological preparations, splenic, lymph nodal, hepatic or bone marrow aspirates may be indicated. Note the plasma cells and prominent Russell bodies. The leishmanial (Montenegro) skin test is of limited value, as are serological and culture procedures. *(H&E)*

**383**

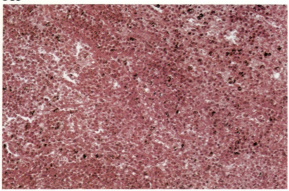

**383 Malaria** Malaria, a protozoal disease contracted from the bite of infected mosquitoes, continues to be the foremost infectious disease in terms of morbidity and mortality. The pathological findings are the result of rupture of parasitised red cells with subsequent phagocytosis of haemoglobin, malarial pigment and parasites by cells of the mononuclear phagocytic series. The lymphoreticular tissues enlarge and show a characteristic slate-grey pigmentation which is particularly evident in liver and spleen, and less so in lymph nodes which frequently remain of normal size. In acute disease the spleen is enlarged, soft and congested with prominence of the red pulp and sinus lining cells at the expense of the lymphoid component as in this field. Note the hyaline vascular change in the walls of the arterioles (see **428**). *(H&E)*

**384**

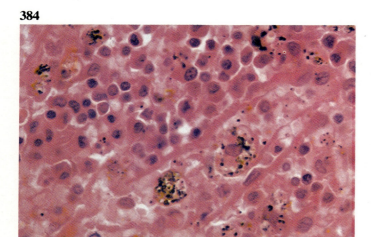

**385**

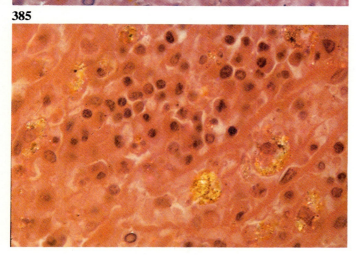

**384 and 385 Malaria** Of the four species infecting man, *Plasmodium falciparum* is the most important and most dangerous but is endemic only in tropical areas. *P. vivax* has a wider geographical distribution and still persists in some countries with a temperate climate. *P. malariae* at one time common in Europe has been largely eradicated and *P. ovale*, the rarest type of all, is limited to parts of Africa and the Far East. With the exception of *P. falciparum* intracellular parasites are not seen. The diagnostic feature permitting the recognition of malaria as a cause of splenic enlargement is the presence of malarial pigment. This pigment is brownish-black, **384**, and except for its presence *within* macrophages is indistinguishable from formalin pigment; also, like formalin pigment, it is birefringent, **385**, when viewed under the polarising microscope. *(384 H&E; 385 H&E (polarised light))*

**386 Histoplasmosis** With the exception of Africa, where the term *histoplasmosis* is used without qualification, histoplasmosis refers to the fungal disease due to infection with *Histoplasma capsulatum*. The disease is widespread in Africa, the Americas and parts of Asia, and is much more common than the disease caused by *H. duboisii*, which occurs only in Africa. At the early stages of infection with *H. capsulatum*, lymphadenitis is generally present either as a bronchopulmonary lymphadenitis in association with a primary lung infection, or as a regional lymphadenopathy at a site draining a skin infection. Lymphadenitis is present also in the chronic visceral form of

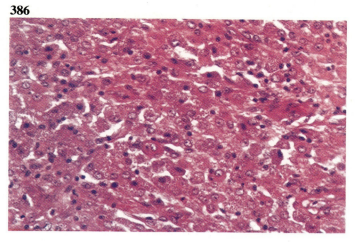

the disease or in the course of generalised haematogenous histoplasmosis which may affect immuno-logically compromised individuals. The lesions found in lymph nodes vary from non-caseating tuberculous granulomas which may fibrose, to extensive areas of caseous necrosis. In some susceptible (non-immune) individuals there is widespread proliferation of macrophages as shown here. Even at this low magnification, innumerable small ovoid encapsulated organisms can be identified. *(H&E)*

**387 and 388 Histoplasmosis** The intracellular organisms which are now easily identified at higher magnification, **387**, may be confused with those of leishmaniasis or *Cryptococcus neoformans*. PAS staining, **388**, is then helpful since like the larger *H. duboisii*, the histoplasmas are coloured red but surrounded by a clear zone due to shrinkage artefact. Leishmaniasis can be differentiated by the demonstration of kinetoplasts, and *Cryptococcus neoformans* by the carminophylia of the cell walls on staining with mucicarmine. Cryptococcal involvement of lymph node is also a very rare event. *(387 H&E; 388 PAS)*

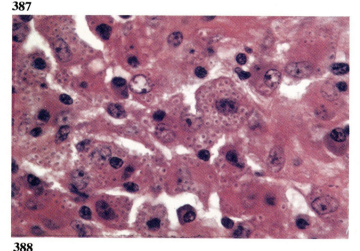

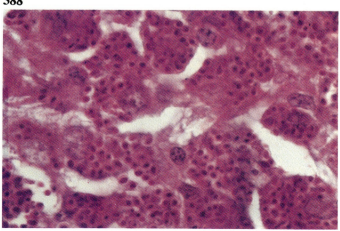

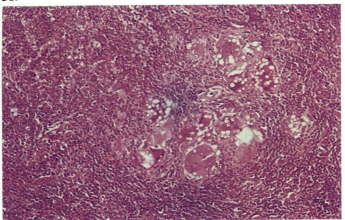

**389 Histoplasmosis of African type** This disease occurs only in the tropical belt of Africa and is due to infection by *Histoplasma duboisii*. Lymphadenitis may accompany a cutaneous lesion or occur as part of a systemic infection. Very occasionally lymphadenopathy may be the only manifestation. At all stages of the disease the most characteristic finding is the presence of foreign body type giant cells containing the causative organism. Focal abscess formation is not a feature but necrosis with suppuration or spreading caseation can occur. In this early lesion discrete giant cells containing many rounded histoplasmas are seen adjacent to a lymphoid follicle. In contrast to the organisms of *H. capsulatum* which are mainly found in macrophages, *H. duboisii* cells are much larger, measuring 10–15 microns, and their double contoured walls are seen easily. *H. duboisii* may be confused sometimes with *Blastomycosis dermatidis*, particularly since both infections are endemic in the same regions of Africa. However *B. dermatidis* differs in that its organism contains multiple nuclei or chromatin condensations and may be extremely difficult to demonstrate. *(H&E)*

390

391

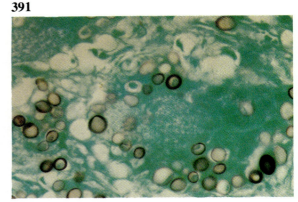

**390 and 391 Histoplasmosis of African type** In epithelioid granulomas or in those cases with extensive necrosis, special fungal stains may be necessary to demonstrate the organism. Particularly useful is the PAS method, **390**, which stains the wall and cytoplasm but leaves a clear space between due to shrinkage artefact and reveals a rare hyphal form, and the Grocott methanamine silver technique, **391**, which silvers (blackens) the large ovoid yeast forms. *(390 PAS; 391 Grocott)*

392

**392 Coccidiomycosis** This infection, which must not be confused with the protozoal intestinal disease coccidiosis, is a deep-seated fungal infection caused by *Coccidioides immitus*. The disease may vary from a clinically inapparent infection to severe and fatal mycosis. The lungs are primarily infected but dissemination may occur to other organs including lymph nodes. In lymph nodes the infection characteristically results in the formation of granulomas. In this example there is early central necrosis and within the giant cells the large spherules of *C. immitus* are easily seen. *(H&E)*

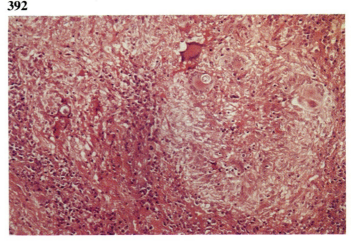

**393 Coccidiomycosis** The endemic areas are Mexico, South Western States of North America and parts of Central South America. Since the granulomas may undergo caseous necrosis, as shown here, and when spherules are not easily detected, the disease is likely to be confused with tuberculosis. *(H&E)*

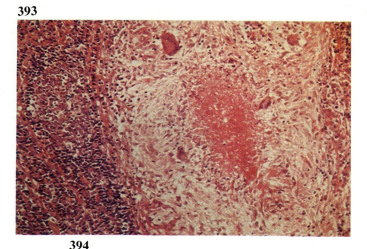

**394 Coccidiomycosis** The spherules or sporangia of *C. immitus* are usually contained within the giant cells of the granulomas. They are characterised by their large size, thick wall and granular content, here showing shrinkage artefact. Notice the very numerous plasma cells adjacent to the epithelioid granuloma. *(H&E)*

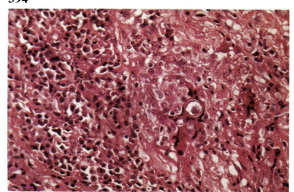

**395 Coccidiomycosis** Replication of the fungus occurs by a process of endosporulation. In this example a mature sporangium in a giant cell contains numerous endospores. Eventually there is rupture of the wall and liberation of endospores into the tissue, an event which initially excites an acute inflammatory response but which later proceeds to granuloma formation. *(H&E)*

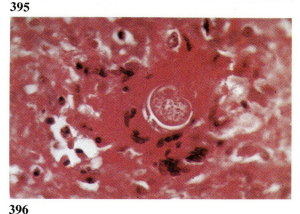

**396 Coccidiomycosis** The spherule shown here is surrounded by a thick eosinophilic proteinaceous material, in some ways resembling the Splendore-Hoeppli phenomenon (see **400**). Such an appearance is, however, much more characteristic of *Sporotrichum schenki*, the causative agent of sporotrichosis, another deep-seated fungal infection which may also involve lymph nodes. *(H&E)*

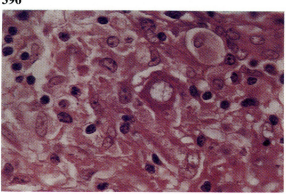

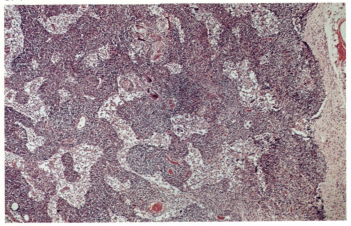

**397**

**397 Schistosomiasis (bilharziasis)** Schistosomiasis or bilharziasis represents an important group of diseases second only to malaria in terms of morbidity and mortality. Unlike malaria, the incidence of schistosomiasis is actually increasing as a result of irrigation programmes. Lymph nodes may be affected at any stage and, in long-standing disease, lymph node involvement may be an incidental finding. In this node several discrete ova are present within the parenchyma. There is capsular thickening and sinus histiocytosis but parenchymal fibrosis is not yet evident. *(H&E)*

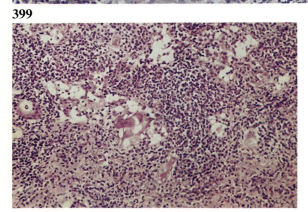

**398**

**398 Schistosomiasis (bilharziasis)** Schistosomiasis is caused by trematodes (flukes) and its incidence is determined by the distribution of fresh water snails (the intermediate host) which inhabit large tracts of Africa, parts of the Middle and Far East and some parts of South America. Following the penetration of the skin by the cercariae and after a latent period, the mature flukes deposit their ova within the venous system and may be found subsequently in various tissues including lymph nodes. These three recently deposited ova have incited a granulomatous response and are surrounded by a histiocytic zone, lymphoid cells and many eosinophils. At this stage the internal structures of the eggs with their miricidiae are well preserved. *(H&E)*

**399**

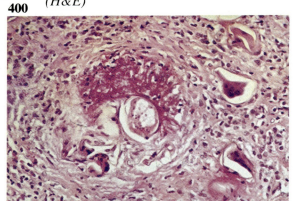

**400**

**399 Schistosomiasis (bilharziasis)** Three serious diseases in man are caused by Schistosomiasis: urinary schistosomiasis due to *S. haematobium*, intestinal schistosomiasis caused by *S. mansoni* and Asian intestinal schistosomiasis resulting from an infection with *S. japonicum*. Apart from the different clinical features and principal organs involved, these three variants of schistosomiasis can be differentiated histopathologically on the basis of the morphology of the ova. The ovum of *S. haematobium* has a terminal spine, *S. japonicum* has a round ovum with no spine, and *S. Mansoni* has an ovoid ovum with a lateral spine as shown here. *(H&E)*

**400 Schistosomiasis (bilharziasis)** The central ovum shown here is partially surrounded by eosinophilic proteinaceous material of an irregular contour. This finding constitutes the Splendore-Hoeppli phenomenon. This phenomenon was thought originally to represent either a new species of sporotrichum or material secreted by the sporotrichum. It is now recognised as an immunological response and is seen in many mycotic, bacterial and helminthic infections – including schistosomiasis. *(H&E)*

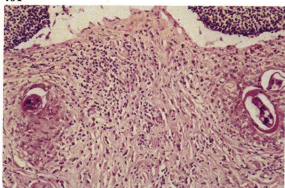

**401** Schistosomiasis (bilharziasis) Ova are found not only in lymph node parenchyma but in capsular tissue. In this example, the subcapsular sinus is preserved but the capsule is considerably thickened and the three ova are surrounded by cellular fibrous tissue in which lymphocytes and eosinophils are conspicuous. *(H&E)*

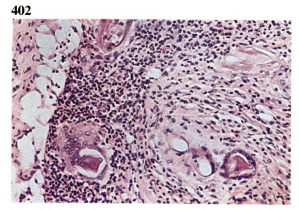

**402** Schistosomiasis (bilharziasis) With chronic diseases many of the ova become progressively destroyed and surrounded by fibrous tissue. Some ova will still retain recognisable morphological characteristics. In this example the two partially destroyed ova within giant cells exhibit the terminal spine of *S. haematobium. (H&E)*

**403** Onchocerciasis This filarial disease due to *Onchocerciasis volvolus* is an important cause of blindness, and is widespread and endemic in tropical Africa, the central areas of South America, Mexico and parts of the Middle East. Superficial and more deeply located lymph nodes may be involved, particularly those draining the skin nodules. Such nodes show a reactive sinus histiocytosis, and increased numbers of plasma cells, eosinophils and histiocytes within the nodal parenchyma. There is also a characteristic perivascular fibrosis. Microfilaria *(arrow)* are usually easily visualised and in established disease usually more apparent in relation to the fibrotic areas and not to the reactive inflammatory infiltrates. *(H&E)*

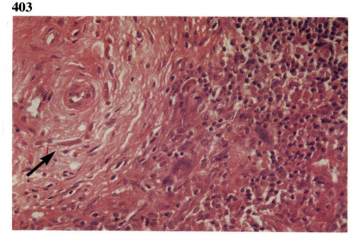

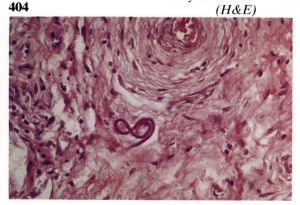

**404** Onchocerciasis In this field an entire coiled *O. volvolus* is seen lying in fibrous tissue in the vicinity of a small vessel. The dark material occupying virtually the whole length of the worm is nuclear chromatin. Note the absence of inflammatory cells in its immediate vicinity. *(H&E)*

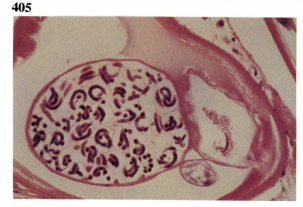

**405** Onchocerciasis A cross-section through the uterus of the gravid female illustrates numerous mature microfilaria. The gravid female is found generally only in skin nodules but occasionally, as shown here, when a lymph node is adherent to an overlying skin nodule they may be present in the adherent associated capsular tissue. *(H&E)*

**406**

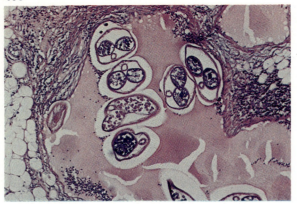

**406 Wuchereria bancroftii lymphadenitis** This filarial disease has a very precise geographical distribution being limited to the North by the 40° latitude and to the South by the Tropic of Capricorn. The infection is responsible for an obstructive lymphangitis and the clinical manifestations of lymphoedema or 'elephantiasis' due to blockage of lymphatics by the adult worm. In this inguinal node a cross-section of a gravid female *W. bancroftii* is seen within the dilated lymphatic. There are numerous microfilaria in the double uterus below which is a transverse section through the intestine. The living worm causes little cellular response but when dead initiates a marked eosinophilic reaction and abscess formation. With the exception of *Brugia malayi*, other filariae rarely involve lymph nodes. *(H&E)*

## Sarcoidosis and other granulomatous diseases of unknown or non-infectious cause

Sarcoidosis is a systemic chronic granulomatous disease with a predeliction for lymphoreticular tissues. The aetiology is unknown although one of the most favoured views is that sarcoidosis represents an altered tissue (immunological) response to infection with *Mycobacterium tuberculosis*. The histological lesions, however, differ from those in tuberculosis in that caseous necrosis of epithelioid granulomatous foci is not a feature. Non-caseating granulomas of course occur as a response to many other agents including pathogenic organisms. Thus, a firm diagnosis of sarcoidosis based solely on the histological appearance of a node should never be made without full clinical details and special information based on radiological and other laboratory investigations, such as a negative Mantoux test and a positive Kveim test.

One interesting aspect of sarcoidosis is the apparent sparing of the small and large intestine and abdominal lymph nodes. In contrast non-caseating granulomas regularly occur at these sites in Crohn's disease (regional enteritis), a condition considered to be a quite separate entity to sarcoidosis – albeit also one of unknown aetiology. Non-caseating granulomas are also a manifestation of a reaction to various allergens of both organic and inorganic type. Thus the products of neoplasms within the drainage area of a lymph node may induce a variety of reactive changes including non-caseating granulomas; exposure to certain inorganic substances such as beryllium can result in granulomatous disease.

Rare but distinctive giant cell granulomatous lesions with or without fully formed epithelioid granulomas occur in certain poorly understood conditions of unknown aetiology which lack defined clinical manifestations. Such conditions include the pure giant cell lymphadenopathy occurring in young and usually fit adults, and the generalised giant cell tuberculoid granulomas developing within lymphoreticular tissue (particularly spleen) in the entity known as Stengel-Wolbach sclerosis.

**407 Sarcoidosis involving lymph nodes** When the superficial groups of nodes are involved it is usually the cervical and axillary nodes which show the greatest enlargement. Each of these two axillary nodes measures more than two cm and is of a firm consistency; they are not bound together by fibrosis, although this may occur with groups of more massively enlarged nodes. Of the deeper seated lymph nodes it is those in the mediastinum which are usually the most extensively affected.

**407**

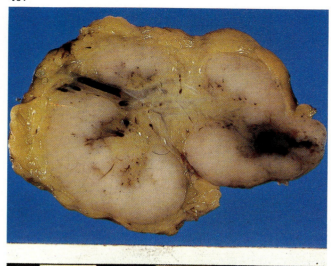

**408**

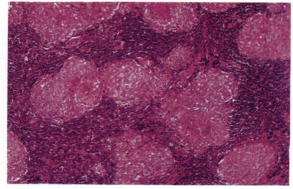

**408 Sarcoidosis in lymph nodes** In established sarcoidosis the histological appearance is characteristic in that there is extensive replacement of nodal architecture by generally rounded epithelioid cell granulomas. Some are discrete but others are coalescing, and a few show minimal central necrosis. Smaller less well developed epithelioid foci sometimes occur, when confusion with toxoplasmosis, brucellosis and drainage reactions to various neoplastic conditions may arise. *(H&E)*

**409**

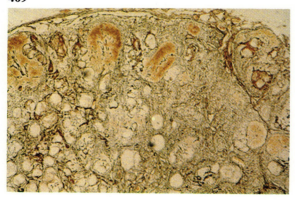

**410**

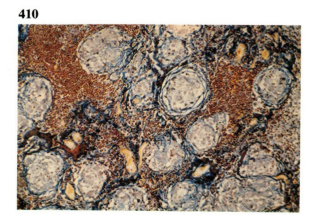

**409 and 410 Sarcoidosis in lymph nodes** A reticulin preparation, **409**, or a trichome, **410**, is useful in delineating the discrete granulomas and emphasising the predominance of the connective tissue fibre at their periphery, and its relative lack in the central parts. (**409** *Gordon & Sweets;* **410** *Mallory's trichome*)

**411**

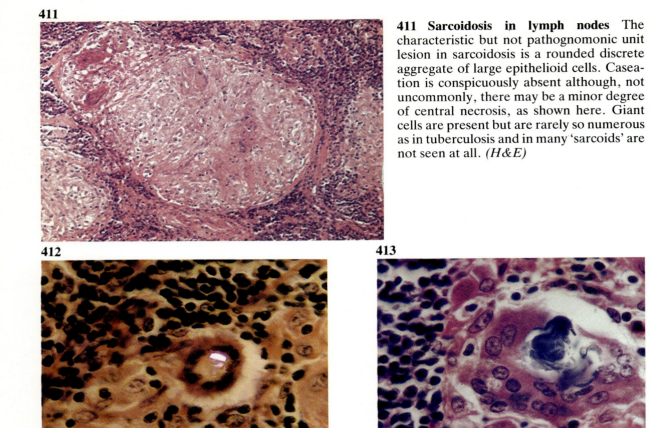

**411 Sarcoidosis in lymph nodes** The characteristic but not pathognomonic unit lesion in sarcoidosis is a rounded discrete aggregate of large epithelioid cells. Caseation is conspicuously absent although, not uncommonly, there may be a minor degree of central necrosis, as shown here. Giant cells are present but are rarely so numerous as in tuberculosis and in many 'sarcoids' are not seen at all. *(H&E)*

**412**

**413**

**414**

**415**

**412, 413, 414 and 415   Sarcoidosis in lymph nodes** A variety of different inclusions may be seen within the giant cells of the sarcoid granulomas. These range from simple crystalline inclusions as seen in **412**, in polarising light, to laminar intensely haematoxyphil structures known as concoid or Schaumann bodies, **413**, which also may exhibit birefringence in polarising light. The very distinctive inclusion in **414** is known as the asteroid body because of the central eosinophilic mass from which radiate delicate elongated spicules. Figure **415** shows a plastic-processed asteroid stained with toluidine blue. None of these inclusions is specific to sarcoidosis since all may be found in other granulomatous lesions, notably tuberculosis, berylliosis and Crohn's disease. *(412 H&E polarising light; 413, 414 H&E; 415 Toluidine blue)*

**416**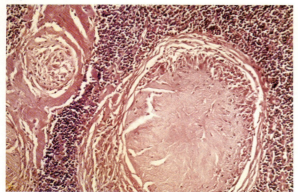

**416 Sarcoidosis in lymph nodes** With progressive disease there is gradual replacement of the cellular elements with mature fibrous tissue. Generally though not here, in any one lymph node the age and degree of fibrosis of the lesions is similar. *(H&E)*

**417**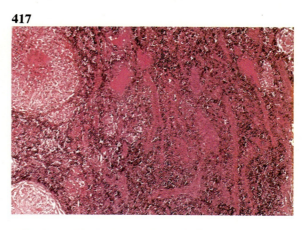

**417 Sarcoidosis in lymph nodes** In the uninvolved portions of the lymph nodes there may be other reactive changes. In this example there is marked proliferation of the postcapillary venules in the paracortex adjacent to the granulomas. *(H&E)*

**418**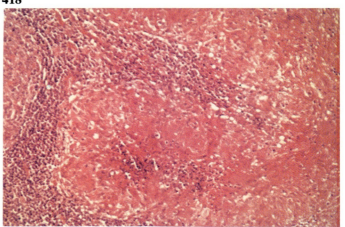

**418 Sarcoidosis in lymph nodes** In occasional lymph nodes there may be prominent necrosis, particularly at the centres of the sarcoid granulomas. This necrosis, which contains much more cellular debris than the bland coagulative necrosis of caseation, may show an eosinophilic appearance that is generally termed fibrinoid necrosis. *(H&E)*

**419 Sarcoidosis involving the spleen** In up to 20 per cent of patients with sarcoidosis, usually those with relatively advanced disease, the spleen is palpably enlarged. It is likely, however, that the spleen is involved in a much higher proportion of patients. This spleen weighed over 2 kg and shows replacement of its substance with coalescing whitish nodules superficially resembling lymphoma.

**419**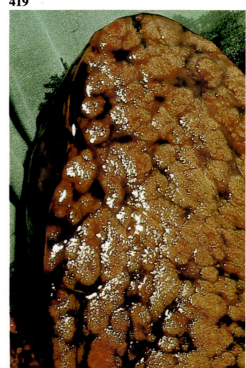

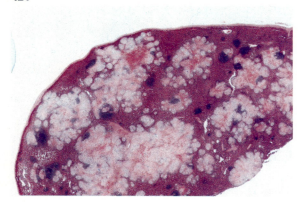

**420  Sarcoidosis involving the spleen** A section of the spleen in **419** shows the presence of variably-sized coalescing nodules of sarcoid tissue. Over half of the splenic parenchyma was replaced by granulomatous tissue. Such spleens are an ideal source for the sarcoid antigen used in the intradermal Kveim test. *(H&E)*

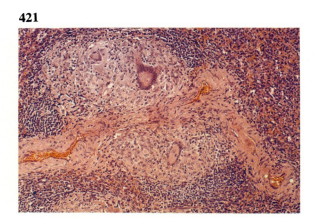

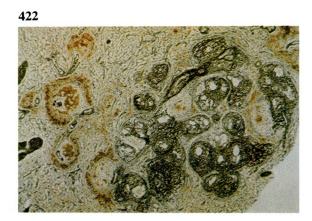

**421 and 422  Sarcoidosis involving the spleen** Non-caseating tubercles, **421**, are present mainly in the T-cell areas aggregated around follicular arterioles in a manner very similar to that seen in the non-specific granulomas developing in the spleen in Hodgkin's disease. Fibrosis is already well established, **422**, and there is an abundance of fibre throughout the granulomas which may be related to site.
*(**421** H&E; **422**  Gordon & Sweets)*

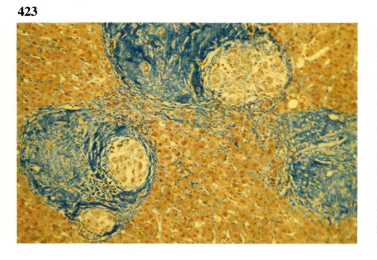

**423  Sarcoidosis involving liver** The liver is another organ frequently involved during the course of sarcoidosis and the granulomas may be found in portal tracts or parenchyma. These scattered discrete non-caseating hepatic granulomas outlined by connective tissue are similar in appearance to those seen in miliary tuberculosis, in patients with inflammatory bowel disease and in primary biliary cirrhosis, and to the sarcoid-like lesions in Hodgkin's disease. The separation of these different entities can be made only by a combination of the pathologist's findings and comprehensive clinical details. *(Mallory's trichrome)*

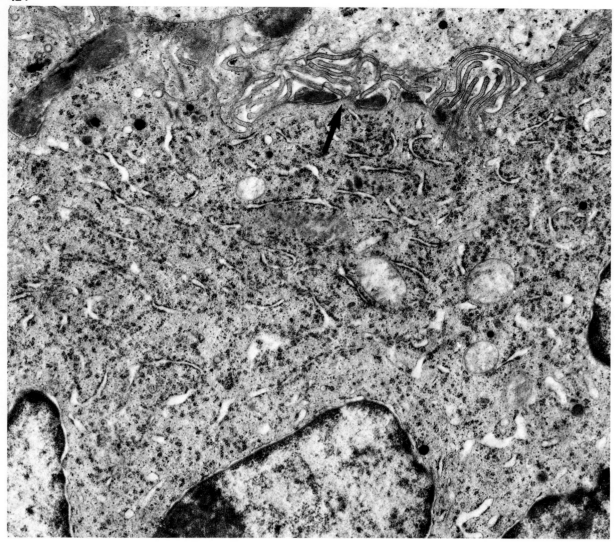

**424 Sarcoid granulomas, ultrastructure** The large epithelioid and giant cells forming the granulomas contain an abundance of ribosomes and short strands of rough endoplasmic reticulum and, therefore, may be quite pyroninophilic. The complex filiform cytoplasmic projections at the periphery, in association with electron dense proteinaceous material (*arrow*), is a noteworthy feature. (× *27,250*)

**425**

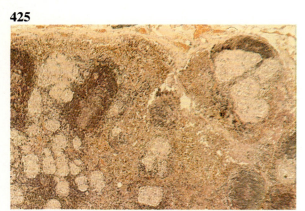

**425 Crohn's disease lymphadenitis** In Crohn's disease (regional enteritis) the regional abdominal lymph nodes show a range of appearances. The changes vary from non-specific reactive changes to non-caseating granulomas indistinguishable from those found in sarcoidosis and other diseases associated with granuloma formation. Like sarcoidosis the granulomas may show central necrosis and, later, a tendency to undergo fibrosis. Caseation is excessively rare but has been described, and in these cases it is essential to exclude tuberculosis. Less commonly, scattered or aggregated Langhans giant cells are found but no epithelioid foci. *(H&E)*

**426**

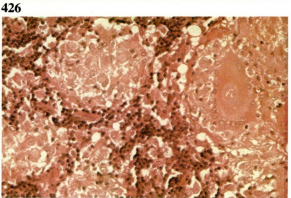

**426 Beryllium lymphadenitis** In the pulmonary and diffuse forms of berylliosis resulting from industrial exposure to beryllium salts, there may be lymph nodal involvement. The classical changes found are discrete giant cell epithelioid granulomas indistinguishable from those seen in sarcoidosis. Like the latter disease, occasionally there may be central necrosis, and the presence of both concentric laminar haematoxyphil bodies essentially similar to the Schaumann bodies, and asteroid bodies such as the early one shown here. In some cases it may be necessary to process the lymph nodes for spectrography when the demonstration of beryllium salts will confirm the diagnosis. *(H&E)*

# Connective tissue disorders involving lymphoreticular tissue

Not surprisingly the connective tissue group of diseases may involve lymphoreticular tissue. The three diseases which commonly induce lymphadenopathy are rheumatoid arthritis (see **222**), systemic lupus erythematosus and polyarteritis nodosa. Lymph node involvement in patients with dermatomyositis, systemic sclerosis, anaphalactoid purpura and polymyalgia rheumatica also occurs, and it is recognised in the less well-defined but related entities such as thrombotic thrombocytopaenic purpura, Wegener's granulomatosis and some of the allergic granulomatoses. Connective tissue diseases may also involve the spleen, particularly polyarteritis nodosa. Important aspects of this group of diseases are the increased incidence of lymphoma, and the association of some, particularly rheumatoid arthritis, with macroglobulinaemia.

**427**

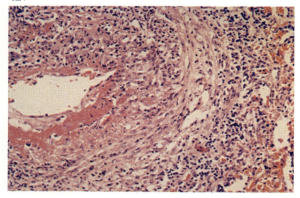

**427 Polyarteritis nodosa** Involvement of splenic vessels may result in multiple foci of necrosis or larger areas of infarction. The vascular changes are similar to those seen in other tissues. This artery shows fibrinoid necrosis, mainly of the inner part of the wall, and a prominent inflammatory infiltrate. *(H&E)*

**428**

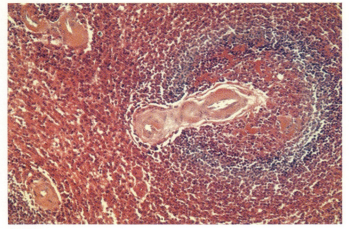

**428 Splenic hyaline vascular change** A common finding in the spleen of elderly individuals, which occurs even in some younger persons, is a diffuse eosinophilic thickening of the walls of the small trabecular arteries and arterioles of the lymphoid tissue. In this example not only do the vessels appear thickened and eosinophilic but there is also proteinaceous exudate in the germinal centre (see **233**). These changes must not be confused with vascular amyloid deposition, or with the fibrinoid degeneration of the connective tissue diseases. There is no correlation with splenic hypertension and hyaline vascular change, which is viewed as a degenerative phenomenon. *(H&E)*

**429**

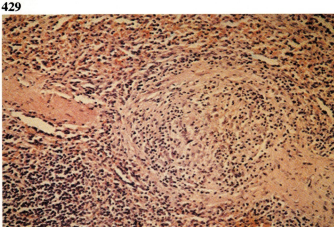

**429 Polyarteritis nodosa** In addition to the vascular changes and areas of parenchymal necrosis, acute inflammation of the connective tissue of capsule and trabeculae may occur. This acute trabeculitis, as shown here, is very characteristic of polyarteritis nodosa, and later may be associated with a histiocytic epithelioid cell response. *(H&E)*

**430**

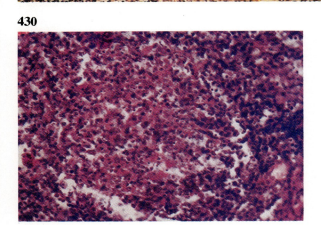

**431**

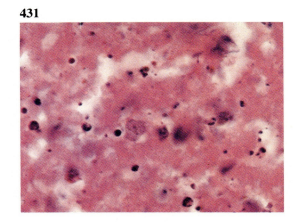

**430 and 431 Systemic lupus erythematosus** Lymph nodes are frequently involved in systemic lupus erythematosus. Indeed lymph node enlargement, particularly of the cervical nodes, may be the presenting feature of this disease. In many instances the changes, like those of rheumatoid arthritis, are those of a non-specific reactive process. In others there is evidence of necrosis, a finding of considerable diagnostic value. These areas of necrosis vary from microscopic foci to much larger areas. Figure **430** illustrates a small area of necrosis with considerable cellular disintegration and formation of nuclear dust. It is particularly difficult in a cellular tissue such as lymph node to identify with certainty the characteristic haematoxyphil bodies, but occasionally they are present, **431**, in large numbers. *(H&E)*

**432**

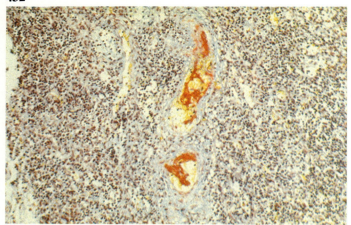

**432 Systemic lupus erythematosus** The vessels of both nodal parenchyma and of the pericapsular tissue may show vascular changes. In this example of a nodal vessel, stained with a trichrome technique, there is early involvement with fibrinoid necrosis (*red*) of the intima. The patient was a young woman who also had features of thrombotic thrombocytopaenic purpura. (*Martins scarlet blue*)

**433 Systemic lupus erythematosus** A curious but helpful finding in lymph nodes, but more often in spleen, is the vascular lesion known as laminar periarteriolar sclerosis in which arterioles, particularly those of the splenic follicles, are the site of a concentric adventitial fibrosis. This 'onion scale' appearance in a small splenic artery is not pathognomonic of SLE. It is seen in some cases of Felty's syndrome and in sarcoidosis. In SLE, in contrast to sarcoidosis, the concentric rings of fibrous tissue are more variable in thickness; there may also be evidence of vascular necrosis. (*PTAH*)

**433**

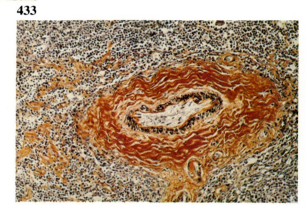

**435**

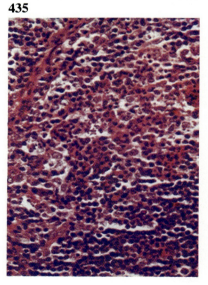

**434**

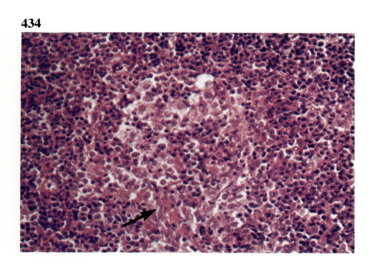

**434 and 435 Dermatomyositis** Lymph nodal changes are described in dermatomyositis but are less well documented and are frequently non-specific. This patient with confirmed dermatomyositis also had features of SLE. There was fever and abdominal lymph node enlargement, and an axillary lymph node showed, in addition to a very marked follicular hyperplasia, microscopic foci of necrosis. Figure **434** shows early fibrinoid necrosis (*arrow*) developing in a germinal centre which lacks tingeable body macrophages; **435** shows a more advanced focus adjacent to a small necrotic vessel. In both foci neutrophils are present. (*H&E*)

# Infiltrative and degenerative disorders involving lymphoreticular tissue

Included in this broad category of miscellaneous conditions are simple degenerative processes such as hyaline vascular degeneration, fatty change, the deposition of a number of pigments of both endogenous and exogenous type, the deposition or accumulation of specific substances as in amyloidosis and the rare storage disorders such as the lipidoses. In this section only amyloidosis and two of the lipidoses, namely Gaucher's disease and Niemann-Pick's disease have been selected for illustration.

**436 and 437 Amyloidosis** The deposition of amyloid, a fibrous protein, may complicate a number of diseases, in which case the resulting amyloidosis is said to be secondary, as distinct from primary amyloidosis which occurs without any known predisposing cause. Among the diseases associated with the secondary form are chronic infective or inflammatory processes, the connective tissue disorders (rheumatoid arthritis in particular) multiple myelomatosis and some lymphomas. There are also a number of familial forms of amyloidosis, and localised amyloid deposits in ageing but otherwise normal individuals is now recognised with increasing frequency. Lymph nodes may be involved in either primary, **436**, or secondary amyloidosis and, very occasionally, lymphadenopathy may be the presenting feature. One cause of secondary amyloidosis is Waldenström's macroglobulinaemia, **437**. This lymph node shows extensive amyloid deposition separating groups of plasma cells. *(H&E)*

**436**

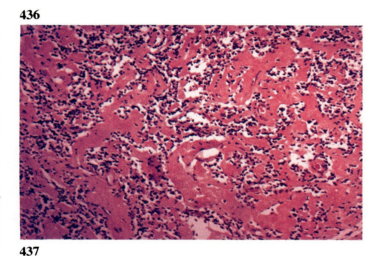

**437**

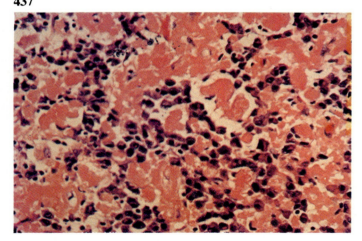

**438** **Amyloidosis** There is usually marked splenic involvement in secondary amyloidosis, but primary amyloidosis also can affect the spleen. The amyloid deposits are at first confined to the walls of small arteries when they need to be distinguished from the degenerative hyaline vascular material so commonly seen in ageing spleens (see **428**). Later, with progressive disease amyloid is seen deposited in a focal or diffuse form: the focal type is more common. Macroscopically the spleen shows innumerable round translucent deposits 2–3 mm in diameter replacing the lymphoid follicles, an appearance for which the term 'Sago' spleen is used. Microscopically the amyloid deposits appear as pink homogenous nodules which have destroyed the lymphocytes of the follicles. The intervening pulp is unaffected. The focal type of splenic amyloidosis results in less enlargement than the diffuse type in which the spleen may be grossly enlarged and characterised by a waxy texture and sharp edge on sectioning. *(H&E)*

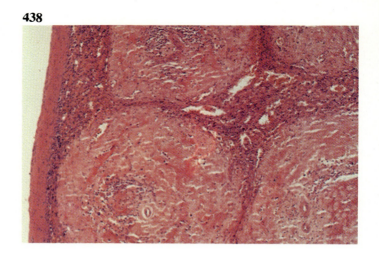

**439 and 440** **Amyloidosis** Although of low antigenicity, the intercellular amyloid deposits sometimes may induce a florid foreign body giant cell response as shown in this lymph node, **439**, from a patient with secondary amyloidosis. This giant cell response is not to be confused with diseases characterised by the formation of giant cell systems in which there may also be amyloid formation, **440**. In this selected field from a lymph node excised from a patient during the course of splenectomy for advanced sarcoidosis, amyloid has been deposited between the non-caseating granulomas. *(H&E)*

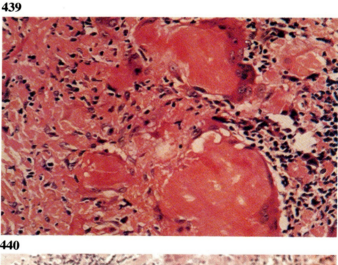

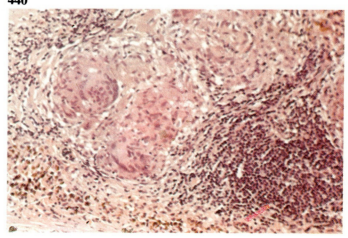

**441 Amyloidosis** There are a number of methods useful in the identification of amyloid. At macroscopical level Lugol's iodine combines with the protein deposits to give a dark brown colour. It was this apparent identity with starch which was responsible for the selection of the term amyloid. Congo red combines with amyloid to give a characteristic pale orange or salmon pink colour, as shown here, and providing the 'stained' material is subsequently viewed in polarising light is the most useful stain at microscopical level. Other less reliable methods include the rosaniline group of dyes employed to demonstrate metachromasia, and thioflavine-T which is a fluorescent dye and requires an ultraviolet light source. *(Congo red)*

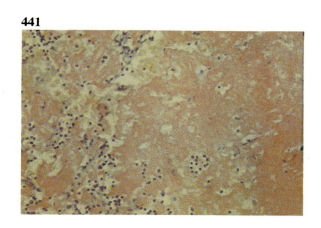
**441**

**442 and 443 Amyloidosis** Congo red binds with the amyloid fibrils in such a way that when viewed in polarising light the combination of dye and protein exhibits a characteristic birefringence, **442**, appearing apple green (*arrow*) in one direction and orange yellow in the other. When the Nicol prism is rotated through 90°, **443**, the tinctorial pattern is reversed. This property is known as dichroism. *(Congo red; viewed in polarised light)*

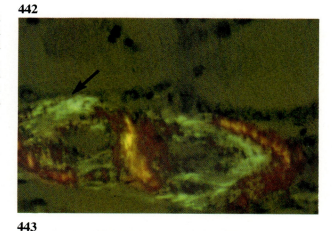
**442**

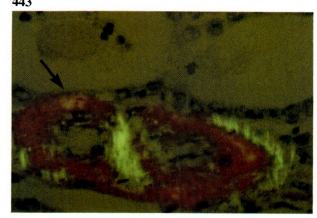
**443**

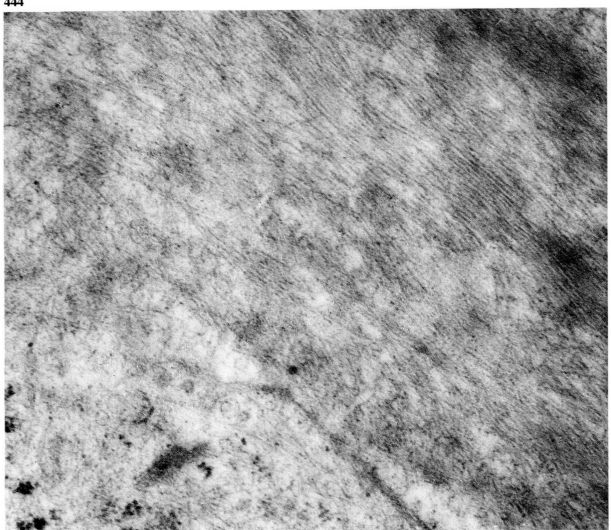

**444 Amyloid, ultrastructure** The fibrous protein of amyloid which is 'primary' or, secondary to multiple myelomatosis, has amino acid sequences suggesting an identity with the whole or part of immunoglobulin light chains. The sequence differs in different individuals and is of either kappa or lambda type, supporting the concept that the amyloid is the product of a clone of plasma cells. In contrast, the major protein constituent of the amyloid of classical secondary type, and in hereditary amyloid disease, appears unrelated to immunoglobulin and has been named Protein A. At ultrastructural level amyloid has a quite specific appearance consisting of either parallel or criss-crossing filaments 7.5 nm in diameter. *(× 60,000)*

**445 Gaucher's disease** This disease belongs to the group of storage disorders known as the sphingolipidoses. The defect is an inborn error of metabolism in which there is a deficiency of the enzyme glucocerebrosidase. As a result, a cerebroside – kerasin – progressively accumulates within the mononuclear phagocytic system of cells, and in the chronic form of the disease affected individuals show enlargement of spleen, liver, bone marrow and, to a lesser degree, lymph nodes. The spleen generally shows the greatest involvement and often weighs several kilogrammes. The normal parenchyma is replaced and expanded by large lipid-containing cells. These cells are usually arranged in groups and accumulate in relation to the splenic sinuses as shown here. This particular example also shows many red cells. *(H&E)*

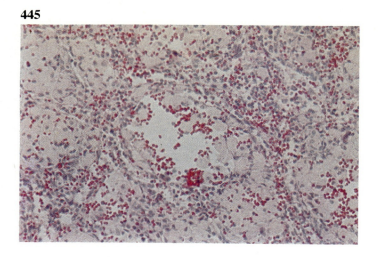

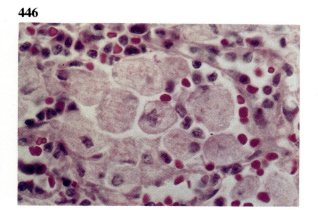

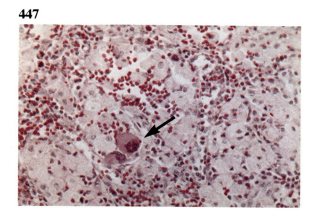

**446 and 447 Gaucher's disease** The disease is hereditary, more common in Jews than other ethnic groups, and presents either as a rapidly fatal disease of infancy or in a more chronic form in children and adults. The diagnosis is made morphologically by the demonstration of the characteristic pale swollen phagocytic cells within the affected organs. These Gaucher cells are pathognomonic with a unique cytoplasmic appearance, **446**, likened to that of ground glass in which there are faint linear streaks or striae. The intracytoplasmic lipid, however, cannot be demonstrated by sudanophilic dyes. In some examples where there is extensive bone marrow involvement, the spleen may show evidence of extramedullary erythropoiesis, **447**, with the presence of megakaryocytes *(arrow)* contrasting strongly with the Gaucher cells. That Gaucher cells are phagocytic is demonstrated by the occasional ingested red cells. *(H&E)*

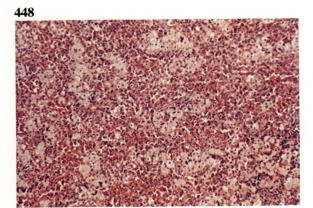

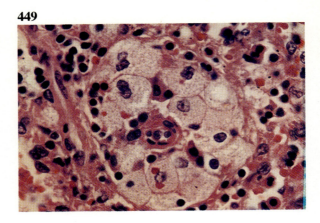

**448 Neimann-Pick disease** This disease is another sphingolipidosis. It is rarer than Gaucher's disease but shows a more marked familial incidence and affects Jews more frequently. It is also extremely rare in adults, usually presenting in infancy with progressive central nervous system involvement. The defective enzyme is a sphingomyelinase and the lipid which accumulates is predominantly a phospholipid. At all stages splenic and often lymph nodal involvement are conspicuous features, but in comparison to Gaucher's disease the liver is proportionately more enlarged than the spleen. The affected organs contain collections of pale macrophages which at low magnification, as seen here, resemble quite closely the appearance of Gaucher's disease. *(H&E)*

**449 Neimann-Pick disease** At high magnification the abnormal cells can now be seen to differ from those of Gaucher cells in that the cytoplasm has a finely divided granular appearance due to the presence of minute vacuoles, and lacks striae. Note the ingested red cells. These vacuolated or Neimann-Pick foam cells are highly characteristic and are found in virtually every tissue, and their presence in bone marrow or lymph node biopsies allow a presumptive diagnosis of this condition to be made. *(H&E)*

# Histiocytos X

This term incorporates Letterer-Siwe disease, Hand-Schüller-Christian disease and eosinophilic granuloma. These three rare and poorly understood conditions with widely differing patterns of behaviour are believed to represent variants of a neoplastic proliferation of cells belonging to the mononuclear phagocytic system. Another term sometimes used to describe these three diseases is 'differentiated progressive histiocytoses' in distinction to the malignant histiocytic proliferations. Lipid accumulation within the abnormal macrophages may occur in long-standing Hand-Schüller-Christian disease and to a lesser extent in eosinophilic granuloma. For this reason Hand-Schüller-Christian disease was formerly grouped with the lipidoses. The lipid accumulation is not, however, a reflection of disordered fat metabolism, and is now viewed as a secondary event.

Lymph node involvement occurs in Letterer-Siwe disease and Hand-Schüller-Christian disease but is rare in eosinophilic granuloma. At histopathological level and in the absence of relevant clinical and radiological data, it may not always be possible to distinguish the lymph node changes in the three conditions since certain features are common to all.

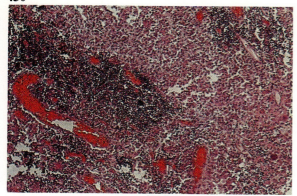

**450 Letterer-Siwe disease** This disease (non-lipid histiocytosis) occurs most commonly in infants and children below three years of age and, in typical cases, is characterised by a rapid and fatal course. It is thus the most 'malignant' member of the histiocytosis X group. The widespread proliferation of abnormal mononuclear phagocytes results in hepatosplenomegaly, generalised lymph node enlargement and bone marrow involvement. Multiple skin nodules are usually present, and fever and anaemia are often conspicuous features of the disease. In early and rapidly fatal cases as in this example of a post-mortem lymph node architecture is preserved but the sinuses are expanded and widened by the pale histiocytic cells contrasting strongly with the lymphocytes. *(H&E)*

**451 Letterer-Siwe disease** As the disease progresses the proliferating histiocytes expand and replace normal structures; in some tissues such as bone, the tumour-like masses result in localised destructive lesions. Multinucleated forms of varying size are sometimes a prominent feature, as in this example, and the multinucleated cells show a range of appearances including those of foreign body – and Langhans giant cells. Eosinophils are usually present though variable in number and, occasionally, there are microscopic foci of necrosis *(arrow)*. The proliferating histiocytes appear mature and well differentiated with irregular indented vesicular nuclei and abundant cytoplasm. Mitotic and phagocytic activity are rarely noted. In atypical cases with a more prolonged course there may be lipid accumulation in the histiocytes and an appearance identical to that of Hand-Schüller-Christian disease. *(H&E)*

451

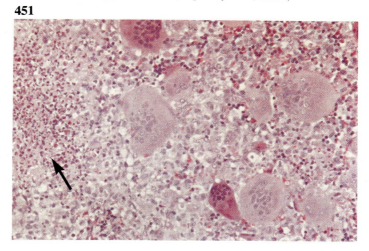

452

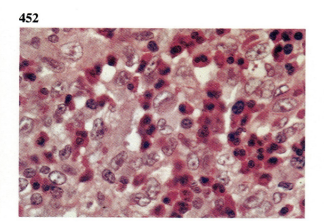

453

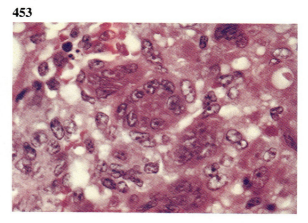

**452 and 453 Letterer-Siwe disease** The majority of mononuclear cells, shown in **452** accompanied by numerous eosinophils, and the giant cells show no nuclear features to indicate a malignant nature. Figure **453** illustrates a group of cells in which some nuclei do show a degree of atypia with prominent indentations producing highly irregular nuclear contours, and moderate hyperchromasia. *(H&E)*

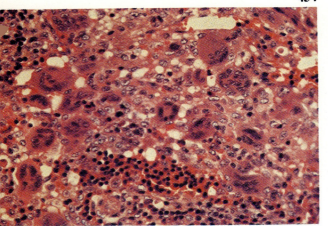

**454 Hand-Schüller-Christian disease** This disease which occurs at all ages but most commonly in children, is generally much more prolonged than Letterer-Siwe disease, with survival of more than ten years in some cases. There is, in addition to hepatic, dermal, splenic and nodal involvement, a very marked tendency for skeletal involvement; if the skull is affected this may result in diabetes insipidus. The pattern of nodal involvement is very similar to Letterer-Siwe disease and in early cases the appearances of the proliferating histiocytes also closely resemble those of the more 'malignant' variants. Giant cells are present and eosinophils are generally abundant and distributed either focally or more diffusely among the histiocytic cells. *(H&E)*

**455**

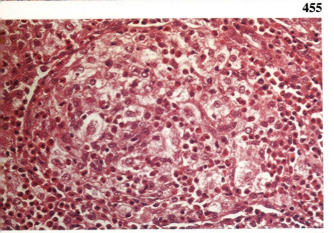

**455 Hand-Schüller-Christian disease** As the disease progresses, and in contrast to Letterer-Siwe disease, the histiocytes become aggregated into clusters, develop a more abundant cytoplasm due to the accumulation of lipid, and exhibit a vacuolar appearance as seen here. The lipid is predominantly cholesterol and its esters, and it is this fatty accumulation which was responsible for the previous designation of Hand-Schüller-Christian disease as 'normo-cholesterolaemic primary cholesterol lipidosis'. In long-standing cases there is a tendency for the 'xanthomatous' areas to undergo fibrosis. *(H&E)*

**456**

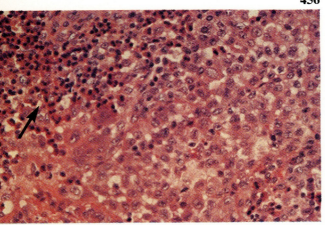

**456 Eosinophilic granuloma of lymph nodes** Eosinophilic granuloma is usually a solitary lesion occurring in the bones of children and adults and generally therefore is referred to as eosinophilic granuloma of bone. Occasionally the lymph nodes are affected also, and rarely a solitary lymph node appears to be the only site of the disease, as shown here. Architecture is generally preserved with retention of lymphoid follicles but the sinuses are widened and infiltrated by histiocytic cells. Eosinophils (*arrow*) vary in number and sometimes occur in the form of lakes and there are also occasional multinucleate forms. The prognosis of this condition is variable with some progressing to a malignant histiocytosis often developing bone lesions, and others remaining localised. *(H&E)*

**457**

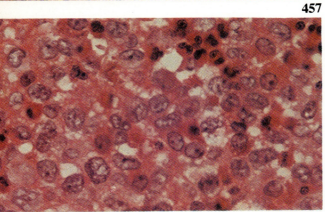

**457 Eosinophilic granuloma of bone** Eosinophilic granuloma occurring in bone has a generally good prognosis, though some progress and develop the features of Hand-Schüller-Christian disease. Morphologically the cellular composition of the lesion is very similar to Hand-Schüller-Christian disease and, like that variant, the histiocytic cells may also contain appreciable amounts of lipid, though not in this example from the humerus of a 14-years-old boy. The unity of the conditions making up histiocytosis X is strengthened by the findings at ultrastructural level (see **459**). *(H&E)*

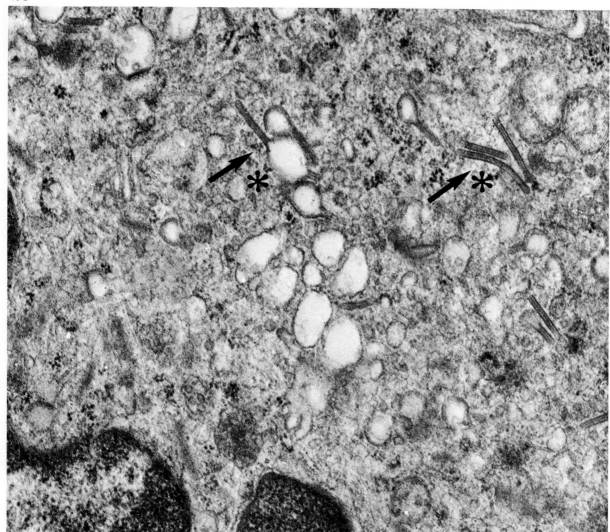

**458 Langerhans' cell, ultrastructure** Within skin is a specialised cell called the Langerhans' cell. Originally considered to be related to the melanocyte it is now believed to belong to an intraepidermal system of mononuclear phagocytic cells. Its importance lies in its content of a specialised cytoplasmic organelle, the Langerhans' granule, which has since been identified in the cytoplasm of histiocytosis X cells (see **459**), some histiocytic tumours and cells in some reactive histiocytic conditions. The granules are characterised by rod shaped, flask shaped or tennis-racket shaped profiles (*arrow*) within which there is a median line. They are considered to represent a specialised type of endocytosis, though often they appear to have a close relationship with the Golgi apparatus. *(× 48,000)*

**459 Histiocytosis X, ultrastructure** Part of a histiocytic cell from an eosinophilic granuloma of bone is shown here. The cytoplasm contains an abundance of organelles including Langerhans' granules (*arrow and inset*) and shows a markedly irregular perimeter. Note the presence of linear densities representing immature Langerhans' granules. Langerhans' granules have been identified also in cases of Hand-Schüller-Christian disease and Letterer-Siwe disease and are strong evidence for the close relationship of the three histiocytic disorders. (× *19,400; inset × 42,200*)

# Hodgkin's disease

Hodgkin's disease is now generally accepted as a malignant lymphoma, and the previous sub-division of the disease into paragranuloma, granuloma and sarcoma by Jackson and Parker is no longer tenable. In 1963 Lukes, Butler and Hicks proposed a classification consisting of six histo-pathological categories. This was later modified at a symposium held in Rye, New York. The Rye classification, as it is now known, subdivides the disease into four types. The interrelationships of the two previous classifications with Rye are shown thus:

| Jackson and Parker | Lukes, Butler and Hicks | Rye | Grade |
|---|---|---|---|
| Paragranuloma | lymphocytic/histiocytic diffuse | lymphocytic predominance | I |
| | lymphocytic/histiocytic nodular | | |
| | nodular sclerosis | nodular sclerosis | |
| Granuloma | | | |
| | mixed | mixed cellularity | II |
| Sarcoma | diffuse fibrosis | lymphocytic depletion | |
| | reticular | | |

The Rye classification has now been universally adopted. The first two types carry a good prognosis (Grade I) while the second two types have a worse prognosis (Grade II). There is a marked difference in the incidence of the four types in different series. In most, however, nodular sclerosis type predominates. In the British National Lymphoma Investigation (BNLI) nodular sclerosis type is the most common, accounting for 71 per cent; the mixed cellularity type is next in frequency at 17 per cent and the lymphocytic predominance and lymphocytic depletion types represent about 8 per cent and 4 per cent respectively. In this trial no children under 15 years are included.

The majority of patients with Hodgkin's disease present in early adult life. In most series the major peak occurs in the 20–30-year-old age group, with a second smaller peak in the 55–65-year-old age group. With the exception of the nodular sclerosis type which is distinctly more common in females, but only following puberty, the other three types are slightly more common in males. The most frequent presentation is unilateral cervical lymph node enlargement but other groups of nodes, spleen and extranodal sites such as liver, bone marrow and lung, may be involved at pre-sentation; mediastinal lymphadenopathy is peculiarly common in nodular sclerosis Hodgkin's disease in females. Splenomegaly and lymphangiography are unreliable in predicting splenic and/or abdominal lymph node enlargement. It is now common practice for patients presenting with clinical stage I and II and often stage III disease to undergo staging laparotomy for the purpose of histopathological staging, when in addition to splenectomy, liver and abdominal lymph nodes are biopsied. It is also convenient at the same time to perform an iliac crest biopsy to obtain a large intact sample of bone marrow. On the basis of these findings patients are placed in one of four staging groups according to the Ann Arbor system.

| Stage | Extent of disease |
|-------|-------------------|
| I | Involvement of a single lymph node region although more than one node may be affected at that anatomical site. |
| (IE | Involvement of a single 'extralymphatic' organ or site.) |
| II | Involvement of two or more lymph node regions on both sides of the diaphragm. |
| (IIE | Localised involvement of an 'extralymphatic' organ or site *and* one or more lymph node regions on the same side of the diaphragm.) |
| III | Involvement of lymph node regions on both sides of the diaphragm, which may be accompanied by localised involvement of an 'extralymphatic' organ or site, or by involvement of spleen or both. |
| IV | Diffuse or disseminated involvement of one or more 'extralymphatic' organs or tissues such as liver, lung, pleura, bone-marrow or skin, with or without associated lymph node enlargement. |

There is a further subdivision into A & B categories according to whether there are systemic symptoms such as fever in the absence of infection, significant weight loss and night sweats. The extent of the disease (clinical or pathological stage) determines therapy, whereas the histopathological stage predicts response to treatment and likely prognosis. It is also recognised that if there is progression from a favourable to a less favourable histopathological type as seen in the change from lymphocytic predominance to mixed cellularity or lymphocytic depletion types, or of mixed cellularity to lymphocytic depletion type, prognosis is adversely affected. Interestingly, nodular sclerosis type does not progress to the Grade II types although there may be considerable variation in the cellular composition of the nodules which may affect prognosis. In other words 'once a Noddy always a Noddy'. It has also become apparent that modern therapy has revolutionised the life expectancy in patients with Hodgkin's disease, which is now 'curable' in the majority of patients, and that one of the major complications now is not the disease itself but the increased susceptibility to infections, often of opportunistic type, exhibited by patients with Hodgkin's disease and in whom there is often a striking and early defect in T-lymphocytic immunity.

460

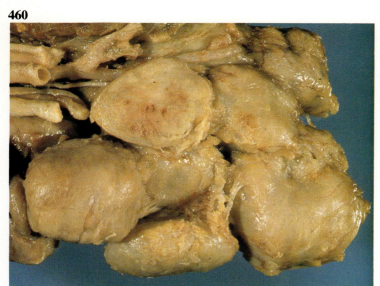

**460 Hodgkin's disease, lymph node enlargement** Enlargement of one group of superficial nodes, most often cervical, is a common presentation in Hodgkin's disease. These axillary lymph nodes although showing considerable enlargement are, in contrast to many inflammatory conditions, discreet – a characteristic of malignant lymphoma. It is most unusual for the nodes to be painful although there may be some tenderness on palpation.

461

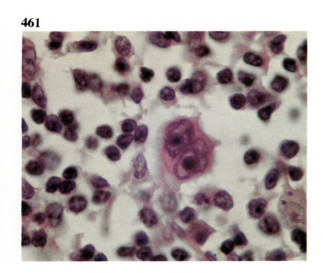

**461 Hodgkin's disease, Reed-Sternberg cell** The identification of Reed-Sternberg cells is mandatory to the diagnosis of Hodgkin's disease and, except in some rare circumstances, such a diagnosis should never be made in their absence. The example shown here is of the classical binucleate, or mirror image type with two similarly sized and shaped nuclei each containing huge, sharply contoured eosinophilic nucleoli. In formalin fixed paraffin processed sections there is clearing of nuclear chromatin around the nucleoli producing a halo effect. The cytoplasm is seldom abundant in relation to nuclear size and in general shows well-defined limits, although in some instances may appear irregular. *(H&E)*

462

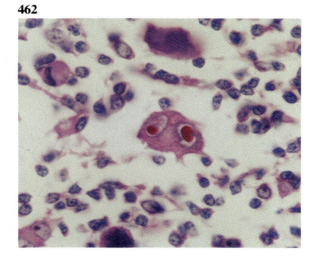

**462 Hodgkin's disease, Reed-Sternberg cell** With methyl green-pyronin (MGP) staining the nucleoli of Reed-Sternberg cells are intensely MGP positive. The cytoplasm stains less intensely and with much more variability. A frequent pattern of staining is where the pyroninophilia is confined to the peripheral portions of the cytoplasm. The MGP stain is useful in the identification of Reed-Sternberg cells, particularly in cases of lymphocyte predominant Hodgkin's disease when they may be sparse. *(MGP)*

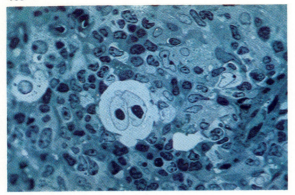

**463 Hodgkin's disease, Reed-Sternberg cell** The morphological features of Reed-Sternberg cells are enhanced in semi-thin sections of plastic-processed material and show considerable cytoplasmic detail. Notice that the perinuclear halo effect is absent, indicating that its presence in conventional paraffin processed material is a fixation processing artefact. *(Toluidine blue)*

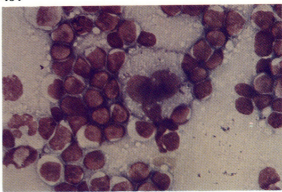

**464 Hodgkin's disease, Reed-Sternberg cell** Imprints of lymph nodes involved in Hodgkin's disease are not always diagnostic since Reed-Sternberg cells are resistant to sampling. In this preparation, however, a classical Reed-Sternberg cell is seen surrounded by closely adherent lymphocytes. Note again the absence of a perinuclear halo and the greater degree of basophilia at the cytoplasmic perimeter. *(May-Grünwald-Giemsa)*

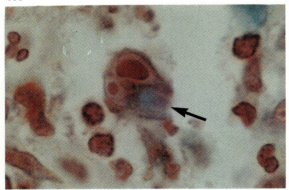

**465 Hodgkin's disease, Reed-Sternberg cell** Enzyme studies in the past to demonstrate lysozymal activity in Reed-Sternberg cells have been generally non-productive, and have been cited as evidence that Reed-Sternberg cells are not of histiocytic origin. In our experience at high magnification it is possible to visualise a positive staining reaction for acid phosphatase and non-specific esterases, but it is focal *(arrow)* and related to the Golgi apparatus and thus not always evident in the plane of section. *(Non-specific esterase)*

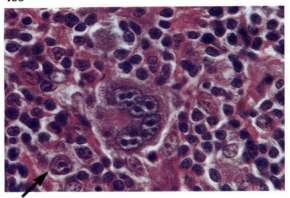

**466 Hodgkin's disease, Reed-Sternberg cell** Reed-Sternberg cells are frequently multi-nucleated. One common form is a large cell with several nuclei arranged in a horseshoe configuration and each containing prominent nucleoli. This type of multinucleated Reed-Sternberg cell is commonly associated with Hodgkin's disease of nodular sclerosing type. Adjacent to it *(arrow)* is an atypical mononucleated cell (see **479** and **480**) with a single non-lobated nucleus of similar appearance to the multinucleated cell nuclei. Reed-Sternberg cells are never seen in mitoses, do not synthesise DNA, and are thus characteristic of non-replicatory or end cells. *(H&E)*

**467**

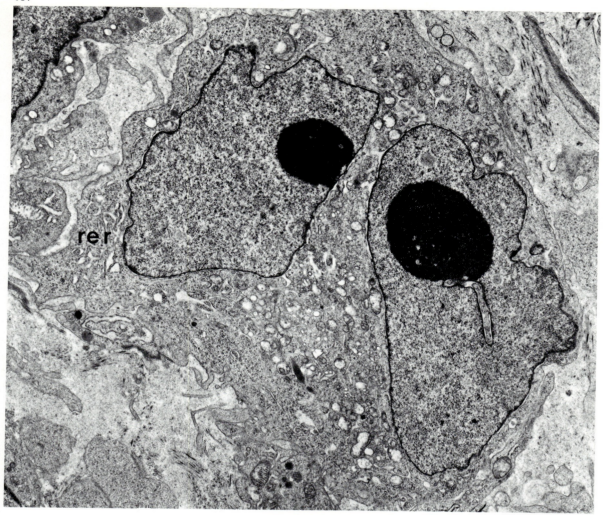

**467 Hodgkin's disease, Reed-Sternberg cell, ultrastructure** This classic mirror image Reed-Sternberg cell shows two nuclear masses, each with a large electron dense nucleolus. Although the nucleus appears binucleate here, often it is possible to discern continuity between what is in reality a single but folded nucleus. The nuclear chromatin is finely and evenly dispersed with some accentuation at the nuclear membrane. The abundant cytoplasm with irregular contour contains various organelles including mitochondria, free ribosomes, short profiles of rough endoplasmic reticulum (rer) and a few electron dense lysosomal structures. This combination of features suggests a histiocytic rather than a lymphoid origin. *(× 7,250)*

**468**

**468 Hodgkin's disease, Reed-Sternberg cell** An atypical mononucleated cell may be designated as a Reed-Sternberg cell at light microscopical level if the nucleus is lobated and shows more than one characteristic nucleolus surrounded by the clear nuclear zone. Such cells are common in lymphocyte predominant Hodgkin's disease. *(H&E)*

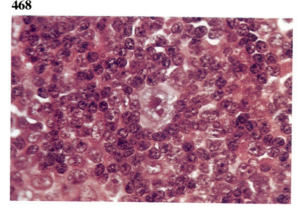

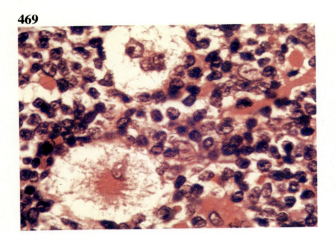

**469**

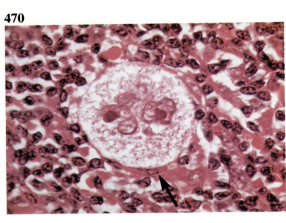

**470**

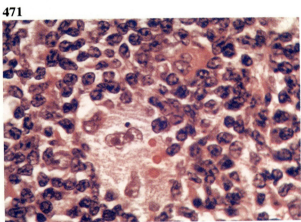

**471**

**469, 470 and 471 Hodgkin's disease, lacunar cells**
Lacunar cells are considered to be variants of the Reed-Sternberg cell but are seen only in the nodular sclerosis type of Hodgkin's disease. They are very large in volume and their typical appearance as seen in paraffin processed formalin sections are those of a shrunken cell lying within a clear space, **469**. The nucleus is multilobated and the nucleoli, although sometimes prominent, are seldom as large or as acidophilic as in the Reed-Sternberg cell. In better fixed preparations, **470**, there is still some contact between the particulate cytoplasm and the surrounding cells and often a very close contact with fibroblasts (*arrow*) as shown here. Occasionally, phagocytosed material is seen within lacunar cells, **471**, here consisting of three red cells and nuclear debris. (*H&E*)

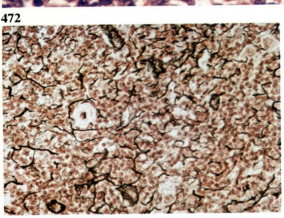

**472**

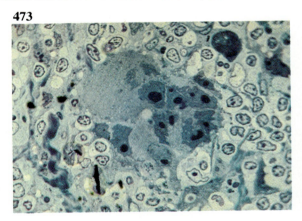

**473**

**472 Hodgkin's disease, lacunar cell** Reticulin fibre is often seen in close association to lacunar cells. In this example a fibroblast nucleus is just visible between a reticulin fibre and the lacuna. It is this 'tethering' of lacunar cells, which also can be observed at ultrastructural level, that affords an explanation for the shrinkage artefact responsible for the appearance of these cells in conventional sections. (*Gordon & Sweets*)

**473 Hodgkin's disease, lacunar cell** Lacunar cells are well preserved in optimally fixed plastic processed material and do not show any shrinkage of the cytoplasm, which is voluminous and appears to flow between the neighbouring cells making intimate contact with them. This example was obtained from a patient with nodular sclerosing Hodgkin's disease involving the mediastinum and thymus. (*Toluidine blue*)

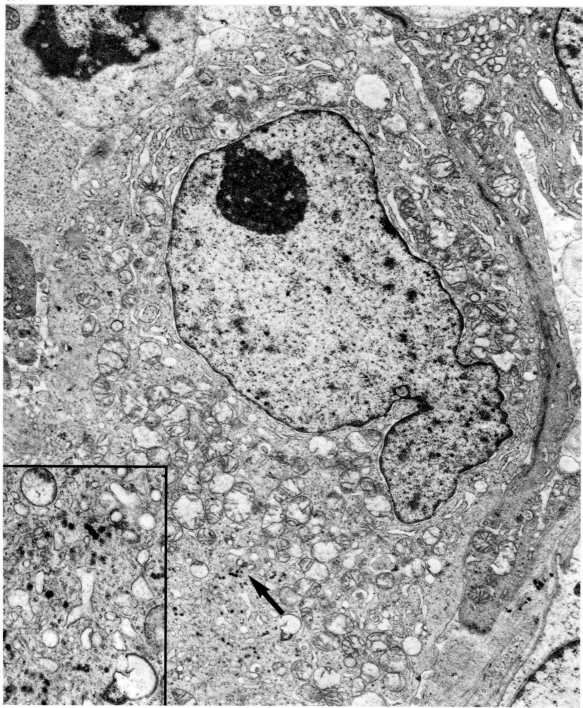

**474  Hodgkin's disease, lacunar cell, ultrastructure** Part of a lacunar cell is shown in intimate contact with the elongated process of a fibroblast on the right. The cytoplasm is voluminous and contains a variety of organelles of which mitochondria are the most conspicuous. There are also numerous small electron dense bodies (*arrow*). The inset is a detail of the cytoplasm showing electron dense granular structures in the vicinity of the vesicles of the Golgi apparatus, and smooth endoplasmic reticulum. (× 7,250; inset × 14,500)

**475**

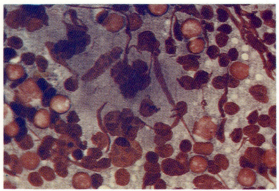

**475  Hodgkin's disease, lacunar cell** Lacunar cells are very fragile but sometimes can be well demonstrated in touch preparations. However because of the abundant but indistinct cytoplasm and the clumped nuclei they are frequently overlooked. *(May-Grünwald-Giemsa)*

**476**

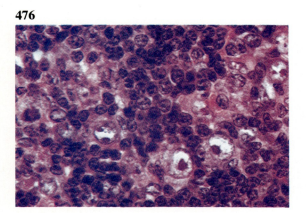

**477**

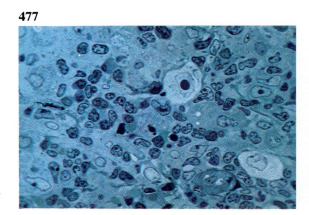

**476 and 477  Hodgkin's disease, atypical mononuclear cell** Large mononucleated cells, also known as atypical reticulum cells, Hodgkin's cells and indeterminate cells, are a common and fairly constant feature of Hodgkin's disease. Their identification is important and their presence should alert the pathologist to the possible diagnosis of Hodgkin's disease. Figure **476** illustrates three such cells adjacent to histiocytes. In the semi-thin section, **477**, one such cell is seen also closely related to a group of histiocytic cells. *(476 H&E; 477 Toluidine blue)*

**478**

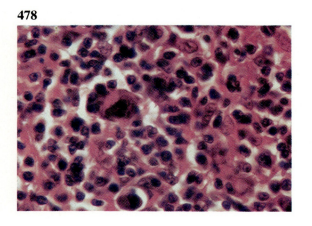

**478  Hodgkin's disease, atypical mononuclear cell** Sometimes it is possible to discern a very close relationship between lymphocytes, Reed-Sternberg cells and, in this instance an atypical mononuclear cell, such that a partial lymphocytic rosette has formed. The atypical mononuclear cell in addition shows early pyknosis, a feature which is particularly common in lymphocytic depleted Hodgkin's disease and which is seen also in Reed-Sternberg and other multinucleated forms. *(H&E)*

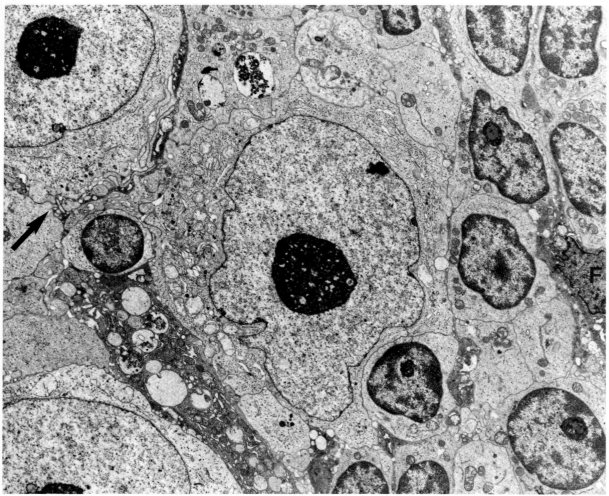

**479 Hodgkin's disease, atypical mononuclear cell, ultrastructure** The large nucleoli and overall nuclear appearances of the atypical Hodgkin's mononuclear cells are very similar to those of Reed-Sternberg cells. There are also cytoplasmic features shared with Reed-Sternberg cells on the one hand and histiocytic cells on the other. Shown here are a group of three atypical mononuclear cells surrounded by lymphocytes and a fibroblast (F). Note the complex peripheral cytoplasmic infolding (*arrow*) of the upper left-hand cell. (× 5,700)

**480 Hodgkin's disease, atypical mononuclear cell, ultrastructure** This is a part of another mononucleated cell. The cytoplasm is rich in organelles including electron dense lysosomal structures, Golgi apparatus, lipid droplets and strands of rough endoplasmic reticulum (rer). A feature frequently seen which may be a fixation artefact is the split in the cytoplasm in the plane of the membranes of the rough endoplasmic reticulum adjacent to cytoplasmic filaments. *(× 14,500)*

**481**

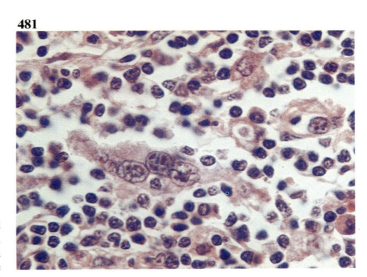

**481 and 482 Hodgkin's disease, atypical multinuclear cell** In addition to classical multinucleated Reed-Sternberg cells a variety of other multinucleated forms are seen. In some examples the nuclei appear septate and contain nuclear structures more suggestive of viral inclusions, **481**, than the classical nucleoli of Reed-Sternberg cells. This appearance is often more striking in sections stained with trichrome procedures, **482**. *(481 H&E; 482 Masson's trichrome)*

**482**

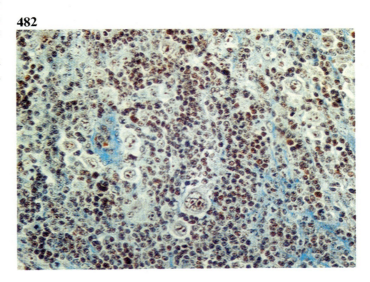

**483 Hodgkin's disease, atypical multi-nuclear cell** Occasionally moruloid structures are found, as shown here, which simulate multinucleated cells. They are however composed of the endothelial cells of the postcapillary venules, which in Hodgkin's disease may be extremely prominent. *(H&E)*

**483**

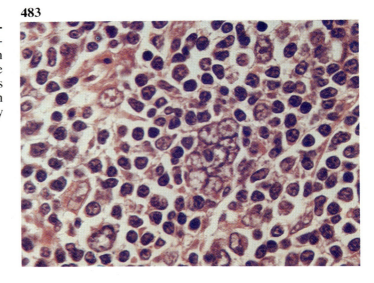

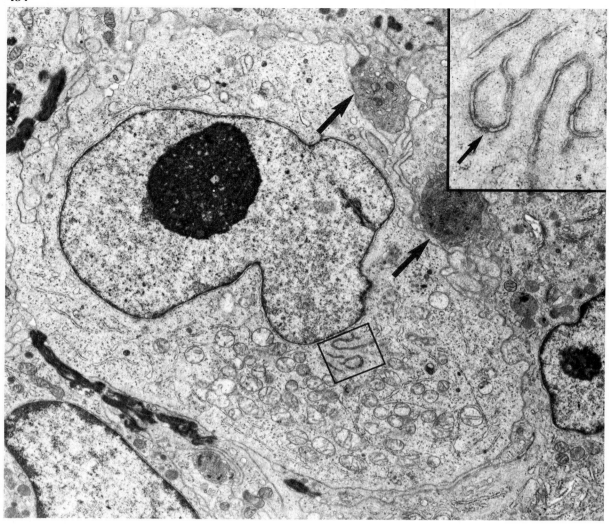

**484   Hodgkin's disease, ultrastructure** The atypical Hodgkin's cells, like Reed-Sternberg and lacunar cells, are in close cytoplasmic contact not only with reactive histiocytes and fibroblasts but also with reticulin and collagen bundles (*arrows*). The cytoplasmic contours show numerous infoldings, and occasional groups of membranes (*boxed, and inset*) bounded by fine filaments *within* the cytoplasm. These represent specialisation to form zonulae occludens (*arrow*). (× 8,000; inset × 27,000)

485

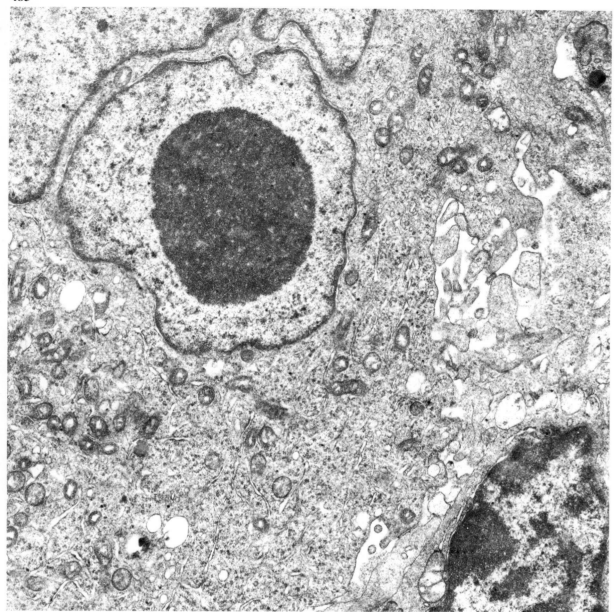

**485 Hodgkin's disease, ultrastructure** Mitochondria in Reed-Sternberg and other atypical cells are sometimes very numerous and may take the form of small lozenge shaped structures as shown here, or long branching mitochondria. Note the undulating peripheral contour and the abundant free RNA, in addition to a few strands of rough endoplasmic reticulum. *(× 14,580)*

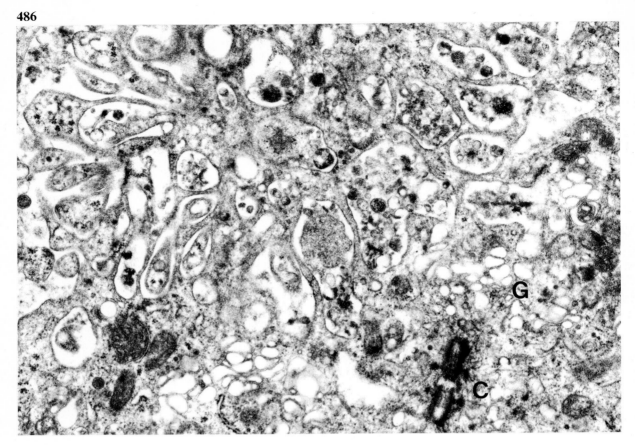

**486 and 487   Hodgkin's disease, ultrastructure** The periphery of many types of Hodgkin's cells may show a complex of cytoplasmic processes. Figure **486** shows a protruding bud of irregular cytoplasmic processes with the vesicular structures lying between the processes containing much particulate debris. Note the Golgi zone (G) and centriole (C). Figure **487** shows arising from the peripheral cytoplasmic membrane (*arrow*) a complex of tubular structures, many of which contain a dense inner core and an appearance somewhat similar to that of the cytoplasmic tubules seen in association with coronavirus infected cells. (**486** × *19,400;* **487** × *30,000*)

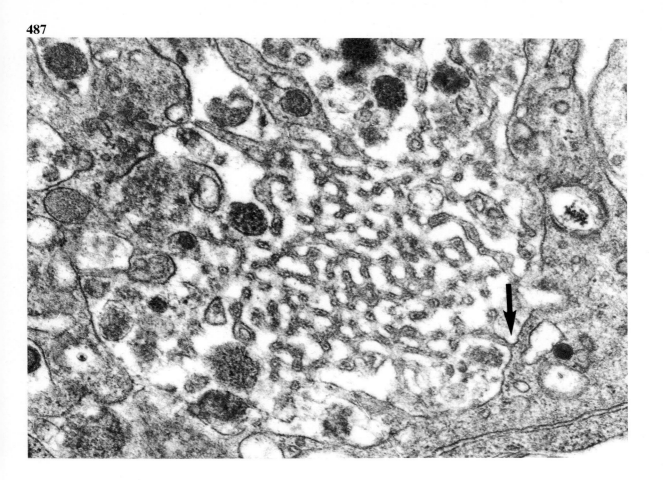

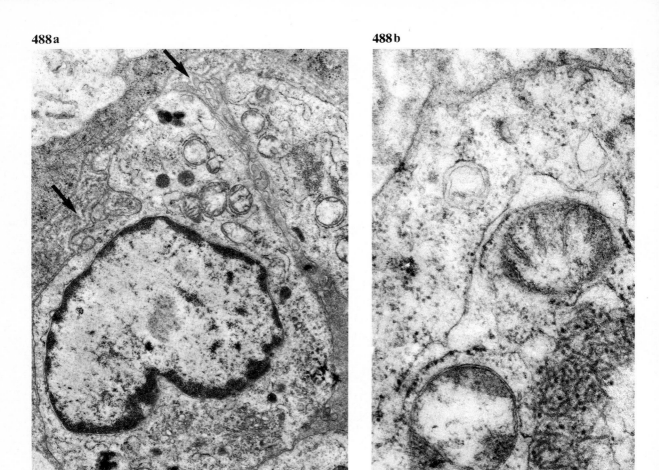

**488a and 488b   Hodgkin's disease, ultrastructure** The vascular component in Hodgkin's disease can be quite prominent and involve postcapillary venules as well as larger vessels, as in many reactive conditions. The surrounding basal lamina (**a**, *arrows*) is usually split into several layers. The endothelial cells are hyperplastic and when viewed at higher magnification (**b**) tubular structures resembling those seen in certain paramyxovirus infections can sometimes be identified in the endothelial cell cytoplasm. This finding is not confined to Hodgkin's disease, for similar structures have also been identified in the histiocytic lymphomas. *(**a** × 12,800; **b** × 40,000)*

**489**

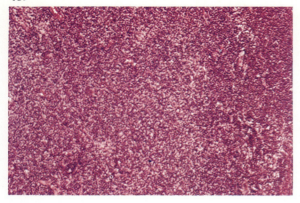

**489 Hodgkin's disease, lymphocytic predominance type** In terms of previous classifications lymphocytic predominance Hodgkin's disease corresponds to the paragranuloma of Jackson and Parker, and to both the nodular and diffuse varieties of the lymphocytic and/or histiocytic categories of Lukes. It is a small group accounting for less than 15 per cent of the total in most series and, in contrast to nodular sclerosis type, the age at presentation is equally spread across the first seven decades of life. It is also more common in males, and includes a high percentage of clinical stage I patients on presentation. This type of Hodgkin's disease may show a diffuse or nodular form of tissue involvement. This example is the more common diffuse variety and shows a monomorphous appearance with effacement of architecture due to replacement with predominantly small lymphocytes. Fibrosis is absent. Such an appearance can be mistaken for a diffuse lymphocytic lymphoma of well differentiated type or CLL. *(H&E)*

**490 Hodgkin's disease, lymphocytic predominance type** In haematoxylin and eosin stained sections Reed-Sternberg cells may be few and difficult to identify. With the aid of methyl green-pyronin staining, however, these cells are much more easily visualised because of the marked pyroninophilia of the large nucleoli. The cytoplasm is generally pyroninophilic but shows much more variation in intensity. *(MGP)*

**490**

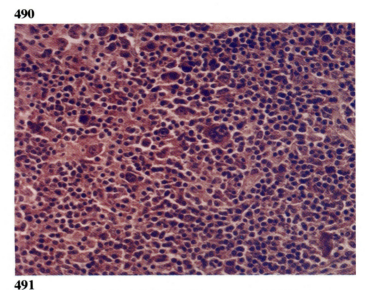

**491 Hodgkin's disease, lymphocytic predominance type** Small lymphocytes are the predominant cell type but it is common to find histiocytes either in small focal aggregates or scattered more diffusely. In this field large atypical mononuclear cells are present in close association with the histiocytes, and there is one lobated Reed-Sternberg cell of the type commonly seen in lymphocytic predominant Hodgkin's disease. Plasma cells are inconspicuous and eosinophils are usually absent. The histiocytic component varies considerably in number and pattern between different lymph nodes in this histological type. *(H&E)*

**491**

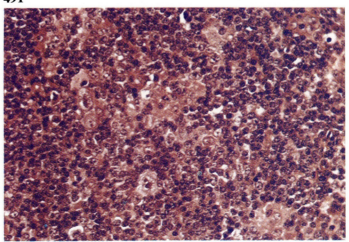

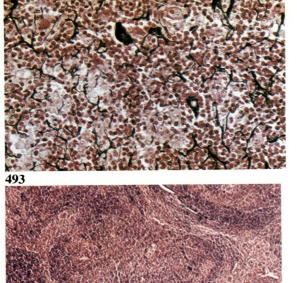

**492** Hodgkin's disease, lymphocytic predominance

**492 Hodgkin's disease, lymphocytic predominance type** Reticulin fibre is generally sparse and most prominent in relation to the small vessels. In this field there is a fairly even admixture of small lymphocytes and histiocytes and which are identified by means of the neutral red nuclear counter stain. *(Gordon & Sweets)*

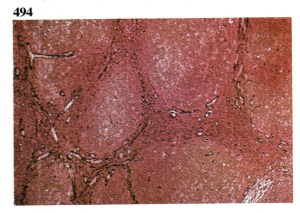

**493 and 494 Hodgkin's disease, lymphocytic predominance type** A not infrequent variant of lymphocytic predominance Hodgkin's disease is a nodular aggregation of the lymphocytic component resulting sometimes in a superficial resemblance to a follicular lymphoma. However the lymphocytic population in these nodular aggregates which sometimes may be very large, **493**, is not consistent with a follicular centre origin. Vessels are usually prominent in the internodular area, a feature which may be emphasised by a reticulin preparation, **494**. These lymphocytic nodules may contain aggregates of histiocytic cells as in the diffuse lymphocytic/histiocytic variant of lymphocytic predominance Hodgkin's disease. Reed-Sternberg cells are generally inconspicuous. (**493** *H&E;* **494** *Gordon & Sweets*)

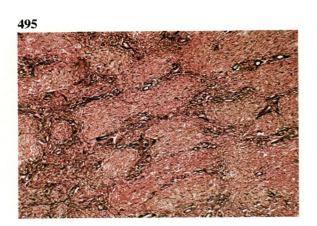

**495 Hodgkin's disease, lymphocytic predominance type** The nodular aggregates are sometimes small as demonstrated by this reticulin preparation. Vessels are again prominent and these and the nodules are well demarcated by the reticulin fibre. There is no evidence to suggest that nodularity confers a better prognosis. *(Gordon & Sweets)*

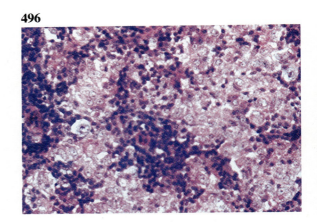

**496 Hodgkin's disease, lymphocytic predominance type** Within the category of Hodgkin's disease of lymphocytic predominance type is recognised a group in which there is a prominent histiocytic component. The histiocytes impart a pink appearance on H&E stained sections – hence the term 'pink Hodgkin's disease'. This histiocytic form may be seen both in the diffuse and nodular variants of lymphocytic predominance Hodgkin's disease. *(H&E)*

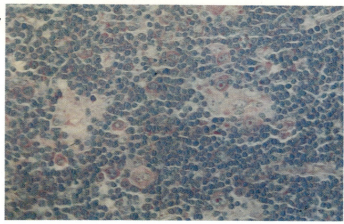

**497 Hodgkin's disease, lymphocytic pre-dominance type** The histiocytic component shows a variable degree of pyroninophilia, as demonstrated by MGP staining. This method also emphasises the presence of forms transitional between typical histiocytes and the atypical mono-nuclear cells which show intermediate degrees of pyroninophilia. *(MGP)*

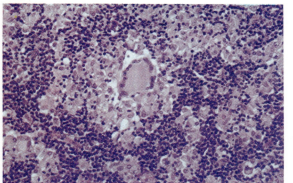

**498 Hodgkin's disease, lymphocytic predominance type** In addition to a more diffuse infiltrate of histio-cytes, scattered ill-defined epithelioid foci with occasional Langhans-type giant cells, as shown here, are a not uncommon finding; occasionally, these aggregates may resemble in every way those of sarcoid granulomas. Infectious agents are rarely in-criminated although it is important to consider and exclude a concomitant infection with tuberculosis or toxoplasmosis. It is equally important to be alerted by this appearance to consider a diagnosis of Hodgkin's disease and search for Reed-Sternberg cells. *(H&E)*

**499 Hodgkin's disease, nodular sclerosis type** Nodular sclerosis as an entity was de-scribed by Lukes in 1963 and thus has no single corresponding group within the Jackson and Parker classification. In most series it forms the largest group with an incidence that has varied from approximately 40 per cent to 70 per cent. Conferring this diagnosis indicates a generally good prog-nosis. The disease occurs predominantly in young individuals with a striking and single peak in the 15–25-year-old age range. Unlike the other types of Hodgkin's disease there is following puberty an increased incidence in females, and a marked pro-pensity for mediastinal involvement. Re-garding clinical stage there is a relatively high incidence of patients presenting with stage II disease. Involvement of lymph nodes often results in a characteristic cut-surface appearance, with white fibrous tissue enclosing nodules of creamy soft tumour. Notice how the tumour has bulged slightly above the areas of fibrosis during the process of fixation.

**500 Hodgkin's disease, nodular sclerosis type** This low power view of the lymph node in **499** emphasises the broad acellular fibrous bands, stained pink, surrounding the cellular nodules of lymphoid tissue. Notice the variable size of the nodules, the varying thickness of the fibrous bands, and the absence of vessels within the bands. *(H&E)*

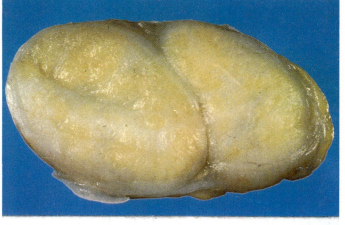

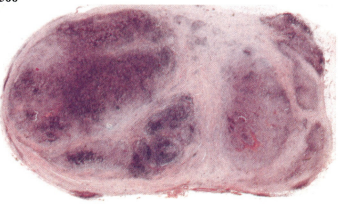

187

**501  Hodgkin's disease, nodular sclerosis type** The cellular nodules of Hodgkin's tissue are here stained intensely with haematoxylin, indicating a high lymphocyte content and that this example of nodular sclerosis Hodgkin's disease is likely to be of a lymphocytic predominant cellular composition. Even at this relatively low magnification occasional lacunar cells are visible (*arrow*). *(H&E)*

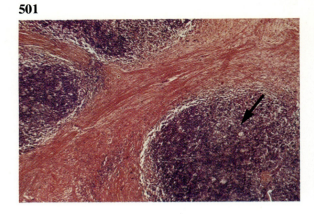

501

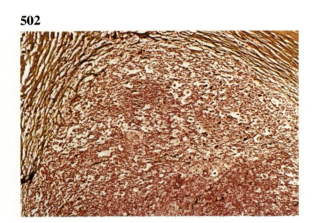

502

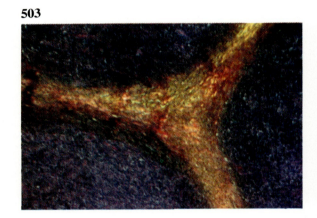

503

**502 and 503  Hodgkin's disease, nodular sclerosis type** Reticulin preparations, **502**, emphasise the coarse, collagenous fibres of the fibrous bands and the relative absence of fibre within the cellular nodules. A characteristic of the collagen is birefringence, **503**, when the H&E stained section is viewed under the polarising microscope. This is a useful feature, since the sclerosis seen in mixed or lymphocytic depleted types of Hodgkin's disease is not normally birefringent. *(502 Gordon & Sweets; 503 H&E, polarised light)*

**504 Hodgkin's disease, nodular sclerosis type** A typical nodule in nodular sclerosis shows lacunar cells which tend to lie mainly toward the centre of the nodule. Occasionally classical Reed-Sternberg cells are hard to find and this is particularly so in nodular sclerosis occurring in the very young and the very old. The numbers of lacunar cells also vary considerably from case to case. Their presence is useful as a diagnostic marker of this type of Hodgkin's disease but, as pointed out previously, their distinctive appearance is the result of fixation artefact. *(H&E)*

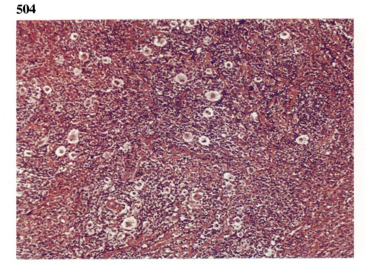

504

**505 Hodgkin's disease, nodular sclerosis type**
Lacunar cells are particularly well visualised in trichrome preparations, the dark staining of the lymphocytic component providing additional contrast for the unstained cytoplasm of the lacunar cells. *(Masson's trichrome)*

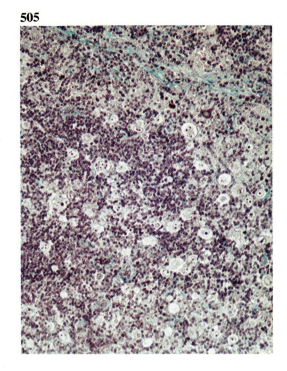

**506, 507 and 508 Hodgkin's disease, nodular sclerosis type** This type of Hodgkin's disease differs from the other types in that it never changes to a different histopathological type, remaining always a nodular sclerosis type. The lymphocytic component and the numbers of other cell types such as plasma cells and eosinophils, however, vary from case to case, quite apart from the variability in number of lacunar cells, Reed-Sternberg cells and other atypical forms. For this reason some pathologists like to subdivide nodular sclerosis into lymphocytic predominance, **506**, mixed cellularity, **507**, and lymphocytic depletion varieties, **508**, described elsewhere in the section, according to the cellular composition of the nodules. These differences in cellular composition and the transition from one type of *nodular* cellularity to another as, for example, lymphocytic predominant nodules to mixed or lymphocytic depleted nodules may have important prognostic implications. *(H&E)*

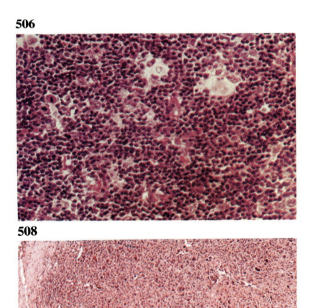

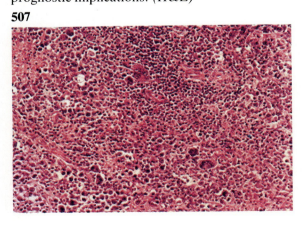

189

**509**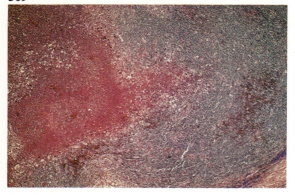

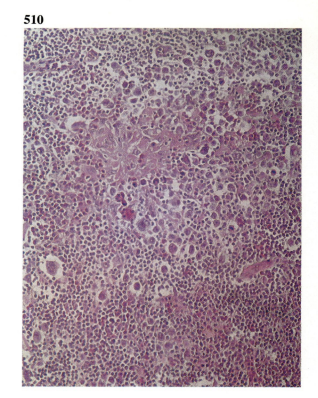
**510**

**509 and 510  Hodgkin's disease, nodular sclerosis type** The cellular component is prone to undergo necrosis. The necrotic foci may vary from extensive areas, **509**, to very small foci, **510**, and usually are accompanied by a marked polymorph neutrophil and, in this example, eosinophil response. A number of lacunar cells are becoming pyknotic (see **532**). *(H&E)*

**511  Hodgkin's disease, nodular sclerosis type** Occasionally, in addition to the coarse collagenous bands there is a diffuse, irregular fibrosis within the nodules. This finding is usually seen in Hodgkin's disease of nodular sclerosing type with a lymphocytic depleted cellularity, and may be the result of previous necrosis. Note the abundant lacunar cells. *(H&E)*

**511**
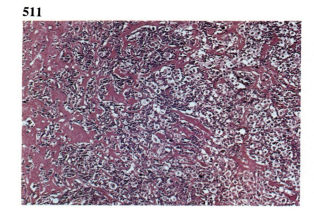

**512  Hodgkin's disease, nodular sclerosis type** The morphological features of this small nodule completely enclosed by a fibrous band are well seen in the semi-thin plastic section. Note the absence of shrinkage artefact. The fibrous bands are relatively acellular and the absence of a vascular component is apparent. *(Toluidine blue)*

**512**
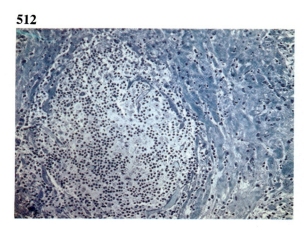

**513**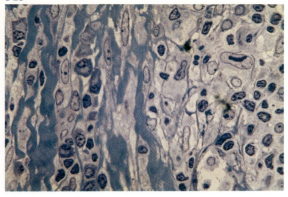

**513 Hodgkin's disease, nodular sclerosis type**
Plasma cells are usually numerous in nodular sclerosis type and tend to be most numerous within the fibrous bands at the edge of the nodule. In toluidine blue-stained plastic sections fibrous tissue appears as wavy blue fibrillar material. *(Toluidine blue)*

**514**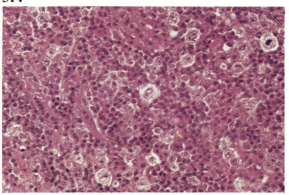

**514 Hodgkin's disease, nodular sclerosis type** The eosinophil content varies from one example to another. In this node they were numerous and were not associated with necrosis. A significant eosinophilia is also seen in a few patients, the cause of which is uncertain and which does not appear to affect prognosis. *(H&E)*

**515**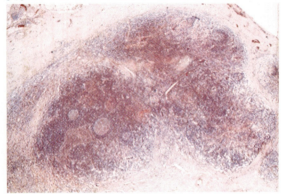

**515 Hodgkin's disease, nodular sclerosis type** In some lymph nodes although banded sclerosis may be advanced, areas are found in which there is partial preservation of architecture – in particular, preservation of lymphoid follicles. *(H&E)*

**516**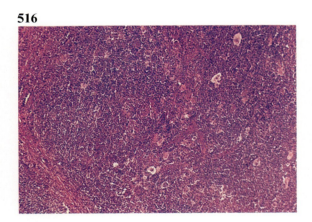

**517**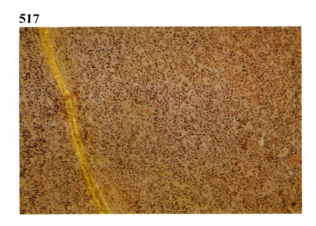

**516 and 517 Hodgkin's disease, nodular sclerosis type** In recent years it has been recognised that in the nodular sclerosis type fibrosis may be minimal although lacunar cells are present: a combination of features now called nodular sclerosis type, cellular phase. In **516**, a few lacunar cells are present and there is early formation of a fibrous band ( *left* ). Such early fibrous band formation is seen more clearly in polarised light, **517**, since the characteristic birefringence is present. (**516** *H&E;* **517** *H&E polarised light*)

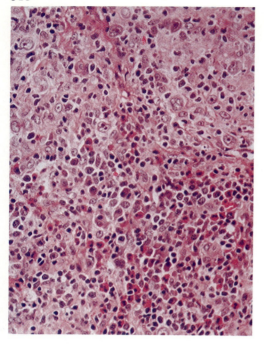

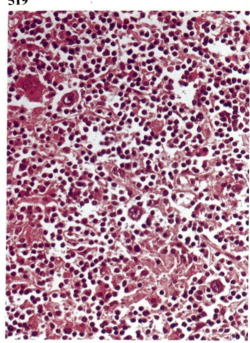

**518  Hodgkin's disease, mixed cellularity type** The incidence of mixed cellularity type has tended to decrease in recent years. Once considered to be the classical form of Hodgkin's disease, in some series it now accounts for only 15–20 per cent of the total number. The reasons for this apparent decrease include a more precise definition of the other three histopathological types, in particular the acceptance of the differing cellularity seen in what is now regarded as classical nodular sclerosis type. Mixed cellularity type presents a much more pleomorphic cellular appearance. There is an absence of nodularity, and fibrosis is seldom extensive. Typically, as here, the mixture of cells consists of lymphocytes, histiocytes, polymorph neutrophils and eosinophils, plasma cells and fibroblasts, seen in association with frequent atypical mononuclear cells and Reed-Sternberg cells. *(H&E)*

**519  Hodgkin's disease, mixed cellularity type** Mixed cellularity type, like lymphocytic predominance, shows a greater incidence in male patients. The age at presentation, however, is later with a distinct peak in the 25–45-year-old age group. There may also be difficulty in deciding whether to designate a given example as lymphocytic predominance or mixed cellularity type. An error in diagnosis has important clinical implications since mixed cellularity types have a much worse prognosis than lymphocytic predominance type. In this example, lymphocytes predominate but there are too many atypical mononuclear forms to permit a diagnosis of lymphocytic predominance type. Note the focal necrosis. *(H&E)*

**520  Hodgkin's disease, mixed cellularity type** Mixed cellularity type is much more often widespread at presentation than lymphocytic predominance type. Reticulin preparations can be useful in distinguishing between lymphocytic predominance type and the mixed cellularity type as shown here, as reticulin is much more abundant and coarser in nature in the latter.
*(Gordon & Sweets)*

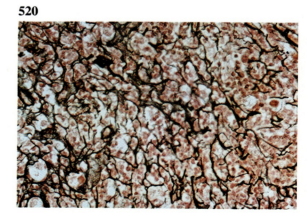

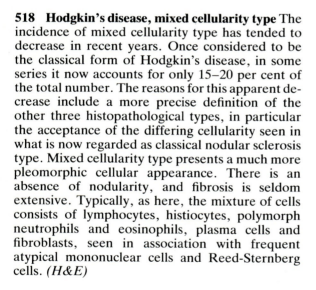

**521 Hodgkin's disease, mixed cellularity type**
This high power field shows several atypical mononucleated cells and a classical Reed-Sternberg cell in addition to histiocytes and fibroblasts. The postcapillary venules are prominent, which may cause diagnostic confusion with angioimmunoblastic lymphadenopathy. Note the early fine fibrosis. *(H&E)*

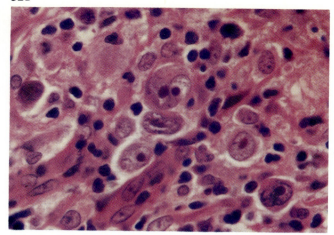

521

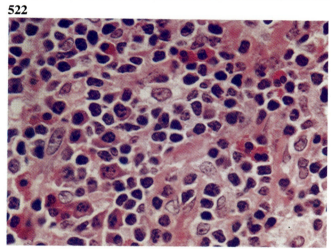

522

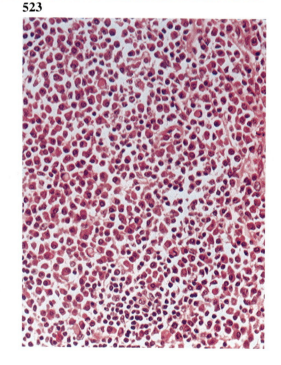

523

**522 and 523 Hodgkin's disease, mixed cellularity type** Intercellular fibrosis is clearly evident in this typical example, **522**, of mixed cellularity type, with numerous eosinophils and plasma cells. Plasma cells may be extremely numerous and form large aggregates as in **523**. *(522 H&E; 523 MGP)*

**524**

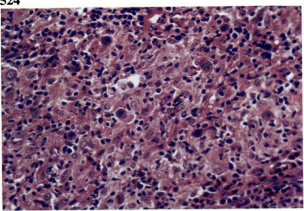

**525**

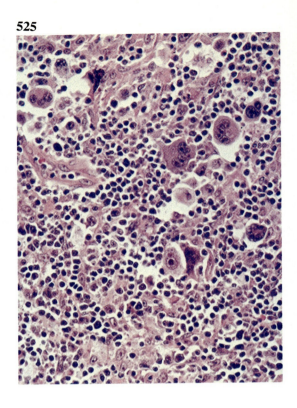

**524 and 525 Hodgkin's disease, mixed cellularity type** Some nodes in this condition show a high histiocytic and fibroblastic content, **524**, at the expense of the lymphocytic component, which may then be confused with the diffuse fibrosis variant of lymphocytic depletion type of Hodgkin's disease. Other nodes, **525**, are seen in which there are large numbers of atypical multinucleated giant cells and Reed-Sternberg cells such that a diagnosis of the reticular variant of lymphocytic depletion Hodgkin's may be considered. Note the fixation artefact around the large cells which must not be mistaken for the lacunae surrounding the shrunken cytoplasm of lacunar cells. *(H&E)*

**526 Hodgkin's disease, lymphocytic depletion type** This term combines Luke's reticular and diffuse fibrosis types of Hodgkin's disease because, despite the very different histopathological appearances, lymphocytic depletion is common to both. Also, examples are seen where both types of histopathology are represented. As a group, the disease is of poor prognosis. It occurs predominantly in males, shows no peak age incidence but is rare below 20 years of age, and on presentation is likely to show widespread disease. Affected nodes commonly show areas of necrosis which is usually most pronounced in the reticular form. In this example of the reticular type there are bizarre multinucleate cells, together with numerous eosinophils and polymorph neutrophils, and fibroblasts. Lymphocytes are markedly reduced. *(H&E)*

**526**

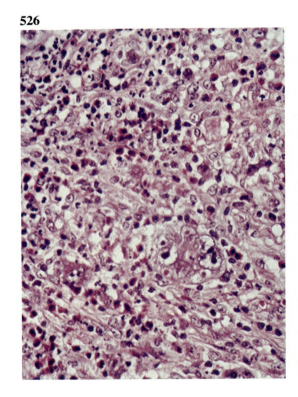

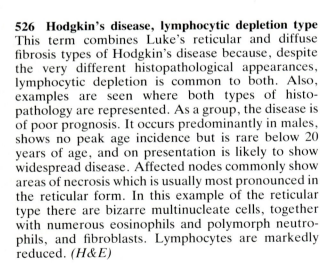

**527**

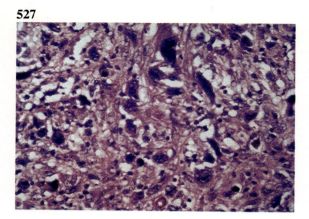

**528**

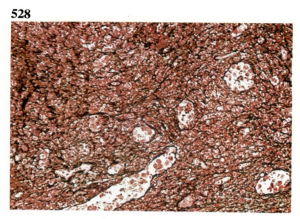

**527 and 528  Hodgkin's disease, lymphocytic depletion type** Many examples of the reticular form were formerly classified as Hodgkin's sarcoma. In addition to numerous Reed-Sternberg cells there are large numbers of bizarre pleomorphic giant cells, **527**, often with markedly hyperchromatic nuclei and showing active mitotis with abnormal forms. Reticulin fibre, **528**, may be very abundant and often runs in fascicles and encloses groups of cells. *(527 H&E; 528 Gordon & Sweets)*

**529**

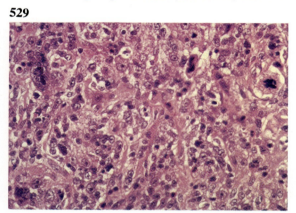

**530**

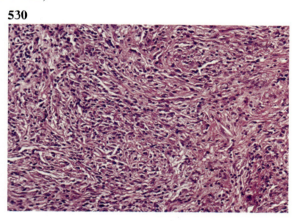

**529 and 530  Hodgkin's disease, lymphocytic depletion type** Another variant of lymphocytic depletion Hodgkin's disease is that showing diffuse fibrosis. Fibroblasts, abnormal mononuclear cells and Reed-Sternberg cells, **529**, result in a polymorphous appearance, and intercellular collagen is conspicuous. Banded fibrosis as in nodular sclerosis Hodgkin's disease is never seen. As in the reticular variety nuclear hyperchromatism and necrosis may be conspicuous features. In other cases, **530**, the fibrous component may predominate and the identification of Reed-Sternberg cells may be extremely difficult. Such diffuse fibrosis is a fairly common finding in autopsy specimens and may be related to treatment. *(H&E)*

**531 Hodgkin's disease, lymphocytic depletion type** In certain instances, as here, the distinction between a lymphocytic depletion type of Hodgkin's disease and a non-Hodgkin's lymphoma of histiocytic type may be extremely difficult. However, this distinction may be of no more than academic interest if the hypothesis that Hodgkin's disease represents a neoplastic proliferation of mononuclear phagocytic cells is proven. Meanwhile controversial cases are in the BNLI series placed in a category called atypical histiocytic Hodgkin's disease (Grade II). *(H&E)*

**531**

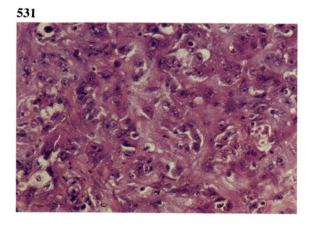

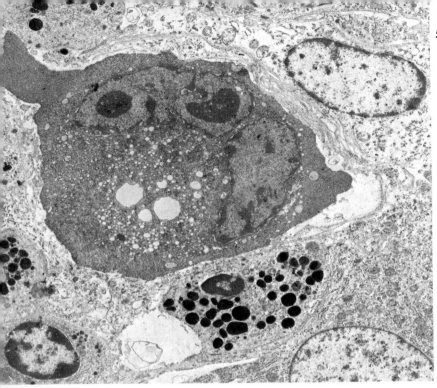

**532 Hodgkin's disease, lymphocytic depletion type, ultrastructure** Not only are the abnormal giant forms with hyperchromatic nuclei a common finding in lymphocytic depletion types, but the mononuclear and Reed-Sternberg cells often shcw nuclear pyknosis and shrinkage of cytoplasm with condensation of cytoplasmic organelles. The apoptotic cell shown here appears electron dense with well defined limits but still shows the nuclear features of a Reed-Sternberg cell. Note the surrounding polymorphs and epithelioid cells. (× 4,800)

**533 Hodgkin's disease, lymphocytic depletion type, ultrastructure** An ultrastructural level the bizarre multinucleated cells often reveal an abundant irregular cytoplasm filled with fine filaments, in addition to a variety of organelles. The nuclei lack the nuclear chromatin arrangement of classical Reed-Sternberg cells being more clumped and more abundant, and there is an absence of the pathognomonic huge nucleolus. This particular example shows in addition (*inset*) annulate lamellae, a structure believed to be derived from the endoplasmic reticulum which has been described in a variety of neoplastic cells. (× 7,800; inset × 33,680)

533

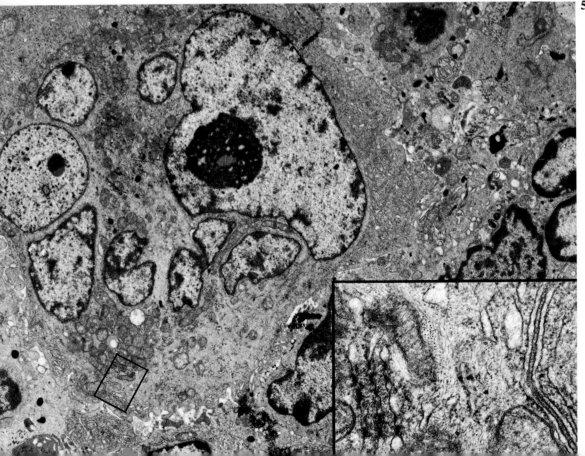

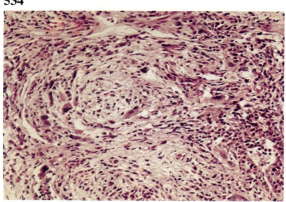

534

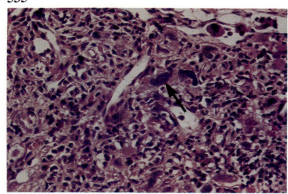

535

**534 and 535  Myelofibrosis simulating Hodgkin's disease** Exceptionally rarely, patients with myelofibrosis may present with lymph node enlargement due to nodal involvement by the myelofibrotic process. If such nodes are biopsied there is a risk of their being interpreted as Hodgkin's disease of lymphocytic depletion type, since there is generally prominent fibrosis and few lymphocytes, **534**, and the giant cells of megakaryocytic origin (*arrow*) may be misinterpreted as Reed-Sternberg cells, **535**. *(H&E)*

**536  Hodgkin's disease, abdominal nodes** In this autopsy specimen there is extensive coeliac and paraaortic lymph node enlargement which extends to the bifurcation into the iliac arteries. It is a remarkable feature in Hodgkin's disease that the firm, rubbery nodes, even in advanced disease, may remain discrete. Such a degree of abdominal lymph node involvement would show a grossly abnormal lymphangiogram picture.

536

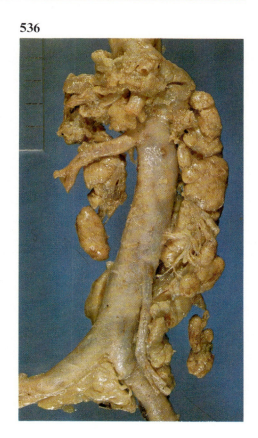

**537 Hodgkin's disease, abdominal lymph nodes**
Although not a common finding, the presence of
Hodgkin's disease – in this example, of mixed
cellularity type – within a lymph node also showing
post-lymphangiogram effects is seen from time to
time in material removed at staging laparotomy.
This involvement, of course, will alter the clinical
staging, and abdominal lymph nodes should be
removed always for histological examination if
they appear enlarged or abnormal. *(H&E)*

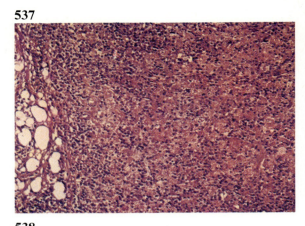

**538 Hodgkin's disease, abdominal lymph nodes** It
is important, where possible, to biopsy abdominal
nodes at staging laparotomy, even if the nodes are
not enlarged and feel normal on palpation, for
there may be focal or partial involvement. In this
example from a patient with classical nodular
sclerosis Hodgkin's disease in the diagnostic
biopsy, the lymph node shows preservation of
architecture and follicular hyperplasia but lacunar
cells are scattered throughout the paracortex
indicating the cellular phase of nodular sclerosis.
*(H&E)*

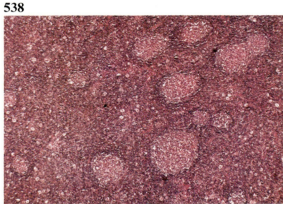

**539 and 540 Hodgkin's disease, abdominal lymph
nodes** Focal, and cellular phase nodular sclerosis
disease often appears to arise in the T-dependent
paracortex and, as shown in **539**, the abnormal
cells are closely related to the postcapillary
venules, which sometimes may be very conspicuous
in Hodgkin's disease. Early nodular sclerosis is not
always confined to the paracortex. Figure **540**
clearly demonstrates the presence of lacunar cells
within the lymphocytic cuff around a germinal
centre, an area which is considered to be B-
lymphocytic. *(H&E)*

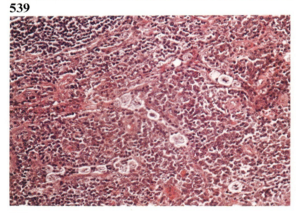

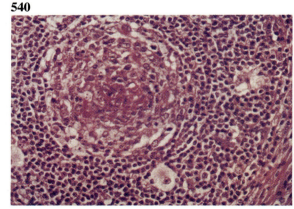

**541 and 542 Hodgkin's disease, abdominal lymph nodes** A common finding in abdominal lymph nodes which are not the site of Hodgkin's disease is the presence of granulomas. These may consist either of collections of foamy macrophages, **541**, or lipogranulomas similar to those seen in the spleen, or may consist of discrete epithelial cell foci with Langhans giant cells resembling those found in sarcoidosis, **542**. Such sarcoid-like granulomas are found also in spleen and liver, and they are important in two respects: firstly, they should not be confused with Hodgkin's disease and secondly, their presence should institute a careful search to exclude early Hodgkin's disease or other causes of non-caseating granulomas. *(H&E)*

**541**

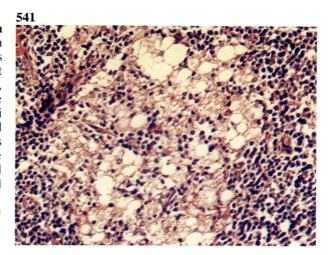

**542**

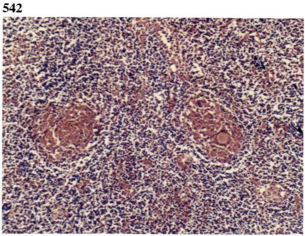

**543 Hodgkin's disease, abdominal lymph nodes** Other nodes may show reactive features such as sinus histiocytosis. In this example not only is there a prominent degree of sinus histiocytosis but there is evidence of erythrophagocytosis, a finding which must not be confused with histiocytic medullary reticulosis. The reason for the erythrophagocytosis is not known, nor its relation to the excess iron deposition in lymph nodes and spleens (see **544, 556**) seen in some cases. *(H&E)*

**543**

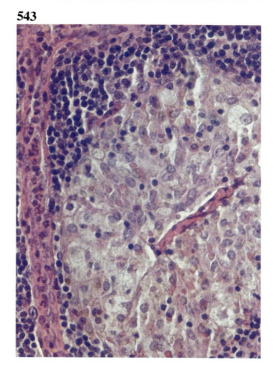

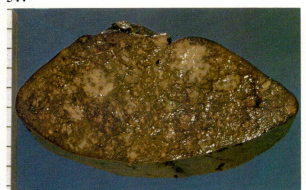

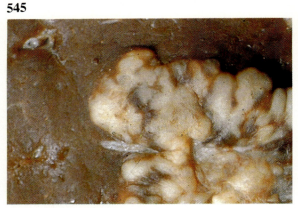

**544 and 545   Hodgkin's disease, spleen** The spleen is commonly involved in Hodgkin's disease, but it is exceptional for it to be the *only* site of the disease. The involved spleen, which may be enlarged or of normal size, shows a number of different macroscopic appearances. The most characteristic is where the cut surface of the fixed spleen, **544**, shows a variegated pattern due to a widespread and irregular infiltrate of whitish tissue – an appearance likened to that of porphyry or at a more mundane level a German sausage. If the spleen is sectioned before fixation, **545**, the tumour deposits bulge above the uninvolved splenic tissue.

**546   Hodgkin's disease, spleen** Splenic size is an unreliable guide as to whether there is likely to be involvement with Hodgkin's disease. Some very large spleens show reactive changes only, with an increased volume of white pulp. This spleen was of normal size but nevertheless on sectioning showed occasional focal deposits (*arrow 1*) measuring only a few millimetres. The hilar lymph node was also involved, and foci of Hodgkin's disease were present in the two splenunculi (*arrow 2*). It is extremely important to section adequately the splenectomy specimens since these early small and focal lesions are easily missed on a more casual inspection. It is our practice to section the spleen transversely into three or four thick slices for the purposes of fixation, and when the specimen is fixed ideally to slice at 0.2–0.3 cm intervals. For this purpose a bacon slicer is invaluable.

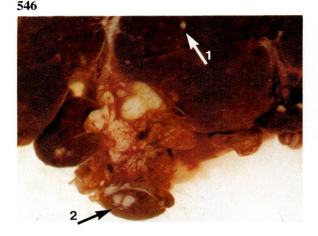

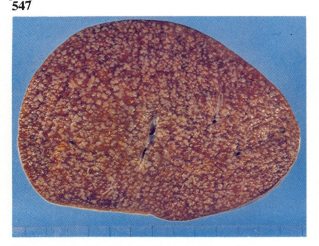

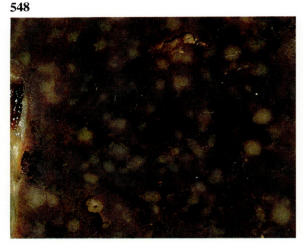

**547 and 548   Hodgkin's disease, spleen** The spleen may be very large and on sectioning in the unfixed state, **547**, show innumerable discrete soft creamy nodules simulating the appearance of a follicular lymphoma. This mode of involvement can also simulate sarcoidosis and miliary tuberculosis. Other examples on close inspection in the fixed state, **548**, show what appears to be hyperplasia of the white pulp with prominent Malpighian corpuscles. It is important to sample adequately such spleens for microscopic evidence of involvement since the earliest lesions are found in the periarteriolar T-dependent lymphoid tissue.

**549 Hodgkin's disease, spleen** In the BNLI series of staging laparotomies 50 per cent of splenectomy specimens have been found to be involved, though the degree of involvement has varied from occasional microscopic foci to more widespread and macroscopically evident disease. In this low power field a small focus of Hodgkin's disease is seen in the periarteriolar lymphoid tissue of the white pulp. *(H&E)*

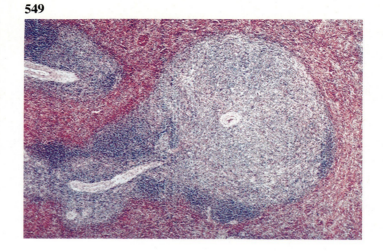

**550 Hodgkin's disease, spleen** Spleens found to be involved at autopsy show a much greater variation in histopathological types as compared with the original, with more frequent examples of lymphocytic depletion Hodgkin's disease. In involved splenectomy specimens the histopathological appearance of the infiltrate is generally similar to that present in the diagnostic lymph node biopsy, though in nodular sclerosis type, the degree of fibrosis is very variable, and the formation of wide collagenous bands enclosing the nodules is not usually a feature. This example shows the distribution of the Hodgkin's tissue in the periarteriolar lymphoid sheath around the follicular arteriole and emphasises the fine sclerosis which tends to be a feature in long-standing cases. *(H&E)*

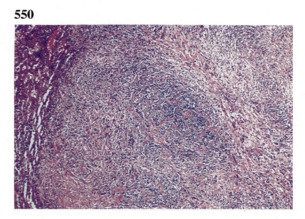

**551 Hodgkin's disease, spleen** Appearances in any one spleen may vary considerably depending on the extent and size of the deposits of Hodgkin's disease. In this example there is very early or microscopical evidence of Hodgkin's disease of nodular sclerosis type in the form of a small lymphocytic nodule containing easily identifiable lacunar cells. Note the absence of fibrosis. *(H&E)*

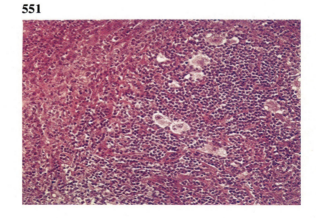

**552 Hodgkin's disease, spleen** A not uncommon finding in spleens removed at staging laparotomy is the presence of sarcoid-like granulomas. These may be seen in association with obvious deposits of Hodgkin's disease or as an isolated phenomenon. Their significance is poorly understood and their main importance lies in that, to the inexperienced pathologist, they may be interpreted as evidence of involvement by Hodgkin's disease. It is wise if granulomas are numerous or if necrosis is present within them to carry out Ziehl-Nielsen staining for acid-fast bacilli. Note how the granulomas develop within the T-dependent periarteriolar lymphoid tissue in a similar manner to sarcoid granulomas. The adjacent B-dependent germinal centre shows eosinophilic change (see **233, 234**). *(H&E)*

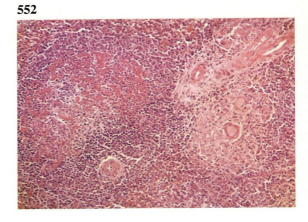

**553 Hodgkin's disease, spleen** In addition to sarcoid-like epithelioid granulomas, small less well developed granulomas are often seen either in involved spleens or in the absence of Hodgkin's disease. Some of these consist almost entirely of fat-containing macrophages – lipogranulomas – similar to those occurring in abdominal lymph nodes. Others contain less striking amounts of fat as shown in this semi-thin plastic section of a collection of histiocytes around a small vessel. In this example there is an atypical mononuclear cell adjacent to the granuloma. *(Toluidine blue)*

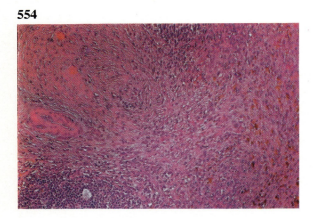

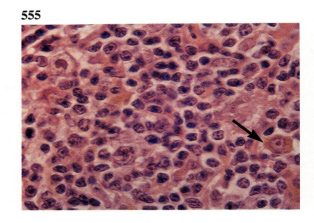

**554 and 555 Hodgkin's disease, spleen** Some spleens show iron deposition in relation to nodules of Hodgkin's disease. Often the iron deposition occurs in the vicinity of areas of fibrosis as in **554**. In other examples, in more cellular areas of Hodgkin's tissue, it is possible sometimes at high magnification, **555**, to identify iron *within* the atypical mononuclear cells (*arrow*) which suggests active phagocytosis. The cause of this accumulation of iron is not clear although it is more likely to be seen in patients who have received treatment. Excessive iron deposition is seen also occasionally in lymph nodes which are not the site of involvement with Hodgkin's disease, and may be the result of haemolysis which is a not uncommon complication. Alternatively, it has been suggested that there is some defect of macrophages in handling iron. *(H&E)*

**556 Gandy-Gamna bodies, spleen** Iron deposition in the spleen in Hodgkin's disease is not to be confused with Gandy-Gamna bodies which are fibrous scars encrusted with both iron and calcium *and* hence haematoxyphil, and which are seen in congestive splenomegalies as a result of focal haemorrhages. *(H&E)*

**556**

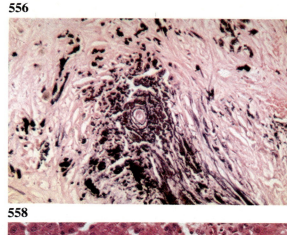

**557**

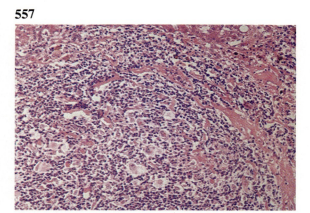

**558**

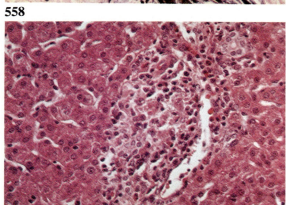

**557 and 558 Hodgkin's disease, liver** It should now be standard practice during staging laparotomy to perform a liver biopsy either as a needle biopsy, wedge biopsy or, preferably, both even if the liver appears macroscopically normal. As in the spleen, the finding of sarcoid-like granulomas usually within portal tracts is not uncommon and should not be confused with evidence of involvement by Hodgkin's disease. When involvement is present it may be evident macroscopically due to the widening of portal tracts with tumour tissue. In **557** the histopathological type is nodular sclerosis; lacunar cells are obvious in the pleomorphic infiltrate. Sometimes, however, early involvement depends upon microscopic examination and, usually, the foci are too small to permit histopathological typing. Reed-Sternberg cells are usually absent, **558**, but may be found after prolonged search in deeper levels. If still absent, it is permissible for small pleomorphic foci in the biopsies of patients with an established diagnosis of Hodgkin's disease, to be interpreted as '*consistent* with a diagnosis of liver involvement in Hodgkin's disease'. In practice one is unlikely to find the liver involved unless disease is present also in the spleen. *(H&E)*

**559**

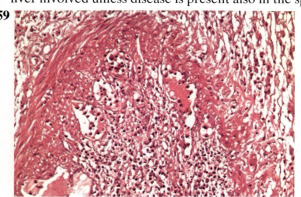

**560**

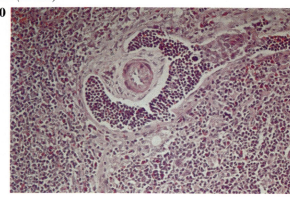

**559 and 560 Hodgkin's disease, vessels** Vascular involvement within lymph nodes by Hodgkin's disease is not at all uncommon but may not be appreciated without the benefit of stains to demonstrate the elastica of blood vessels. In these two examples the vascular involvement is obvious. In **559** the vein is obliterated by Hodgkin's tissue, while in **560** clumps of tumour tissue lie free within the lumen. The relationship of vascular involvement to the spread of Hodgkin's disease has not been defined clearly, and there are some who believe that when more than one site is involved, Hodgkin's disease is of multifocal origin rather than a disease occurring in one primary site which later metastasises. *(H&E)*

**561 Hodgkin's disease, vessels** Involvement of sinuses is rare in Hodgkin's disease. Occasionally, in cases where there is preservation of sinuses typical Hodgkin's cells may be seen within them. The significance of this finding in terms of prognosis is not known. *(H&E)*

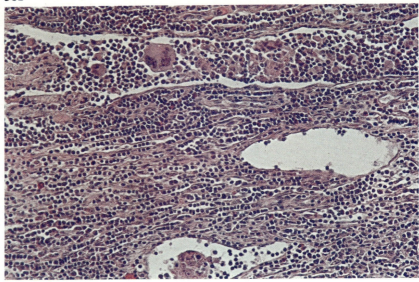

**562 Hodgkin's disease, bone marrow** Bone marrow biopsy in patients with Hodgkin's disease is now part of the routine staging procedure and can be performed either prior to or, preferably, during the staging laparotomy in the form of an iliac crest biopsy. The trephine biopsy here shows a pleomorphic infiltrate in which Reed-Sternberg cells are readily identifiable. However, many false positives are reported by the inexperienced pathologist since the bone marrow in patients with Hodgkin's disease may be cellular, show a shift to the left and contain numerous megakaryocytes. It may also show focal granulomas. *(H&E)*

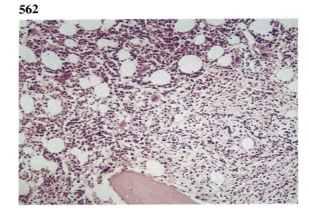

**563 Hodgkin's disease, bone marrow** The technique of plastic processing followed by semi-thin sections is very valuable in resolving whether the bone marrow is involved in Hodgkin's disease in doubtful cases. In this example the large cells present in the hypercellular bone marrow are now clearly evident as megakaryocytes and it is not necessary to proceed to ultrastructural level. The technique also has the merit of excellent fixation and, since bone is easily sectioned by the glass knives used in ultramicrotomes, the trephine biopsies need no decalcification (see also section on technical aspects). *(Toluidine blue)*

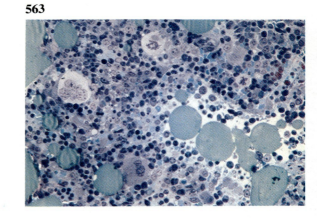

# Lymphomas other than Hodgkin's disease

## The non-Hodgkin's lymphomas

Until relatively recently there has been no general agreement between pathologists on the categorisation of lymphomas other than Hodgkin's disease. The traditional Gall and Mallory classification (*Chart 1*) was replaced in many countries by that of Rappaport (*Chart 2*) proposed in 1956. In the early seventies, however, it became apparent that neither of these two classifications was sufficiently comprehensive nor appropriate in the light of recent advances in the understanding of the lymphoreticular and mononuclear phagocytic systems (LRMPS). Consequently several new approaches to the classification of non-Hodgkin's lymphomas were proposed: British National Lymphoma Investigation (BNLI) – *Chart 1*, Lukes and Collins – *Chart 3*, Kiel – *Chart 4*, Dorfman – *Chart 5*, W.H.O. – *Chart 6*, each in a different way trying to accommodate the new concepts relating to the cells of origin of tumours of the LRMPS. Unfortunately not only was the terminology used widely divergent but, while some of the classifications emphasised morphological features, others concentrated on functional aspects. As a result, it appeared to clinicians that there was no agreement among pathologists working in this field. Though this was very far from the truth, the need remained for international agreement as to terminology and a working classification acceptable to both clinicians and pathologists. Thus in 1976, under the auspices of the National Cancer Institute (NCI), a clinical and pathological retrospective international study was initiated to test the various newer classifications against survival. The histopathological material from patients fulfilling rigid staging requirements was studied retrospectively by a number of pathologists, experts and panelists, and the individual results of the different classifications were then related to actuarial survival, relapse-free periods, and other clinical data. It emerged that in every classification there were well defined non-Hodgkin's lymphoma types which fell into different prognostic categories, with a good measure of cross correlation between the different classifications. Thus it was possible to achieve a working formulation for the categorisation of the lymphomas (*Chart 7*). Those workers who wished to continue with individual classifications – such as Kiel – could do so but, at the same time by reference to the Stanford 'formulation', comparisons between defined histopathological groups would be achieved easily.

Meanwhile, since 1973 the (BNLI) classification has been used in a prospective clinical trial of the non-Hodgkin's lymphoma in patients treated in many radiotherapy centres throughout Great Britain and Northern Ireland. The basic outline of the BNLI classification is presented in *Chart 1* alongside that of Gall and Mallory. An important aspect for the clinician is the separation of the different pathological groups into Grade I (lower) and Grade II (higher) malignant categories. Follicular lymphomas are considered a separate entity but have been subdivided into three groups. The diffuse lymphomas are broken down into seven categories based on the degree of differentiation and the putative cell of origin. All but one of the seven types of the diffuse tumours are considered to derive from lymphoid cells, and thus include plasma cell tumours. However, plasma cell lymphomas are separately categorised because it seems more logical that tumours composed predominantly of plasma cells (extramedullary plasmacytomas) and/or their immediate precursors should be so-called and separated from predominantly lymphocytic tumours showing only some degree of plasma cell differentiation. The remaining seventh type of diffuse lymphoma, the true histiocytic lymphoma, has been included in this classification of non-Hodgkin's lymphomas since it has been shown that cells of the mononuclear phagocytic system are an integral and functionally essential component of the lymphoreticular system, and because recent ultrastructural studies have confirmed the existence of true histiocytic lymphomas. Tumours derived from dendritic cells, and fibre-forming cells (fibroblasts or myofibroblasts) have been identified but since, to date, they appear to be very uncommon, no provision has been made yet for their separate categorisation. It must be emphasised, however, that in diagnosing a diffuse malignant lymphoma, and especially in the case of plasma cell and histiocytic cell tumours, it is important to establish that the disease is arising in the first instance in peripheral lymphoreticular tissue. Inevitably, there remains a small group of unclassifiable tumours.

With regard to the categories used in the Stanford 'formulation', the BNLI categories are very similar (see *Chart 7*). However, the 'formulation' recognises three prognostic categories. The lymphocytic well differentiated group of the Stanford 'formulation' heads the list, but this is for convenience only in order not to break up the sequence of follicular lymphomas, which appear next. The follicular lymphomas are subdivided and, since there was some evidence for the differences in behaviour of the follicular large cell group, this entity is placed in the intermediate grade prognostic category. The diffuse small cleaved cell lymphoma of the 'formulation' corresponds to the diffuse lymphocytic intermediate of the BNLI. The mixed small and large cell lymphoma of the 'formulation' is not, however, identical to the 'mixed' small and large cell category of the BNLI since it accepts some mixtures of reactive cells with the neoplastic lymphocytes – as, for example, the 'epithelioid' variant. The large cell group of the BNLI has been subdivided into two groups in the Stanford 'formulation' since in the NCI studies large cells of follicular centre origin, which were separately catered for in some classifications such as Luke's, did appear to have an improved prognosis. The heterogeneous lymphocytic poorly differentiated group of the BNLI also has been separated into two major categories – though both of poor prognosis. Because of the lack of information on the BNLI plasma cell and histiocytic groups since not all classifications had recognised these as separate entities, and because of conceptual difficulties they appear in the miscellaneous category of the 'formulation'.

In this Atlas the individual categories of the non-Hodgkin's lymphomas will be described in terms of the BNLI classification with a short introductory text to each type preceding the illustrations. Alternative terminology will be included where indicated. The non-Hodgkin's lymphomas form just over half of all lymphomas, with the two largest subgroups being the follicular lymphomas and the large cell lymphomas. The majority of patients are middle-aged to elderly with the important exceptions of the diffuse lymphocytic poorly differentiated group and the histiocytic lymphomas which affect children and young adults more commonly. Unlike Hodgkin's disease, there is no universal adoption of a staging system and patients who undergo staging laparotomy with splenectomy, abdominal lymph node and liver biopsy are in the minority. However, most patients are subjected to lymphangiography, bone marrow and liver biopsy.

The histopathological findings in terms of Grade I or Grade II disease is all important in relation to the selection of treatment, a decision which has been supported by the actuarial survival curves in over 500 patients so treated.

*Chart 1*

| *Gall and Mallory (traditional) Classification (1942)* | *British National Lymphoma Investigation Classification (BNLI) (1974, 1978)* | |
|---|---|---|
| | *Follicular lymphoma*<br>Follicle cells predominantly small<br>Follicle cells mixed small and large<br>Follicle cells predominantly large | |
| Follicular lymphoma | | Grade I |
| Lymphosarcoma, Lymphocytic | *Diffuse lymphoma*<br>Lymphocytic, well differentiated (small round lymphocyte)<br>Lymphocytic, intermediate differentiated (small follicle lymphocyte) | |
| Lymphosarcoma, Lymphoblastic | Lymphocytic, poorly differentiated (lymphoblast)<br>a Non-Burkitt's lymphoma<br>b Burkitt's tumour<br>c Convoluted cell (mediastinal) lymphoma | Grade II |
| Reticulum cell sarcoma | Lymphocytic, mixed small and large cell (mixed follicle cells)<br>'Undifferentiated' large cell (large lymphoid cells) | |
| | Histiocytic cell (mononuclear phagocytic cells)<br>Plasma cell (extramedullary plasma cell) | Grade I and II |
| | Unclassified | |

Plasmacytoid differentiation in lymphocytic tumours, and banded or fine sclerosis are noted.

*Chart 2*
*Rappaport Classification*

Nodular (follicular – diffuse)*


Undifferentiated (stem cell lymphoma)

Histiocytic (reticulum cell sarcoma)

Mixed cell ('histiocytic' – lymphocytic)

Lymphocytic, poorly differentiated
(lymphoblastic lymphosarcoma)

Lymphocytic, well differentiated

*Malignant lymphomas that have follicular (nodular)
 patterns are designated by addition of 'follicular'
 ('nodular') to the cytologically appropriate terms.

*Chart 3*
*Lukes and Collins (1975)*

I   U-cell (undefined cell type)

II  T-cell types
    1 Mycosis fungoides and Sézary's syndrome
    2 Convoluted lymphocyte
    3 Immunoblastic sarcoma of T-cells

III B-cell types
    1 Small lymphocyte (CLL)
    2 Plasmacytoid lymphocyte
    3 Follicular centre cell (FCC) types
      a Small cleaved
      b Large cleaved
      c Small non-cleaved – Burkitt's
      d Large non-cleaved
    4 Immunoblastic sarcoma of B-cells

IV Histiocytic types

V  Cell of uncertain origin
       Hodgkin's disease origin of neoplastic
       cell uncertain

Unclassifiable


*Chart 4*
*Kiel Classification (1974)*

Low-grade malignancy

    Malignant lymphoma (ML) – lymphocytic (CLL and others)

    ML – lymphoplasmacytoid (immunocytic)

    ML – centrocytic

    ML – centroblastic – centrocytic { follicular
                                       follicular and diffuse
                                       diffuse

High-grade malignancy

    ML – centroblastic

    ML – lymphoblastic
         Burkitt type

         convoluted-cell type
         others

    ML – immunoblastic

*Chart 5*
*Working Classification of non-Hodgkin's Lymphomas (Dorfman, 1974)*

*Follicular lymphomas*\*
(follicular or follicular and diffuse)

*Diffuse lymphomas*\*

Small lymphoid

Small lymphocytic (S.L.) (C.L.L.)
S.L. with plasmacytoid differentiation

Mixed small and large lymphoid

Atypical small lymphocytic
Convoluted lymphocytic (thymic)

Large lymphoid

Large lymphoid (pyroninophilic)
Mixed small and large lymphoid
Histiocytic
Burkitt's lymphoma
Mycosis fungoides
Undefined

\*Composite lymphomas, comprising two well-defined and apparently different types of lymphoma within
the same tissue and lymphomas associated with sclerosis, are suitably designated.

*Chart 6*
*WHO Classification (1975, 1976)*

Nodular lymphosarcoma
   Prolymphocytic or polymphocytic and lymphoblastic
      Cleaved cells      { Small cells
                        { Mixed cells
      Non-cleaved cells  { Large cells

Diffuse lymphosarcoma
   Lymphocytic
   Lymphoplasmacytic
   Prolymphocytic or polymphocytic and lymphoblastic
      Cleaved cells      { Small cells
                        { Mixed cells
      Non-cleaved cells  { Large cells
   Lymphoblastic
     including the convoluted type
   Immunoblastic
   Burkitt's tumour
   Mycosis fungoides

Plasmacytoma

Reticulosarcoma

*Chart 7*
*A working formulation of non-Hodgkin's lymphoma*

| Recommendations of an expert international panel (Stanford, 1980) | BNLI equivalents |
|---|---|
| **Low grade** | |
| A  *Malignant Lymphoma*<br>　　*Small Lymphocytic*<br>　　　consistent with C.L.L.<br>　　　plasmacytoid | *Diffuse Lymphoma*<br>　*Lymphocytic, well differentiated*<br>　(small round lymphocyte)<br>　plasmacytoid differentiation |
| B  *Malignant Lymphoma, follicular*<br>　　*Predominantly small cleaved cell*<br>　　　diffuse areas<br>　　　sclerosis | *Follicular Lymphoma*<br>　*Follicle cells predominantly small*<br><br>　　banded or fine sclerosis |
| C  *Malignant Lymphoma, follicular*<br>　　*Mixed, small cleaved and large cell*<br>　　　diffuse areas<br>　　　sclerosis | *Follicular Lymphoma*<br>　*Follicle cells mixed small and large*<br><br>　　banded or fine sclerosis |
| **Intermediate grade** | |
| D  *Malignant Lymphoma, follicular*<br>　　*Predominantly large cell*<br>　　　diffuse areas<br>　　　sclerosis | *Follicular Lymphoma*<br>　*Follicle cells predominantly large*<br><br>　　banded or fine sclerosis |
| E  *Malignant Lymphoma, diffuse*<br>　　*Small cleaved cell*<br><br>　　　sclerosis | *Diffuse Lymphoma*<br>　*Lymphocytic, intermediate differentiation*<br>　(small follicle lymphocyte)<br>　　banded or fine sclerosis |
| F  *Malignant Lymphoma, diffuse*<br>　　*Mixed, small and large cell*<br><br>　　　sclerosis<br>　　　epithelioid cell component* | *Diffuse Lymphoma*<br>　*Lymphocytic, mixed small and large cell*<br>　(mixed follicle cells)<br>　　banded or fine sclerosis |
| G  *Malignant Lymphoma, diffuse*<br>　　*Large cell*<br><br>　　　cleaved cell<br>　　　non-cleaved cell<br>　　　sclerosis | *Diffuse Lymphoma*<br>　*'Undifferentiated' large cell*<br>　(large lymphoid cell)<br>　　large irregularly nucleated follicle cells<br>　　large and small regularly nucleated follicle cells<br>　　banded or fine sclerosis |
| **High grade** | |
| H  *Malignant Lymphoma*<br>　　*Large cell, immunoblastic*<br><br>　　　plasmacytoid<br><br>　　　clear cell<br>　　　polymorphous<br>　　　epithelioid cell component | *Diffuse Lymphoma*<br>　*'Undifferentiated' large cell*<br>　(large lymphoid cell)<br>　　plasma cell differentiation and some<br>　　examples of plasma cell lymphoma |
| I  *Malignant Lymphoma*<br>　　*Lymphoblastic*<br><br>　　　convoluted cell<br>　　　non-convoluted cell | *Diffuse Lymphoma*<br>　*Lymphocytic, poorly differentiated*<br>　(lymphoblast)<br>　　convoluted mediastinal lymphoma<br>　　non-Burkitt's lymphoma |
| J  *Malignant Lymphoma*<br>　　*Small non-cleaved cell*<br><br>　　　Burkitt's<br>　　　follicular areas | *Diffuse Lymphoma*<br>　*Lymphocytic, poorly differentiated*<br>　(lymphoblast)<br>　　Burkitt's lymphoma |

Miscellaneous
    Composite
    Mycosis Fungoides

    Histiocytic
    Extramedullary Plasmacytoma
    Unclassifiable
    Other

No equivalent
Cutaneous T-cell lymphoma (not included in
BNLI classification)
Histiocytic cell (mononuclear phagocytic cells)
Plasma cell (extramedullary plasma cells)
Unclassified
Other –

*Reactive elements are not accepted as criteria for mixed lymphomas in BNLI classification.

## Follicular lymphoma

Follicular lymphomas are among the more common types of the non-Hodgkin's lymphomas, though their incidence varies considerably according to age and ethnic origin. For example they are exceptionally rare in children, very uncommon below 20 years-of-age but occur with increasing frequency in older individuals. They are practically non-existent in the negro races and they are rare in the Chinese. In the BNLI series they constitute approximately 48 per cent of adults included in the trials. It is important to separate this group from the diffuse non-Hodgkin's lymphomas since their prognosis is generally better and, even without treatment, progression of the disease may be extremely slow. It should be understood also that in designating a lymphoma as of follicular type one is implying a B-cell lymphoma since it is now accepted that the germinal centres are B-lymphocytic structures.

Follicular lymphomas may be subdivided into a further three sub-types according to the cellular composition of the neoplastic follicles. The most common is the follicular lymphoma of predominantly small (follicle) cell type. Large cells are generally not numerous, but even if they form up to 1/3rd of the total cellular population, the lymphoma will still be designated as predominantly small cell type. When small and large follicle centre cells are present in approximately equal numbers, the follicular lymphoma is designated as mixed cell type. The least common type, accounting for less than 10 per cent of all follicular lymphomas, is the predominantly large cell type with large cells accounting for more than 2/3rds (66 per cent) of the total cells. It should be stressed also that a lymphoma is still classified as follicular even if only a small portion of the node retains a follicular pattern, the rest being diffuse. In approximately 25 per cent of patients notched nuclear (small cleaved) cells are present in peripheral blood.

**564 Follicular lymphoma** Follicular lymphomas are among the most common forms of lymphoma in Caucasian races. They are rare below 20 years-of-age and are most frequent in elderly males in the 55–65-year-old age group. They derive from the cells of the germinal centre and are thus B-lymphocytic in type. In most cases, the follicle-like structures are clearly delineated, and usually lack lymphocytic mantles, as shown here. These features when taken together with the cellular composition result in a structure more closely resembling a germinal centre than the lymphoid follicle as a whole. However, given the limitations of the term, 'follicular' is convenient and widely understood. (*H&E*)

564

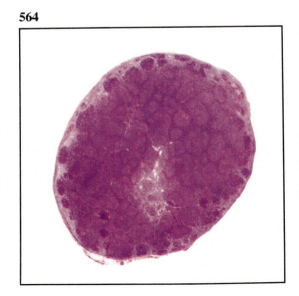

**565 Follicular lymphoma** This follicular lymphoma is atypical in that there are still prominent residual darkly staining lymphocytic cuffs. This finding, particularly when seen in combination with variably sized and shaped 'follicles' can lead sometimes to a diagnosis of reactive follicular hyperplasia, since it is widely taught that neoplastic follicles in contrast to reactive follicles lack a mantle of small lymphocytes, and are generally of similar size and shape. Note the shrinkage artefact around the neoplastic follicles. (H&E)

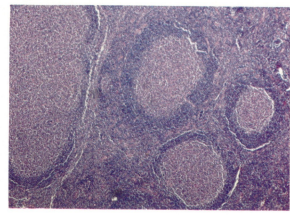

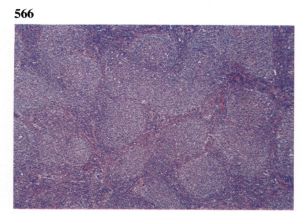

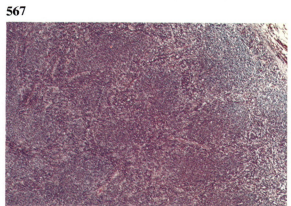

**566 and 567 Follicular lymphoma** In **566** the follicles, while lacking well defined lymphocytic mantles, are rather poorly demarcated from the background and some are already coalescing to form larger irregular nodules. Figure **567** shows follicular structures which are even more indistinct. In such cases reticulin stains are helpful, since the follicular structures are more readily visualised. Note the prominence of the postcapillary venules. (H&E)

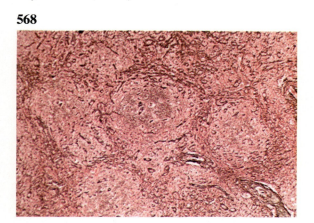

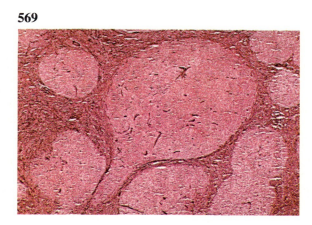

**568 and 569 Follicular lymphoma** Reticulin preparations are often extremely useful in delineating more clearly ill-defined neoplastic follicles, **568**, since these structures are relatively deficient in reticulin fibre, whereas reticulin fibre is increased and condensed in the interfollicular areas, often in relation to postcapillary venules. This method also illustrates more clearly the variation in size of the follicles for while in many cases the neoplastic follicles tend to approximate to each other in size, there are others, **569**, with a wide variation from small to very large follicles. (Gordon & Sweets)

**570 Follicular lymphoma** Extension of the follicular neoplastic process into the perinodal fat, in this case at the hilum, is a not uncommon and extremely helpful finding since this feature is very rarely found in reactive follicular hyperplasias. It is also important to appreciate that such involvement of perinodal tissue at presentation does not indicate a more sinister prognosis nor progression to a diffuse lymphoma. *(H&E)*

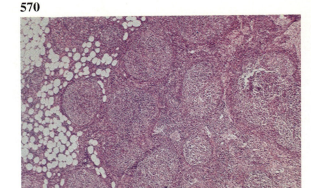

**571 Follicular lymphoma** In this example there is extension of the neoplastic process into the capsule which is greatly thickened and which shows the presence of one ill-defined follicular structure. Note that there is still preservation of the subcapsular sinus which can be seen clearly between the capsule and the follicular structures in the upper part of the field. Note also that in this example interfollicular reticulin fibre is only slightly increased and is not condensed. *(Gordon & Sweets)*

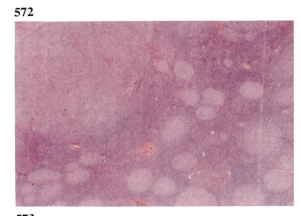

**572 Follicular lymphoma** It is not uncommon for a follicular lymphoma to show diffuse areas within the same node, and for the proportion of follicularity to diffuseness to vary considerably. Such cases may be designated malignant lymphoma, follicular *and* diffuse type, but should never be designated as a diffuse lymphoma, particularly as there is little evidence to indicate that a combination of a follicular and diffuse pattern indicates a worse prognosis. *(H&E)*

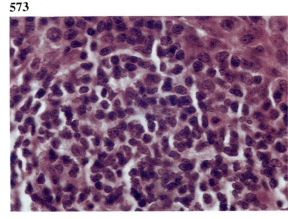

**573 Follicular lymphoma, predominantly small** The majority of follicular lymphomas, as in this example, are composed predominantly of the small irregular follicle centre type lymphocytes (intermediate lymphocytes, small cleaved lymphocytes, centrocytes). There is, however, always a population of larger cells although these vary considerably from case to case, and in this rather thick section are hard to discern. *(H&E)*

**574 Follicular lymphoma, predominantly small** In this high power field of a predominantly small cell follicle, there are large follicle centre cells of both regular and irregular nuclear contour, together with smaller regularly nucleated (centroblastic) cells (*arrow*). Only when such large cells form $^1/_3-^2/_3$rds of the total number of cells will a follicular lymphoma be designated as of mixed type. Note the prominent mitotic activity which is seen in some follicular lymphomas, a fact not generally appreciated. *(H&E)*

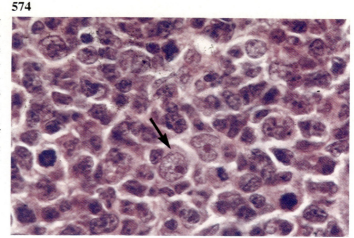

**575 Follicular lymphoma, predominantly small** Methyl green-pyronin staining will often emphasise the presence of large follicle centre cells because of their pyroninophilic cytoplasm. In this example these larger cells are centroblastic (small and large non-cleaved cells) and it is this mixture which is the basis for the term malignant lymphoma centroblastic/centrocytic follicular (see Kiel, Chart 4). Note the pyronin-negative cytoplasm of the predominantly small irregularly nucleated lymphocytes. *(MGP)*

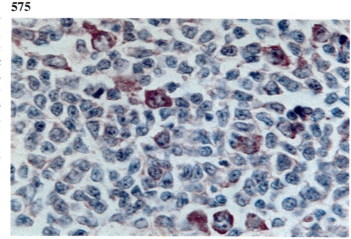

**576 Follicular lymphoma, predominantly small cell type** In this rather ill-defined follicle, although the predominating cell is the small irregularly nucleated cell, there are a number of large cells. Some of these are large follicle centre lymphocytes, but others are dendritic or mononuclear phagocytic in origin). It is important not to confuse this appearance with that of Hodgkin's disease or with a reactive germinal centre. *(H&E)*

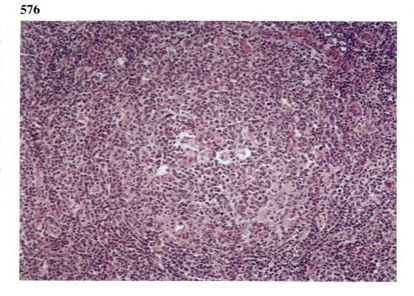

577

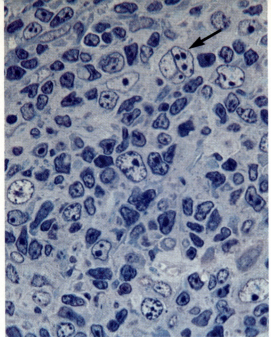

578

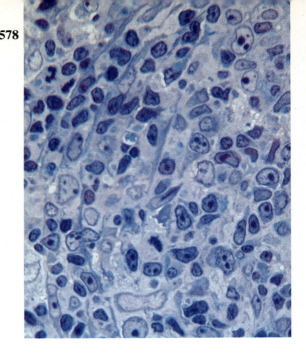

**577 and 578 Follicular lymphoma, predominantly small cell type** Plastic processing, because of the superior fixation and lack of artefact not only shows clearly the marked nuclear irregularity of the small lymphoid population, but also readily permits the identification of the larger lymphoid cells. It now becomes evident, **577**, that many of the smaller lymphoid cells possess nucleoli, and that there is a gradual progression of small to larger cells with increasingly dispersed chromatin. Note also how some of the large irregularly nucleated cells appear septate (*arrow*). The intercellular pale blue material largely consists of the cytoplasm of the dendritic cells. Semi-thin plastic sections are also useful in assessing whether there is interfollicular involvement. In **578**, the early breaching of the limiting reticular fibre by the follicle centre cells is easily seen where both large and small irregular follicle centre cells are seen *'en passage'. (Toluidine blue)*

**579 Follicular lymphoma, circulating cells** In this air dried haematological preparation there is a group of abnormal small lymphoid cells. These cells have long been known to be associated with follicular lymphoma and previously have been called hae-matogones. Other terms currently in usage are notched-nucleus cells, cleaved cells, centrocytes and intermediate lymphocytes. It is in smear preparations that nuclear cleavage or notching is seen most convincingly. Even more characteristic are the straight sides and angulation of the nuclei. These nuclear features directly result from the irregular or cerebroid nuclear contour. The terms convoluted and cerebroid should be avoided, however, since they have come to be associated with a particular type of nuclear irregularity seen in some types of T-lymphocytes, whereas the notched nucleus cells are derived from the follicle centre and are of B-lymphocyte origin. *(May-Grünwald-Giemsa)*

**580 Follicular lymphoma, touch or imprint preparation** The diagnosis of follicular lymphoma may be made on imprint or touch preparation although the value of this technique will vary considerably according to the experience of the investigator. Notching or cleavage is present but is never as striking as in haematological preparations. *(Giemsa)*

579

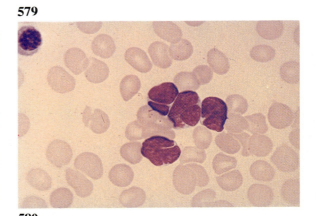

580

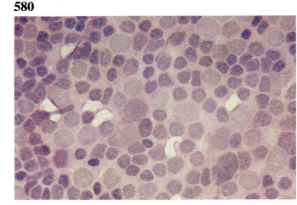

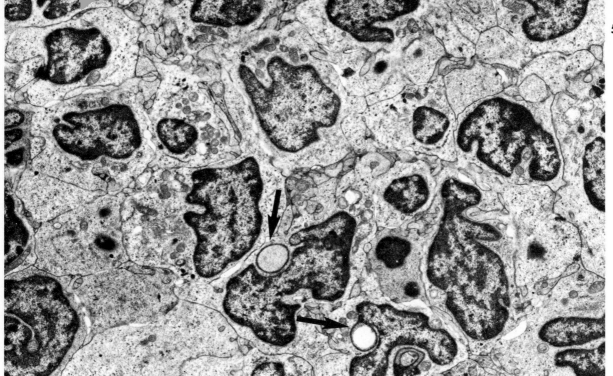

**581 and 582** **Follicular lymphoma, predominantly small cell type, ultrastructure** In these two examples of predominantly small cell type of follicular lymphoma, it is evident that the nuclei are not so much cleaved as irregular, with frequent indentations and protrusions, and prominent nuclear pockets (*arrows*). Compared to small mature lymphocytes the nuclear heterochromatin is less dense and the cytoplasm, which is more abundant, is of an irregular contour since there are close communications between both the lymphoid cells and the interdigitating processes of the dendritic reticular cells. The neoplastic small follicle centre cells thus closely resemble their normal and reactive counterparts. Not shown here are desmosomal attachments between processes of the dendritic cells, which are invariably present. (× 4,800)

**582**

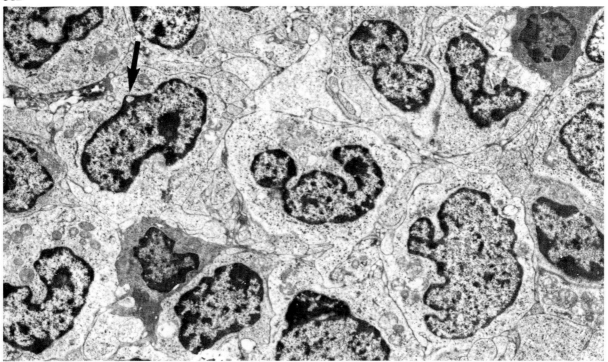

583

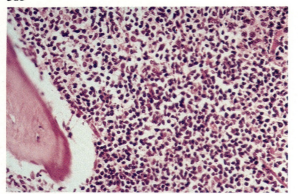

584

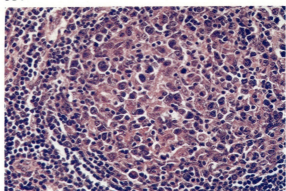

**583  Follicular lymphoma, bone marrow** The bone marrow of patients with follicular lymphoma commonly shows focal infiltration with follicle centre (intermediate) lymphocytes which may be arranged diffusely or less commonly as recognisable follicles. As with the finding of follicular lymphoma (notched nuclear) cells in peripheral blood, the significance of this feature in terms of prognosis is not yet fully understood; available evidence suggests that despite the apparent stage IV disease prognosis is not necessarily adversely affected. When the arrangement is diffuse as shown here it is not possible on the appearances of the bone marrow infiltrate alone to distinguish a *follicular* lymphoma with bone marrow involvement from a *diffuse* lymphoma of follicle centre origin. *(H&E)*

**586  Follicular lymphoma, mixed cell type** In this semi-thin plastic section of a follicular lymphoma of mixed cell type, the large cell component is predominantly of the irregularly nucleated form *(arrow)*. The extreme variation in the shapes of these cells with the coarsely lobated nuclei is well shown, and the nuclear chromatin which is finely dispersed is in marked contrast to the chromatin of the small irregular (intermediate) lymphocytes. Another feature of these large irregularly nucleated lymphocytes which is not clearly seen with routine preparations, is the location of the nucleoli at the nuclear membrane. *(Toluidine blue)*

586

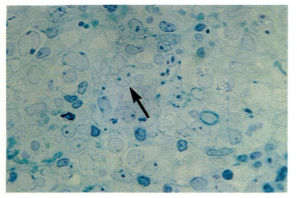

**584  Follicular lymphoma, mixed cell type** This neoplastic follicle is composed of a more pleomorphic population of cells with a mixture of large and small forms in approximately equal numbers. The small cells are the small irregularly nucleated follicle centre cells, but the large cells include both regular and irregularly nucleated cells. Only when large cells account for more than 66 per cent of the total population will a follicular lymphoma be called large cell type. *(H&E)*

585

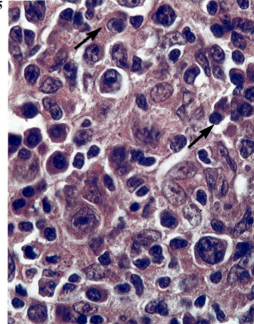

**585  Follicular lymphoma, mixed cell type** Admixed with the small irregular follicle centre lymphocytes are approximately equal numbers of large follicle centre cells of variable morphology. A cell which is not uncommonly found in follicular lymphomas of any type is the plasma cell *(arrow)* which occurs in variable numbers. In occasional follicular lymphomas they are very numerous; when the cytoplasmic immunoglobulin has leached out during processing the plasma cells may show a 'signet ring' appearance. *(H&E)*

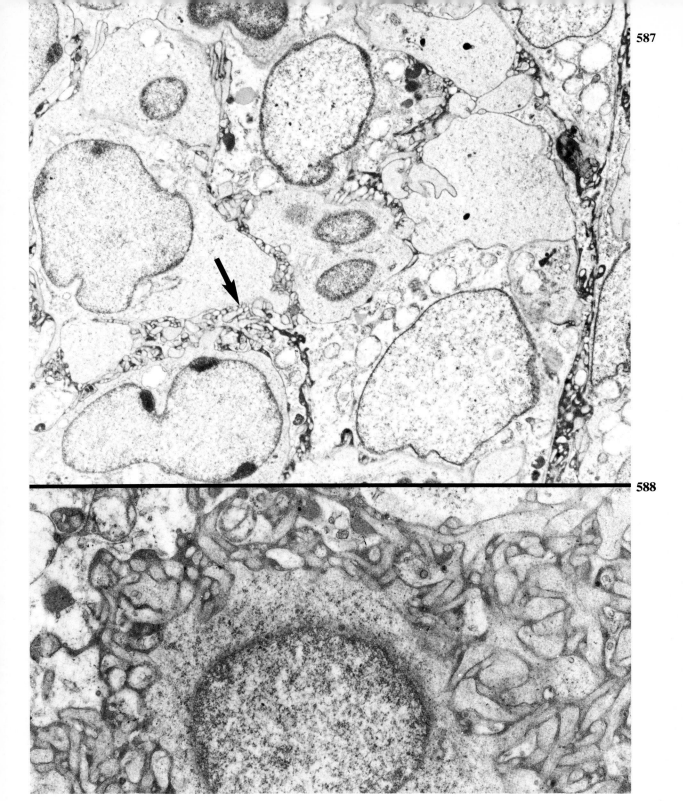

**587 and 588   Follicular lymphoma, mixed cell type, ultrastructure** Part of a poorly fixed neoplastic follicle of mixed cell type is shown in **587** with large irregularly nucleated (cleaved) lymphocytes in the left field and parts of large regularly nucleated (non-cleaved) lymphocytes on the right. Note the presence of nucleoli at the nuclear membrane of the irregular nucleus at the left, and the complex processes (*arrow*) of the dendritic cell. Few, small irregularly nucleated lymphocytes are present in this selected area. Figure **588** shows a dendritic cell with innumerable cytoplasmic extensions interdigitating with those of other dendritic cells. The nucleus shows a very finely dispersed nuclear chromatin, and the cytoplasm in the plane of section is devoid of organelles. (**587** × *5,500;* **588** × *16,200*)

**589 Follicular lymphoma, large cell type** The large lymphoid cells are similar to immunoblasts with an open vesicular nucleus, central and peripheral nucleoli, and sparse cytoplasm. Notice the presence of a few macrophages, and the residual cuff of small mixed lymphocytes at the bottom right corner. Large cell follicular lymphomas are rare, and form less than 10 per cent of all follicular lymphomas in the BNLI series. *(H&E)*

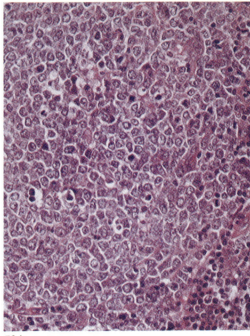

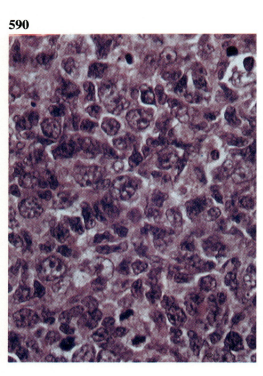

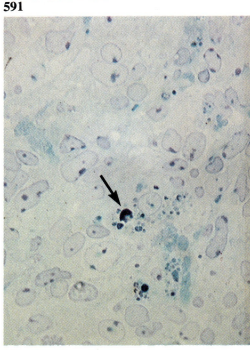

**590 Follicular lymphoma, large cell type** The cellular composition of the large cell type may be predominantly that of the large irregularly nucleated (large cleaved) follicle centre cell or large regularly nucleated cells. Mitotic activity is very variable in follicular lymphomas. Only when seen involving the large cell component does it appear to indicate a worse prognosis. *(H&E)*

**591 Follicular lymphoma, large cell type** Like mitotic activity, it is generally stated that in contrast to reactive germinal centres, the follicles of follicular lymphoma lack the presence of tingeable body macrophages. This statement is incorrect since a significant number of follicular lymphomas do show the presence of scattered tingeable body macrophages, as seen (*arrow*) in this predominantly large irregularly nucleated type. *(Toluidine blue)*

592

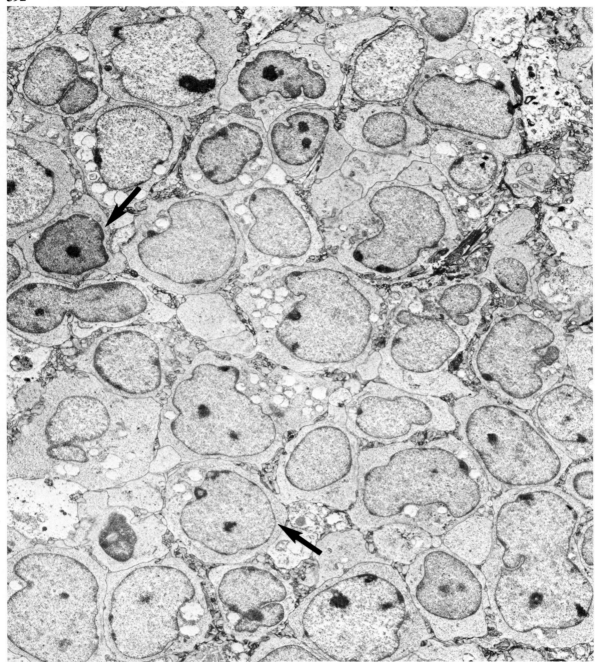

**592 Follicular lymphoma, large cell type, ultrastructure** This is a follicular lymphoma of predominantly large cell type in which small irregular follicle cells (*arrow*) are scanty and large irregular follicle cells outnumber the regularly contoured lymphoid cells (*arrow*). In between the RNA-rich cytoplasm of the large cells can be seen the interweaving processes of the dendritic cells. Note again the affinity of the nucleoli for the nuclear membrane, a characteristic of actively proliferating or secreting cells, and commonly seen in many types of neoplastic cells. (× 3,250)

**593**      **594**      **595**

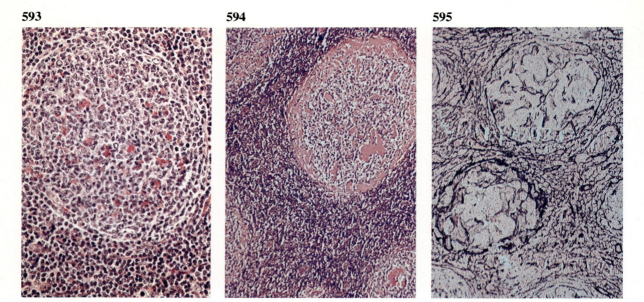

**593, 594 and 595   Follicular lymphoma, eosinophilic change** Eosinophilic material within the neoplastic follicles similar to that seen in post-reactive germinal centres is a not uncommon finding. The amount, however, varies considerably. Figure **593** shows a predominantly small cell type of follicular lymphoma in which there are scattered aggregates of eosinophilic material. Figure **594** shows abundant eosinophilic material, again in a small cell type, which has localised mainly at the periphery and is undergoing organisation and sclerosis as seen in **595**. It is the presence of intercellular material with increased reticulin fibre which accounts for some follicular lymphomas showing reticulin condensation at the junction of the neoplastic follicles with the interfollicular areas. *(593, 594 H&E; 595 Gordon & Sweets)*

**596   Follicular lymphoma** Follicular lymphoma is associated occasionally with a histiocytic response and the formation not only of epithelioid foci, which here can be seen ringing the neoplastic follicle, but also of an occasional non-caseating giant cell granuloma, part of one of which is seen in the lower right-hand field. This is yet another example of the development of sarcoid-like granulomas in response to various neoplastic conditions, but it should be stressed that this reaction is unusual and is much more common in Hodgkin's disease. *(H&E)*

**596**

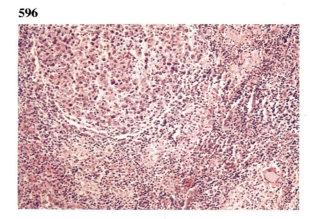

**597   Follicular lymphoma** Postcapillary venule proliferation is a frequent and sometimes prominent finding in the interfollicular areas of a follicular lymphoma. In this example a proliferating vessel is seen in association with interfollicular lymphomatous permeation. *(Toluidine blue)*

**597**

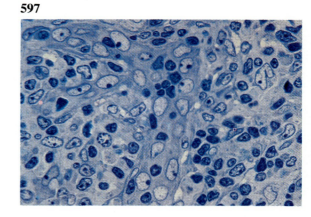

**598 and 599  Follicular lymphoma, fibrosis** A common finding in follicular lymphomas involving groin or abdominal lymph nodes is the presence of fibrosis. Most characteristically, **598**, this occurs at the periphery

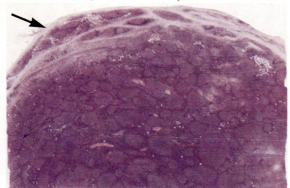

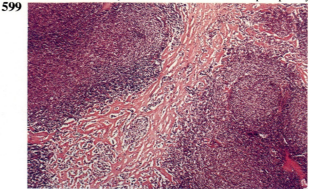

of the lymph node and is arranged in broad bands enclosing lymphoid tissue in which follicular structures may be present (*arrow*); **599** shows less condensed fibrous tissue. Occasional follicular lymphomas show a diffuse fine sclerosis similar to that seen in the diffuse lymphomas of follicular centre origin. This fibrous response is important because the appearances may be interpreted as nodular sclerosis Hodgkin's disease and because follicular lymphomas showing fibrosis have behaved in some series in a more indolent fashion. *(H&E)*

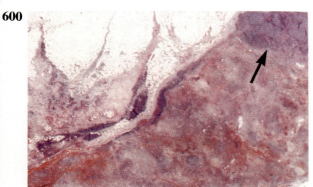

**600  Follicular lymphoma** Necrosis is a complication of many lymphomas. Massive necrosis is most common in groin glands, as in this example of an inguinal node. Only a small area of viable tissue (*arrow*) remains in which follicles can be discerned, the remainder being the site of widespread infarction extending to the perinodal fat. *(H&E)*

**601  Follicular lymphoma, alimentary system** Follicular lymphomas may arise in many extra-nodal sites such as the oropharyngeal lymphoid tissue, skin, spleen, salivary gland and, as here, the gastrointestinal tract, but are rare in comparison to their frequency in lymph node. Diffuse lymphomas of follicle centre origin are more common at this site, and the reason for the low incidence of those showing a follicular pattern is not clear. In this example of a predominantly small cell type arising in the ileum the neoplastic follicles have extended into the submucosae and muscularis propria. *(H&E)*

**602 Lymphoid Polyps alimentary system** It is very important not to confuse reactive follicles occurring in Waldeyer's ring or gastrointestinal tract with a follicular lymphoma. Sometimes in the colon, particularly in rectum, the reactive tissue may appear as a large polypoid mass – the so-called inflammatory polyp – when the likelihood of confusion with a lymphoma is even greater. This example shows such reactive lymphoid polyps. The diagnostic differential feature is the presence of follicles with active germinal centres. *(H&E)*

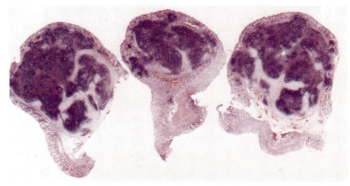

# Diffuse lymphoma, lymphocytic well differentiated

This category, which makes up 10 per cent of the BNLI non-Hodgkin's lymphomas, includes a spectrum of clinical disorders with a similar histopathological appearance in lymph nodes. Such disorders range from the common chronic lymphocytic leukaemia (CLL) with nodal involvement, to the nodal lymphomas of lymphocytic well differentiated type. If CLL – a disease almost exclusively of older age groups – can be excluded, these Grade I lymphomas are uncommon and show a much wider age range. Some of these lymphomas may show plasmacytoid features with or without the production of clinically detectable immunoglobulin. This variant, which some workers (Lennert) place in a separate category – the LP immunocytoma and subdivide into three subtypes – occurs more commonly in the elderly and is more likely on presentation to show generalised lymphadenopathy, and splenic and bone marrow involvement. Extra-nodal sites also may be primarily involved. When the immunoglobulin produced is IgM the lymphoma is often commonly associated with Waldenström's disease. It should be stressed again that despite lymphoplasmacytoid features there may be no clinically detectable immunoglobulin. We should like to emphasise also that when such lymphoplasmacytoid tumours consist *predominantly* of plasma – and lymphoplasmacytoid cells and their immediate precursors - they are placed within the extramedullary plasmacytoma group. Thus, our criteria for the diagnosis of extramedullary plasmacytomas differs from that of others in that we do not demand a pure population of well differentiated plasma cells. The majority of lymphocytic well differentiated lymphomas are of B-lymphocytic origin and, while generally are of slow progression, do not usually have such a good prognosis as the majority of follicular lymphomas. An increasing number of T-lymphocytic well differentiated types are now being defined and there is evidence that these have a worse prognosis. Another condition which may cause diagnostic confusion is lymph node involvement in prolymphocytic leukaemia; usually, however, massive splenic and sometimes hepatic enlargement dominate the clinical picture.

**603 Malignant lymphoma, diffuse lymphocytic well differentiated and CLL** The distinction between a lymph node which is the site of a malignant lymphoma of diffuse well differentiated type and one which is infiltrated with chronic lymphocytic leukaemia (CLL) cells is probably not possible on histopathological grounds alone. Clinically, while they may overlap, there are differences in that CLL is common and affects predominantly elderly individuals, whereas a diffuse lymphocytic well differentiated lymphoma is a rare entity, has a greater age range, and does not carry quite such a good prognosis. Lymph nodes show an infiltrate of small lymphocytes which results in loss of normal architecture and obliteration of the peripheral sinus. In this example capsular invasion is minimal, though there is some involvement of perinodal tissue. (*H&E*)

**603**

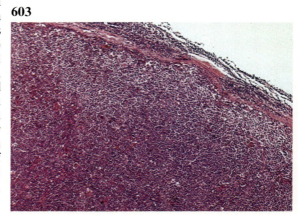

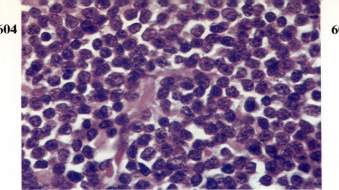

**604**

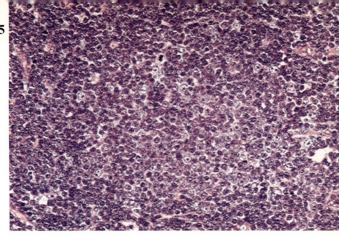

**605**

**604 Malignant lymphoma, diffuse lymphocytic well differentiated and CLL** The infiltrating lymphocytes are about the same size, or slightly larger than normal well differentiated lymphocytes. The majority of lymphomas composed of well differentiated lymphocytes are, like CLL, of B-cell type. (It is very much rarer for lymph nodes to be involved in the infrequent T-cell leukaemias, and their diagnosis on morphological grounds alone is difficult.) The nuclei in contrast to follicular centre lymphocytes are generally round and regularly contoured, and there is more abundant and coarsely aggregated chromatin. Nucleoli are inconspicuous except in prolymphocyte nuclei and there is a lack of mitotic activity. *(H&E)*

**605 Malignant lymphoma, diffuse lymphocytic well differentiated and CLL** A characteristic feature of this type of lymphoma and lymph nodes involved in CLL is the presence throughout of paler areas composed of more primitive lymphoid cells. These pale areas are referred to generally as proliferation centres and when they are very prominent they are an important source of confusion with a follicular lymphoma. Reticulin stains however fail to·delineate them, the reticulin fibre pattern being similar within and outside the centres. *(H&E)*

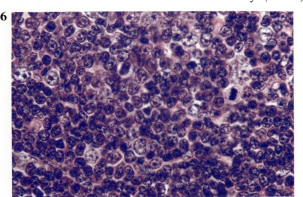

**606**

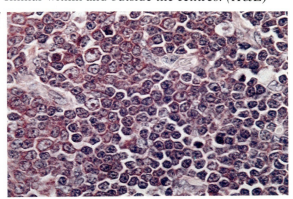

**607**

**606 and 607 Malignant lymphoma, diffuse lymphocytic well differentiated and CLL** The cells comprising a proliferation centre range from nucleated prolymphocytes to larger cells with the characteristics of immunoblasts. In contrast to the lymphocytes around the centres, mitotic activity is usually pronounced, **606**. The cells within a proliferation centre show variable degrees of pyroninophilia depending upon the amount of cytoplasmic-RNA, **607**. Typical plasma cells are seldom recognised within these centres; neither are there irregularly nucleated lymphocytes of follicle centre type. *(606 H&E; 607 MGP)*

**608 Malignant lymphoma, diffuse lymphocytic well differentiated and CLL** In this plastic processed lymph node the component cells of a well differentiated lymphocytic lymphoma show a much greater variation in size, ranging from small mature well differentiated lymphoid cells to large nucleated 'blast' cells – with cells intermediate in size between the two approximating to prolymphocytes. In contrast to T-lymphocytes, B-well differentiated lymphocytes contain very little demonstrable acid phosphatase, non-specific esterase or ß-glucuronidase. *(Toluidine blue)*

**608**

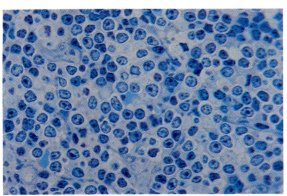

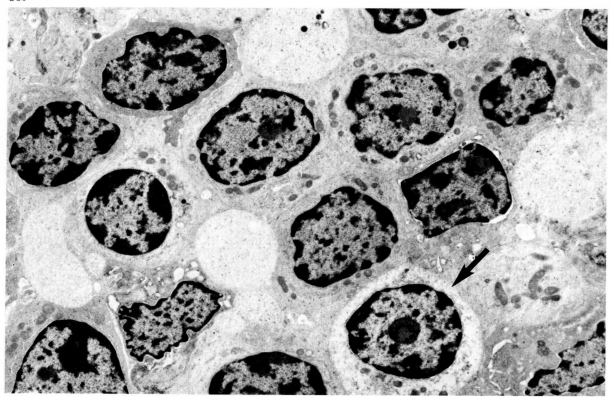

**609 and 610   Malignant lymphoma, diffuse lymphocytic well differentiated and CLL, ultrastructure** At ultrastructural level the cells of a diffuse well differentiated lymphocytic lymphoma do not differ from those of CLL in that the predominant cell is a small relatively mature lymphocyte. The nuclei are rounded or only slightly indented, and the heterochromatin is coarsely aggregated. Nucleoli are only conspicuous in the larger prolymphocytes (*arrows*). Figure **609** shows chronic lymphocytic leukaemia; **610** is from a patient with lymphocytic lymphoma in whom there were no leukaemic manifestations. *(609, 610 × 4,800)*

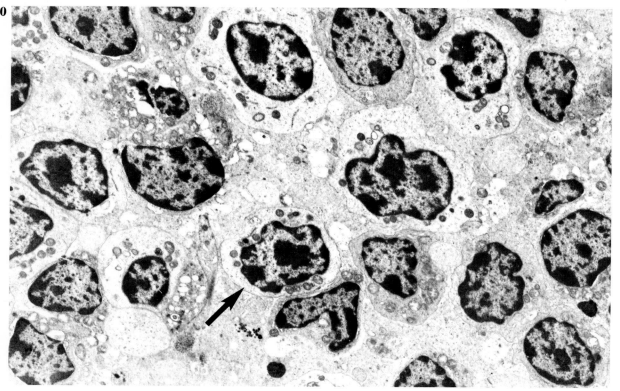

**611**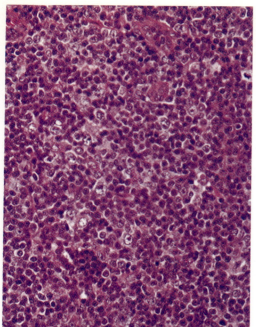

**612**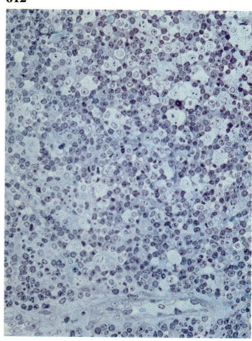

**611 and 612  Malignant lymphoma, lymphocytic well differentiated and CLL** In some instances instead of discrete proliferation centres, blast cells are focally scattered among the population of small well differentiated lymphocytes. In this example of a lymph node resected during the course of CLL, there are many large immunoblasts, **611**. These are more numerous and are better visualised in plastic processed semi-thin sections of the resected spleen, **612**. Such an appearance is consistent with the development of a large lymphoid cell lymphoma (high grade) or Richter's syndrome. A transformation of CLL into a *lympho-blastic* phase is much less common.
*(611 H&E; 612 Toluidine blue)*

**613  Malignant lymphoma, diffuse lymphocytic well differentiated and CLL** Maligant lymphoma of lymphocytic well differentiated type can occur in extra-nodal sites without any leukaemic manifestation but are infrequent. This lymphoma was excised on the presumptive diagnosis of a gastric carcinoma. In contrast to lymph nodes, proliferation centres are absent and prolymphocytes and 'blast' forms were very rare among the monomorphous population of small well differentiated lymphocytes. There is no plasmacytoid differentiation. Such lymphomas formed 4 per cent of our series of gastrointestinal lymphomas. *(H&E)*

**613**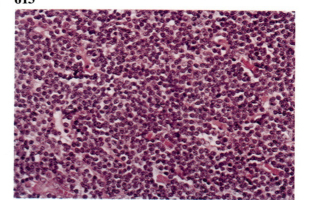

**614  Prolymphocytic leukaemia** This is viewed as a rare variant of CLL. Clinically, the disease like CLL affects mainly elderly males but is manifested by systemic symptoms, massive enlargement of the spleen and to a lesser extent liver, and absent or inconspicuous lymph node enlargement. Patients are often diagnosed initially as suffering from acute lymphoblastic leukaemia. Occasionally lymph nodes are excised for diagnostic purposes. One such node, **614**, shows a monomorphous proliferation of cells larger than those seen in CLL, but with a less dense nuclear chromatin content and easily visible nucleoli. Prolymphocytic leukaemias are predominantly of B-lymphocytic type, very few being of proven T-cell origin. *(H&E)*

**614**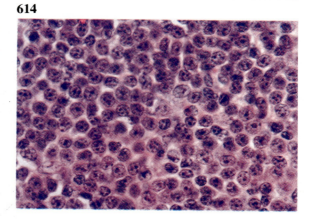

**615**

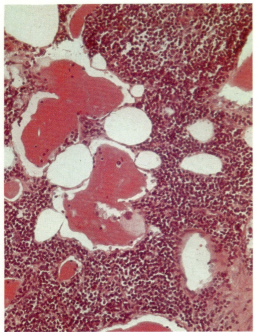

**616a**

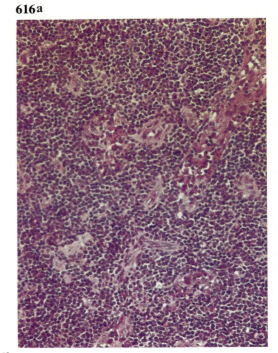

**616b**

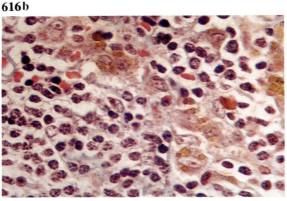

**615, 616a and 616b  Malignant lymphoma, diffuse lymphocytic well differentiated with plasma cell differentiation** Lymphomas (and leukaemias) showing such plasma cell differentiation are by definition B-cell neoplasias. The BNLI classification does not subdivide these tumours into sub-types. However, if the majority of cells are manifestly of plasmacytic type the lymphoma will be designated as a plasma cell lymphoma. Lymphomas showing plasma cell differentiation may or may not be accompanied by the presence of a paraprotein. If a paraprotein is present in the serum, it is usually IgM. In these examples from two patients with Waldenström's macroglobulinaemia lymph node architecture is partially retained. Figure 615 shows preservation of sinuses which are filled with eosinophilic protein (immunoglobulin), while **616a** shows in addition sinusoidal preservation, conspicuous PCVs and small epithelioid clusters. Haemosiderin is sometimes a conspicuous feature, **616b**. Amyloid deposition may also be found (see **437**). (**615, 616a** *H&E;* **616b** *Masson's trichrome*)

**617 and 618  Malignant lymphoma, diffuse lymphocytic well differentiated with plasma cell differentiation** In this example of macroglobulinaemia the majority of cells, **617**, appear to be lymphocytic and only a few plasma cells are evident. Cells with features intermediate between lymphocytes and plasma cells (lymphoplasmacytoid cells) are also present, and there are occasional nuclei containing vacuoles ( *arrow* ). These intranuclear inclusions, **618**, known as Dutcher bodies, are PAS positive (*arrow 1*) and similar inclusions are also present in the cytoplasm (*arrow 2*), see also **623**). They are not unique to IgM secreting cells, for they also occur in IgA producing lymphoproliferative disorders as well as in some reactive plasma cell proliferations. (**617** *H&E;* **618** *PAS*)

**617**

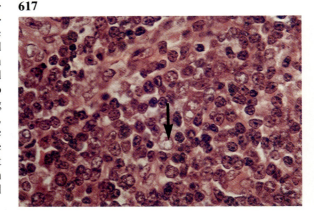

**618**

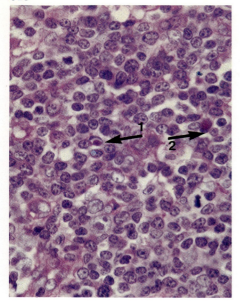

**619**

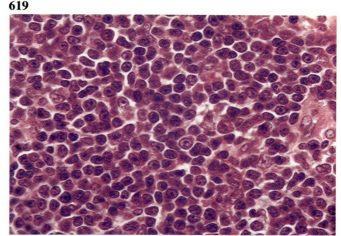

**619 Malignant lymphoma, diffuse lymphocytic well dif-ferentiated with plasmacytoid differentiation** In this lymphoma showing plasma cell differentiation, there was complete replacement of the lymph node with an infiltrate consisting of small lymphocytes admixed with a few typical plasma cells and many lymphoplasmacytoid cells – cells with nuclei superficially resembling lymphocytes or prolymphocytes, but slightly eccentrically placed, and with a more abundant pyroninophilic cytoplasm. Such tumours lack typical proliferation centres. They may progress to more malignant Grade II lymphomas or develop a leukaemic phase; there is a greater involvement of extranodal sites than in diffuse lymphomas of well dif-ferentiated type *without* plasma cell differentiation. *(H&E)*

**620**

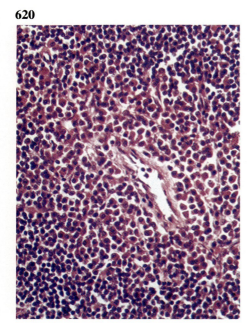

**621**

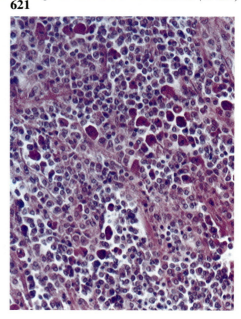

**620 and 621   Malignant lymphoma, diffuse lymphocytic with plasma cell differentiation** In some of these tumours there may be focal areas, often in a perivascular distribution, consisting entirely of well differentiated plasma cells, **620**. Note the *eosinophilic* appearance of the cytoplasm due to the presence of immuno-globulin. Cytoplasmic immunoglobulin is often dramatically revealed by PAS positivity, **621**, where the globules of immunoglobulin or Russell bodies are intensely stained, as in this IgM secreting gastric lymphoma. Cytoplasmic immunoglobulin can be demonstrated also by immunoperoxidase techniques or by electronmicroscopy. *(620 H&E; 621 PAS)*

622

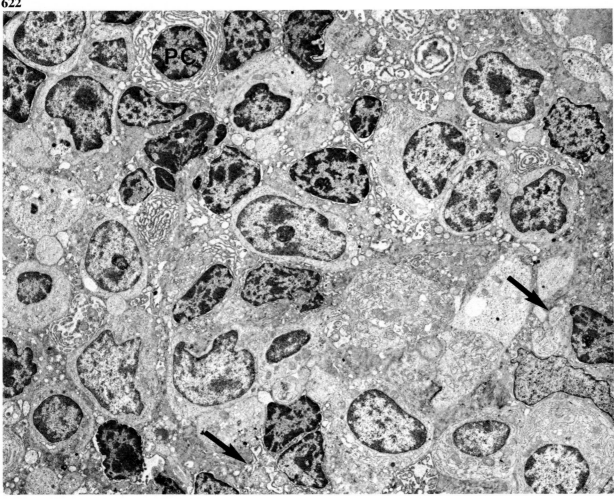

**622 Malignant lymphoma, diffuse lymphocytic well differentiated with plasma cell differentiation, ultra-structure** In this patient with Waldenström's macroglobulinaemia, at ultrastructural level the neoplastic cells show a much more varied appearance than suggested in the paraffin sections. In this field there are many cells with lymphocytic nuclei but plasmacytic cytoplasm (*arrows*), mature plasma cells (PC) and several indeterminate blast cells. A feature not shown here but readily demonstrated with special stains or EM (see **265** and **266**) is a prominent mast cell component. (× 3,250)

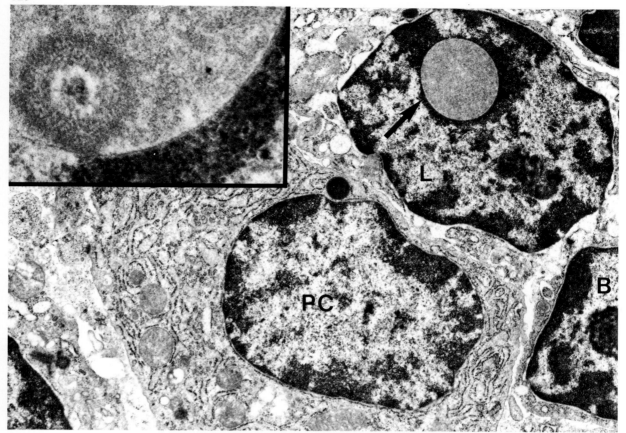

**623  Malignant lymphoma, diffuse lymphocytic well differentiated with plasma cell differentiation, ultrastructure** Contained within the cytoplasm of the group of lymphoid cells shown here are dilated cisternae of rough endoplasmic reticulum containing electron dense secretory products. This feature is most obvious in the mature plasma cell (PC) but is apparent in the cells with lymphocytic nuclei (L) and in the blast cell (B). The PAS positive intranuclear inclusions or Dutcher bodies consist of invaginated cytoplasmic immunoglobulin. Part of one such body is seen in greater detail in the inset, which shows an intranuclear inclusion containing in addition to immunoglobulin a ribosomal lamellae complex. *(× 12,000; inset × 30,450)*

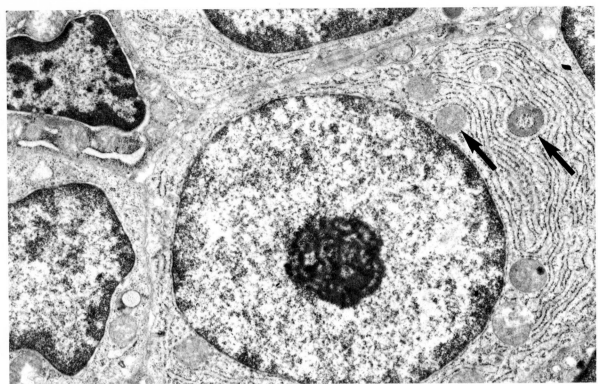

**624 and 625   Malignant lymphoma, lymphocytic well differentiated with plasma cell differentiation, ultrastructure** Figure **624** shows that some of the blast cells are plasmablasts with abundant formation of rough endoplasmic reticulum. The rounded structures (*arrows*) are ribosomal lamellae complexes, and are seen in greater detail in **625** cut transversely and in longitudinal sections. These structures are similar to those seen in hairy cell leukaemia. They consist of ribosomes and parallel arrays of membrane in relation to rough endoplasmic reticulum. The central core is continuous with the cytoplasm. (**624** × *11,580;* **625** × *40,000)*

**625**

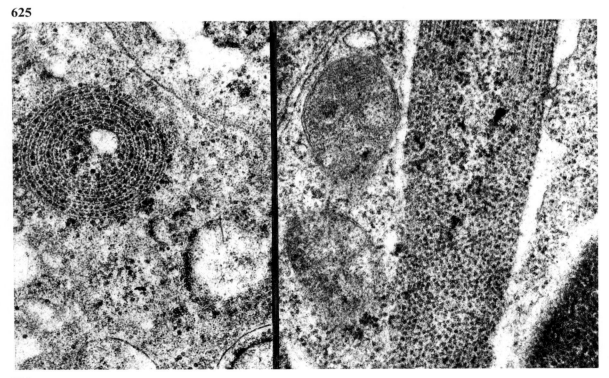

# Diffuse lymphoma, lymphocytic intermediate differentiated

This entity has been recognised only recently. Formerly it was included within the lymphosarcoma, lymphocytic group of Gall and Mallory, and the poorly differentiated lymphocytic group of Rappaport. In the Stanford formulation it is called malignant lymphoma, diffuse – small cleaved cell. Diffuse lymphomas of intermediate type represent the diffuse counterpart of the predominant small cell follicular lymphoma and are of B-cell origin. Unlike follicular lymphoma they form only 4 per cent of the non-Hodgkin's lymphomas, and often at the time of presentation are more likely to be widely disseminated with generalised lymphadenopathy and splenomegaly. The age distribution is, however, similar to follicular lymphoma, being most common in the elderly, and there may be also (approximately 10 per cent of cases) circulating 'notched nuclear' cells. In terms of behaviour, while still falling within the Grade I prognostic category, they do not generally pursue quite such a benign course as the majority of follicular lymphomas; in some, the behaviour is extremely unpredictable.

**626**

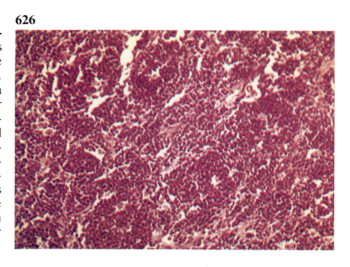

**626 Malignant lymphoma diffuse, lymphocytic, intermediate** This Grade I lymphoma has been recognised only recently and is one of the less common types of non-Hodgkin's lymphoma. It is viewed as the diffuse counterpart of a predominantly small follicle cell follicular lymphoma. At presentation complete replacement of lymph node architecture is usual and the neoplastic infiltrate is diffuse from the outset. At low power it may be difficult to differentiate these tumours from a diffuse lymphocytic well differentiated lymphoma. Others, as in this example, show a 'nodular' appearance due to ill-defined aggregates of cells, which should not be confused with a follicular lymphoma. Proliferation centres do not occur. (H&E)

**627**

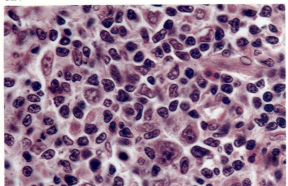

**628**

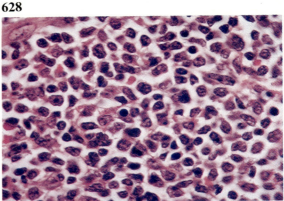

**627 and 628   Malignant lymphoma diffuse, lymphocytic intermediate** High magnification, **627**, shows the irregularly contoured nuclei characteristic of small follicle centre or intermediate lymphocytes. An invariable finding is the presence of large cells scattered among the small cell population, which usually are similar in appearance to the large follicle centre cells of both regularly and irregularly nucleated type (centroblast, immunoblast, large and small cleaved cells). Dendritic cells are also present. The numbers of large cells are variable; they are never aggregated, a feature which, together with the nuclear irregularity, is helpful in distinguishing between a diffuse lymphoma of intermediate type and a diffuse lymphoma of well differentiated type with proliferation centres. Figure **628** shows a lymphoma of intermediate type in which the large cell component is very scarce. Note also the mitotic activity. Since these lymphomas are of B-lymphocytic origin plasma cell differentiation may be present as in any other types of B-lymphoma. *(H&E)*

**629 Malignant lymphoma diffuse, lymphocytic intermediate** A fairly common and helpful finding in this type of diffuse lymphoma is the presence of banded sclerosis both within the involved node and outside, similar to that seen in follicular lymphomas. Another characteristic feature related to fibrosis is the finding of hyalinised material lying between the tumour cells as here, which is often in continuity with vessel walls. *(H&E)*

**630 and 631   Malignant lymphoma diffuse, lymphocytic intermediate** Two uncommon reactive features may be seen, which can lead to diagnostic difficulties. Figure **630** shows reactive tingeable body macrophages. When seen in relation to the sometimes prominent mitotic activity, this finding should not lead to a diagnosis of a malignant lymphoma of poorly differentiated type, for despite evidence of rapid proliferation these tumours generally behave clinically as Grade I lymphomas. Some, however, develop into high

**629**

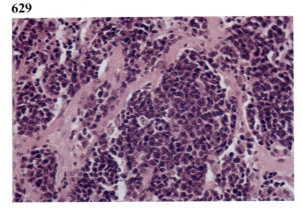

grade (II) lymphomas. The other reactive feature, **631**, is the presence of loose epithelioid aggregates and even sarcoid-like lesions. (**630** *plastic section H&E;* **631** *H&E*)

**630**

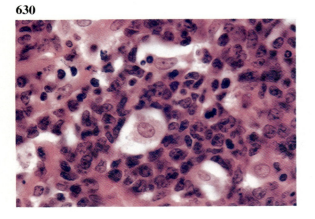

**631**

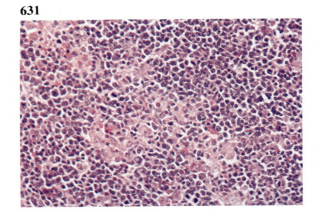

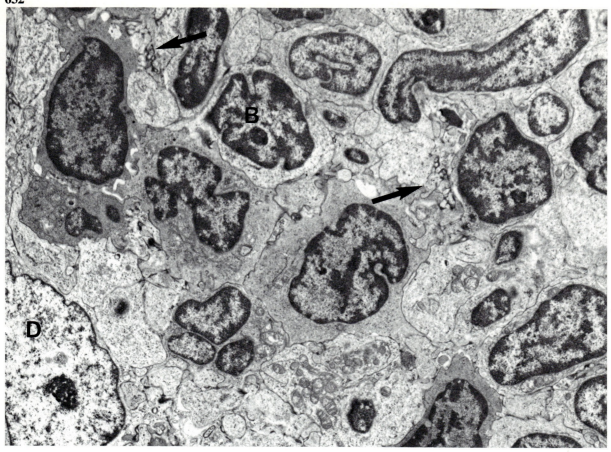

**632  Malignant lymphoma, diffuse lymphocytic intermediate, ultrastructure** Electron microscopy confirms the follicle centre origin of this group of tumours since the appearances are essentially similar to follicular lymphomas of predominantly small cell type. Invariably, between the proliferating cells can be seen the interdigitating processes of dendritic cells (*arrows*) and if searched for desmosomes usually can be demonstrated. Note the dendritic cell nucleus (D) and long cytoplasmic process, and the presence of a few nucleolated blast cells (B). *(× 5,000)*

**633 Malignant lymphoma, diffuse lymphocytic intermediate** As in its follicular counterpart bone marrow involvement is not unusual but is of less prognostic significance than liver involvement, as shown here. The portal tract is expanded by small follicle centre cells but residual structures such as bile ducts (*arrow*) are intact. Because of prognostic implications it is important to distinguish between genuine lymphomatous involvement of liver and reactive lymphocytic hepatic infiltration. *(H&E)*

**633**

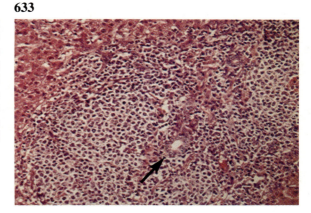

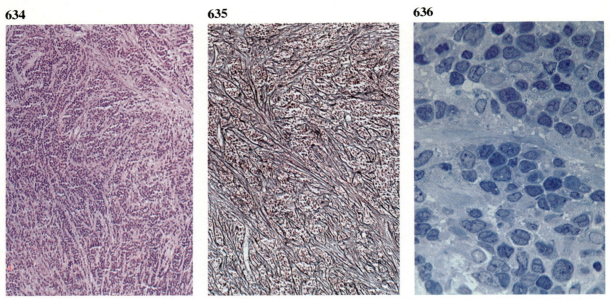

**634, 635 and 636 Malignant lymphoma, diffuse lymphocytic poorly differentiated intermediate** This large abdominal mass of nodes was replaced by a monotonous infiltrate of small lymphoid cells, **634**, with prominent compartmentalising fibrosis, well seen in this reticulin preparation, **635**. A semi-thin section of plastic processed material, **636**, shows a high degree of nuclear irregularity in relatively small, often nucleolated, lymphoid cells. Mitotic activity was also extremely prominent. *(634 H&E; 635 Gordon & Sweets; 636 Toluidine blue)*. **637 Ultrastructure** The atypical appearance at L.M. level is now apparent. There are unusual numbers of nuclear lobes, pockets and bridges, prominent nucleoli and many mitochondria. This lymphoma should be typed Grade II. *(× 16,800)*

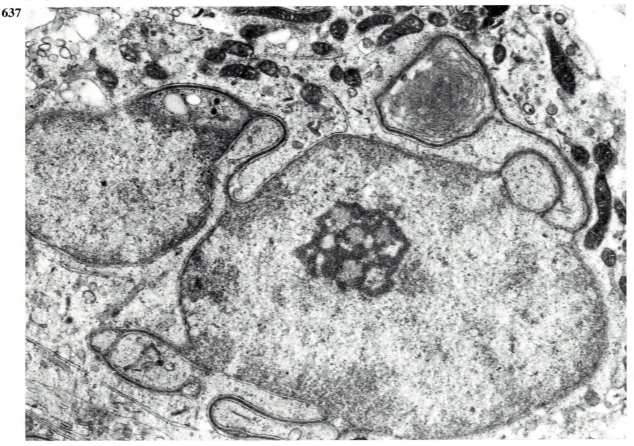

# Malignant lymphoma, diffuse lymphocytic poorly differentiated (lymphoblastic)

Diffuse lymphocytic poorly differentiated (lymphoblastic) lymphoma is a *heterogeneous* category (9 per cent in the BNLI non-Hodgkin's trial) of high grade malignancy (Grade II). It incorporates a number of different entities such as the convoluted cell lymphoma, Burkitt's tumour, and the non-Burkitt poorly differentiated lymphocytic lymphomas which form the largest group of non-Hodgkin's lymphomas seen in children; and a proportion of which show a Burkitt-like appearance. Also, many of the tumours categorised as a lymphocytic poorly differentiated (lymphoblastic) lymphoma represent the tissue phase of acute lymphoblastic leukaemia (ALL) but, since poorly differentiated lymphomas readily exfoliate cells into the blood stream, it may not be possible always to distinguish between the two conditions. There may be difficulties also in differentiating lymphocytic poorly differentiated lymphomas from tumour masses composed of prolymphocytes (see **614**) or other types of blast cells, as in acute myeloid or myelomonocytic leukaemia.

On the basis of marker studies it is now known that the majority of these lymphomas are of B-cell origin. Even Burkitt's tumour, at one time regarded as a lymphoma of undifferentiated lymphoreticular cell type, is now accepted as a B-cell tumour of poorly differentiated lymphocytic or lymphoblastic origin. Indeed, some authorities believe that Burkitt's tumour represents a neoplasm of the non-cleaved follicle centre cell (centroblast). The less common lymphocytic poorly differentiated lymphoma of convoluted type is of T-lymphocytic origin. It usually presents in childhood and adolescence with a mediastinal mass involving the thymus; there may be leukaemic manifestations. This lymphoma is known also as the Sternberg sarcoma and T-cell lymphoblastic lymphoma or lymphosarcoma. Enzyme histochemistry has also supported a T-cell origin, giving similar results as in other lymphoproliferative disorders involving T-cells – such as the Sézary syndrome and mycosis fungoides. These latter conditions predominantly involve skin. However, since lymph nodes may be affected, these T-cell cutaneous lymphomas will be discussed in the miscellaneous category *(see pages 289-293)*.

The Stanford formulation separates the BNLI lymphocytic poorly differentiated (lymphoblastic) lymphomas into two separate categories; the malignant lymphoma lymphoblastic type incorporating the convoluted and non-convoluted variants, and the malignant lymphomas of non-cleaved cell type which includes Burkitt's tumour.

**638 Malignant lymphoma, diffuse lymphocytic poorly differentiated (lymphoblastic) – Burkitt's lymphoma** Burkitt's tumour is common in certain parts of Africa and frequent in Papua, New Guinea. Sporadic cases have been described throughout the world which show similar morphological and/ or clinical features. It is wise, however, to restrict the term Burkitt's lymphoma to those examples in which there is evidence of exposure to the Epstein-Barr (EB) virus. In the typical African cases, children are most commonly affected and usually present with involvement of jaw, kidneys, gonads, liver, retroperitoneum and endocrine glands. The relative sparing of superficial lymph nodes and spleen is very characteristic. The usual histopathological appearance at low power is a diffuse cellular lymphoid tumour with numerous scattered macrophages resulting in the so called 'starry sky' appearance. *(H&E)*

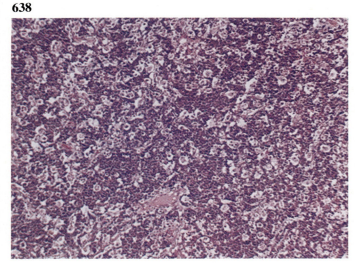

638

**639**

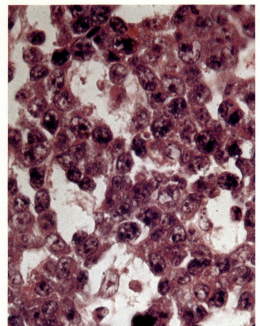

**640**

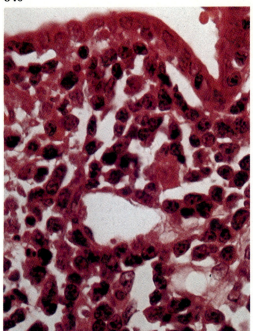

**639 and 640 Malignant lymphoma, diffuse lymphocytic poorly differentiated (lymphoblastic) – Burkitt's lymphoma** The proliferating lymphoid cells in a typical example of African Burkitt's lymphoma as in this jaw tumour usually present in routine paraffin processed material a monomorphic cohesive appearance, **639**. The component cells are rounded, with round or indented nuclei and with chromatin which varies from a finely clumped to a granular appearance. Nucleoli are very variable and may number from one to five. The cytoplasm is scanty though relatively well defined. Tingeable body macrophages with abundant clear cytoplasm containing pyknotic nuclear debris are scattered among the tumour cells. In really well fixed material, but not here, it is sometimes possible to visualise fine vacuoles in the cytoplasm. All these features, however, are influenced very much by fixation and degeneration, as shown in an example of Burkitt's lymphoma involving fallopian tube, **640**. *(H&E)*

**641**

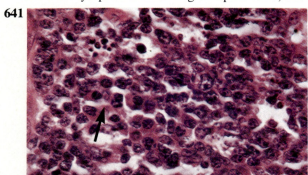

**642**

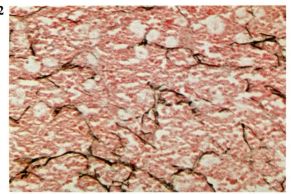

**641 Malignant lymphoma, diffuse lymphocytic poorly differentiated (lymphoblastic) – Burkitt's lymphoma** Like other poorly differentiated lymphomas mitotic figures are frequent and the cytoplasm is rich in RNA and intensely pyroninophilic (see **647**). Indeed it is debatable whether a diagnosis of Burkitt's lymphoma should ever be made in the absence of pyroninophilia. It has been suggested that Burkitt's lymphoma – now accepted as a B-lymphoblastic tumour – is derived from follicle cells, specifically centroblasts. Thus, the finding of occasional foci of plasma cells *(arrow)* among the otherwise monomorphic cells of this jaw tumour in an African child is not surprising.*(H&E)*

**642 Malignant lymphoma, diffuse lymphocytic poorly differentiated (lymphoblastic) – Burkitt's lymphoma** Reticulin preparations are of little value in the diagnosis of this tumour since the pattern will vary considerably according to the type of tissue involved. In this ovarian tumour in a child there is little increase in the amount of reticulin, and tingeable body macrophages are not particularly numerous. *(Gordon & Sweets)*

236

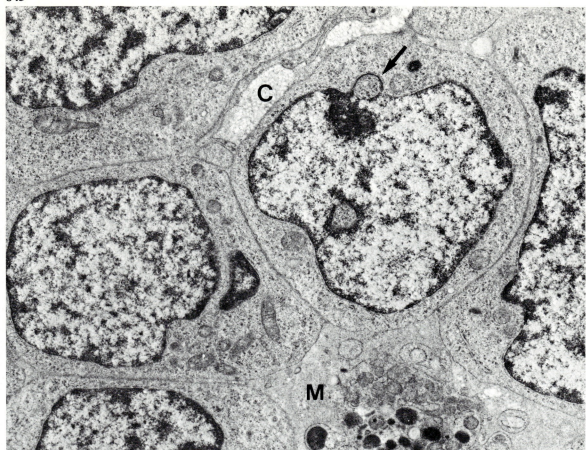

**643    Malignant lymphoma, diffuse lymphocytic poorly differentiated (lymphoblastic) – Burkitt's lymphoma, ultrastructure** Electronmicrograph of a Ugandan Burkitt's lymphoma showing the typical uniform lymphoblasts composing the tumour. The cells are rounded and have large nuclei with prominent nucleoli; a nuclear projection (*arrow*) enclosing cytoplasmic material is present in one cell. The cytoplasm is packed with free ribosomes and contains scanty mitochondria and rare elements of the rough endoplasmic reticulum. A portion of the cytoplasm of a macrophage (M) with numerous dense digestive vacuoles, and bundles of collagen (C) in an intercellular space are also seen. (× 9,100)

**644 and 645 Malignant lymphoma, diffuse lymphocytic poorly differentiated (lymphoblastic) – Burkitt-like** Such lymphomas occur at all ages. They are one of the commonest forms of childhood lymphoma, often presenting with gastrointestinal involvement. In this example from a 12-year-old Caucasian boy there was diffuse involvement of the ileocaecal valve and terminal ileum, **644**. The tumour was localised to gut with the exception of one mesenteric lymph node which showed, **645**, partial involvement by lymphoma. In both the intestinal and lymph node tumours, the morphological appearance of the tumour cells was very similar to a true Burkitt tumour including a prominent 'starry sky' effect. It is important to bear in mind that a 'starry sky' pattern is seen in at least 20 per cent of non-Burkitt poorly differentiated lymphomas and that, despite morphological similarities to Burkitt's lymphoma, a tumour should not be designated as such in the absence of specific (E-B) viral antigen (see **862**). (*H&E*)

**644**

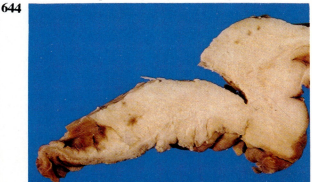

**645**

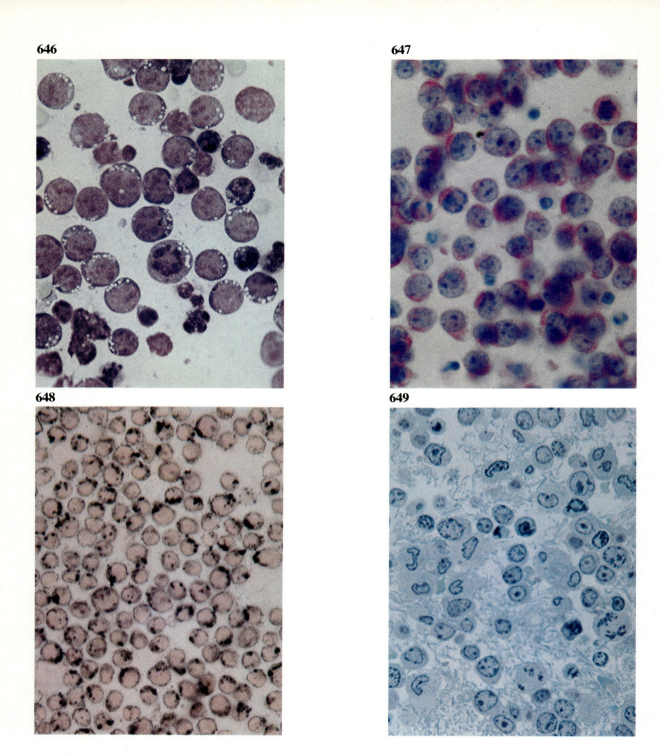

**646, 647, 648 and 649  Malignant lymphoma, diffuse lymphocytic poorly differentiated (lymphoblastic) – Burkitt-like** These preparations were prepared from the ascitic fluid of a child with abdominal involvement two years following treatment for a cervical lymphocytic lymphoblastic lymphoma. The cells, which were not distinguishable morphologically from those of a Burkitt's lymphoma, are well visualised in the air-dried Giemsa preparation, **646**, which enhances the nuclear and cytoplasmic detail and reveals the presence of vacuoles within the cytoplasm. Figure **647** shows the marked pyroninophilia of the cytoplasm which here appears less in quantity due to wet fixation. Figure **648** stained with Sudan black reveals the abundant lipid present within the cells, and **649** is a semi-thin section of a pellet of centrifuged cells processed in resin, which shows the nuclear and cytoplasmic detail with great clarity. (**646** *May-Grünwald-Giemsa;* **647** *Methyl green-pyronin;* **648** *Sudan black;* **649** *Toluidine blue*)

650

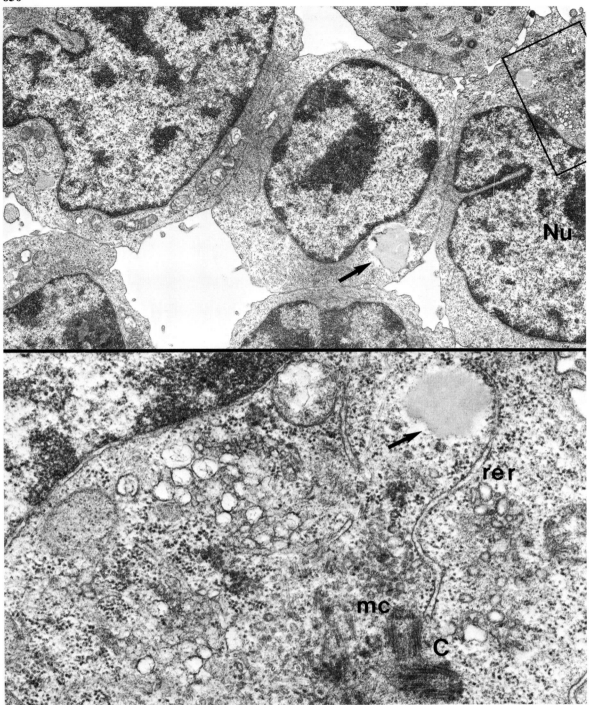

**650 Malignant lymphoma, diffuse lymphocytic poorly differentiated (lymphoblastic), Burkitt-like, ultrastructure** The ultrastructural features of the ascitic fluid cells in **646-649** are those of lymphoblasts with large rounded or indented nuclei and prominent nucleoli (Nu). The cytoplasm contains an abundance of free ribosomes but a sparsity of rough endoplasmic reticulum. Note the presence of lipid droplets (*arrows*). The lower high power view is a detail of the boxed area in one of the cells, showing numerous vesicles of variable size, a centriole (C) and microtubules (MC). A few strands of rough endoplasmic reticulum (rer) are present in addition to the numerous ribosomes. (*upper × 8,400; lower × 25,000*)

**651**

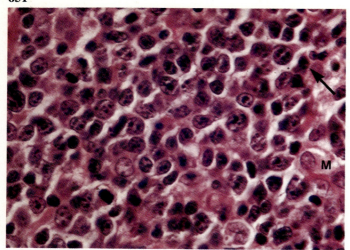

**651  Malignant lymphoma, diffuse lymphocytic poorly differentiated (lymphoblastic/centroblastic)** The majority of cells present the morphological features of germinal centre 'blast' cells (centroblasts). The nuclei are round, regular or slightly indented. The chromatin is evenly distributed with some nuclear accentuation and most of the cells show the presence of three or more nucleoli often in association with the nuclear membrane, The cytoplasm is scanty in amount but clearly delineated and evenly distributed around the nuclei. There are also more conventional 'lymphoblasts' with centrally placed nucleoli and small irregularly nucleated follicle lymphocytes (*arrow*) and there are occasional macrophages (M). *(H&E)*

**652**

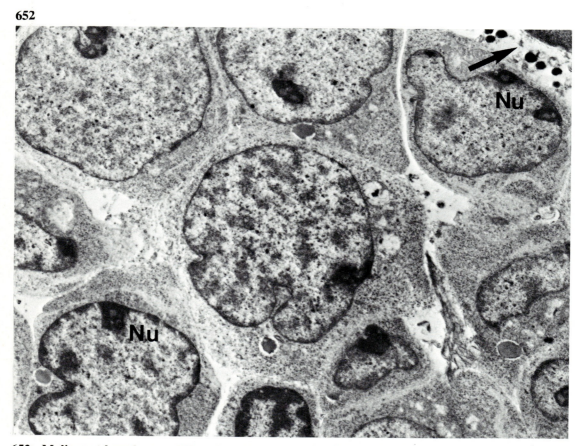

**652  Malignant lymphoma, diffuse lymphocytic poorly differentiated (lymphoblastic/centroblastic), ultrastructure** This lymphoma was abdominal and poorly fixed. Nevertheless the tumour cells show the features of medium sized to large lymphoblasts or centroblasts with single or several nucleoli (Nu), mainly in association with the nuclear margin. The nuclear chromatin, in the rounded or indented nuclei, is dispersed but not to such an extent as in immunoblasts. The cytoplasm is scanty but filled with ribosomes. The granulated cell (*arrow*) seen in the upper right corner is a reactive macrophage. A few small lymphocytes are also included in the field. *(× 8,400)*

**653**

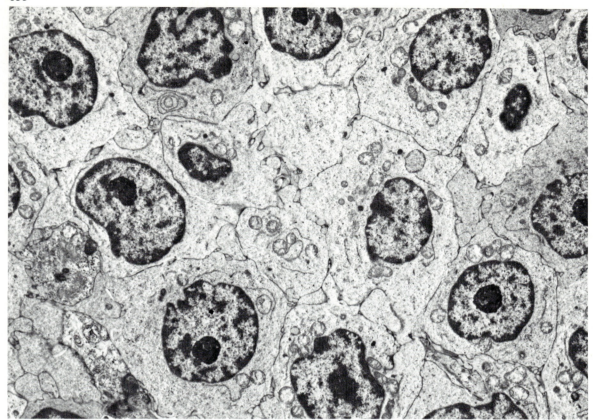

**653 Malignant lymphoma, diffuse lymphocytic, poorly differentiated (lymphoblastic), ultrastructure**
This lymphoma was involving abdominal lymph nodes, the patient having first presented with a cervical lymph node showing a follicular lymphoma of predominantly small cell type. The component cells have undergone 'blastic' transformation but are not centroblasts or immunoblasts. the nuclear chromatin still shows some aggregation and there are prominent single central nucleoli. The cytoplasm is relatively abundant and contains only a modicum of rough endoplasmic reticulum. Between some lymphoma cells can be seen processes of dendritic reticulum cells. *(× 3,950)*

**654** **655**

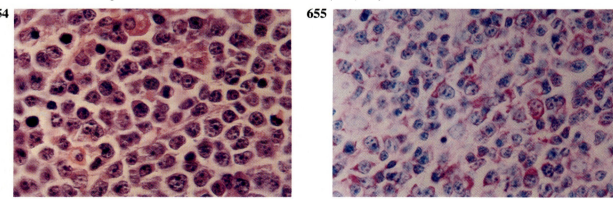

**654 and 655 Malignant lymphoma, diffuse lymphocytic poorly differentiated (lymphoblastic), with plasma cell differentiation** In this gut lymphoma the infiltrating cells show a range of appearances, **654**. There are lymphoblasts and larger cells with a round regular nucleus, coarsely clumped chromatin and the presence of an easily visualised central nucleoli in addition to plasma cells. The cytoplasm of the larger cells (plasmablasts) is more abundant and shows the presence of a perinuclear hof. This lymphoma is an example of a poorly differentiated lymphocytic lymphoma with plasmoblastic and plasmacytic differentiation. Figure **655** illustrates the pyroninophilia of the lymphoid cells and emphasises the perinuclear hofs.
*(654 H&E; 655 MGP)*

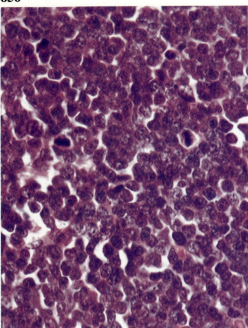
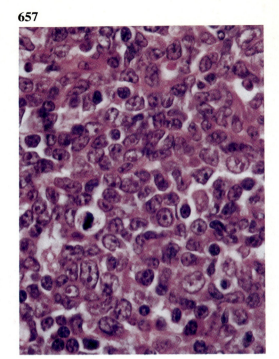

**656 and 657    Malignant lymphoma, diffuse lymphocytic poorly differentiated (lymphoblastic)** A number of tumours are included in this category, some of which are morphologically consistent with a B-cell origin but which show a somewhat different appearance from Burkitt or Burkitt-like lymphomas, lymphomas of obvious follicle centre origin and poorly differentiated lymphocytic lymphomas with plasmacytic differentiation. Such tumours may also lack T- or B-lymphocytic markers. They are most common in childhood. These two examples show tumours composed of non-cohesive lymphoid cells which lack a tingeable body macrophage component. Figure **656** shows a lymphoma composed of relatively small CLL-like cells with rounded nuclei, a rather coarse nuclear chromatin pattern and inconspicuous nucleoli, but with prominent mitotic activity and a cytoplasm showing moderate pyroninophilia. Figure **657** shows a lymphoma from an African child which developed in the lymph nodes already involved by Kaposi's sarcoma. The actively proliferating cells are larger than in **656**, the nuclei are rather more irregular with a more dispersed chromatin, and the nucleoli are more prominent. The cytoplasm also is more abundant and there are occasional plasma cell forms. It is likely that this tumour is of follicle centre origin. *(H&E)*

**658    Malignant lymphoma, diffuse lympho-cytic poorly differentiated (lymphoblastic) and acute lymphoblastic leukaemia (ALL)** ALL is usually diagnosed on clinical (including haematological) data. There are occasions, however, when it may be difficult to distinguish in a blood preparation ALL cells from cells exfoliated into the bloodstream from a poorly differentiated (lymphoblastic) lymphoma, as shown here. The cells have rounded or slightly indented nuclei, the nucleoli are conspicuous, and the cytoplasm appears as a thin bluish rim. *(May-Grünwald-Giemsa)*

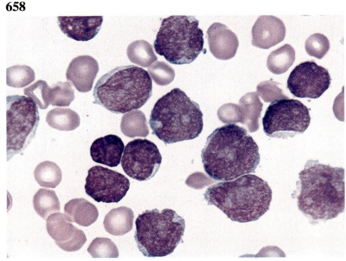

**659** **Acute lymphoblastic leukaemia** Acute lympho-cytic leukaemias have been shown by rosette tech-niques (see **860**) to consist of three types: those derived from B-lymphocytes (the minority), those of T-lymphocytic type (about 25 per cent), and most commonly (70 per cent) those composed of cells lacking any detectable surface markers. How-ever, with specific anti-T serum some of these ap-parently null cells have been redefined as of T-cell origin. Nevertheless, null cell ALL, which may be a stem cell leukaemia, is still the commonest form of ALL. When lymph nodes are involved in ALL it is difficult on purely morphological grounds to distinguish it from a lymphoblastic leukaemia. This is such an example. The lymph node was completely replaced by proliferating lymphoblasts. There is some cohesion of cells but an absence of tingeable body macrophages. *(H&E)*

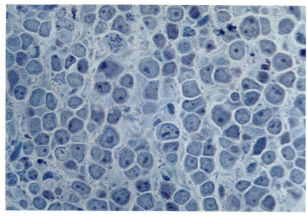

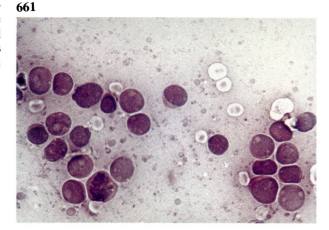

**660 and 661 Acute lymphoblastic leukaemia** Semi-thin sections of plastic processed material, **660**, show better cellular detail. The tumour cells show a greater range in size from small to medium sized lymphocytes and nucleoli are prominent in the generally rounded nuclei. There are no nuclear features to suggest a T-cell origin and imprint pre-parations, **661**, of the ALL cells did not show the presence of acid phosphatase activity. Note the cell in mitoses and the large nucleoli. Marker studies identified the cells as of null-cell type (common ALL). *(**660** Toluidine blue; **661** H&E imprint)*

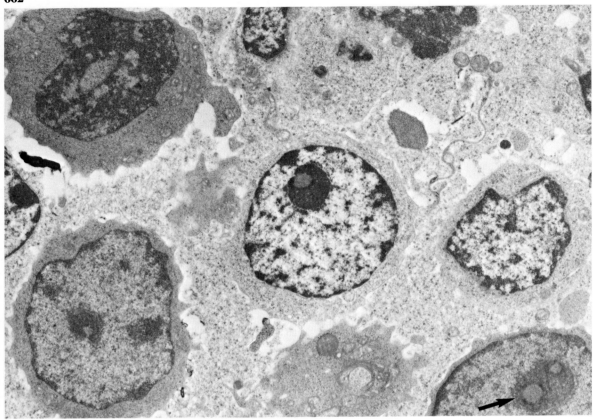

**662   Acute lymphoblastic leukaemia, ultrastructure** The rounded nuclear contour of the poorly differentiated lymphoid cells in **659–661** is confirmed and the large often centrally placed nucleoli which include ring forms (*arrow*) are accentuated. The cytoplasm lacks rough endoplasmic reticulum and lysosomes, and is filled with free RNA mostly in single form. *(× 8,100)*

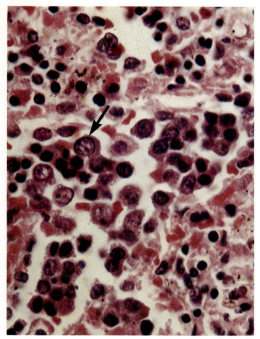

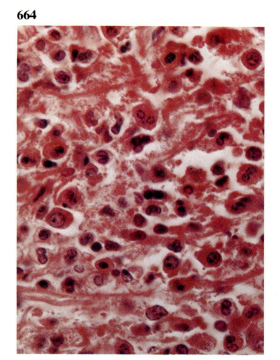

**663 and 664  Myeloid leukaemia** Diagnostic difficulties are encountered occasionally in differentiating tissues infiltrated by an acute myeloblastic leukaemia, **663**. It is however nearly always possible to identify a few granulocytic cells (*arrow*) which will also show chloroacetate esterase positivity (see **857a**). Figure **664** shows an area from another myeloid leukaemia in which there is the helpful finding of eosinophil and eosinophil precursors. *(H&E)*

**665  Extramedullary erythropoiesis** Another diagnostic problem, usually seen in spleen as shown here, can be a florid extramedullary erythropoiesis. The proliferating cells usually occur in groups and in addition to lymphocytic and granulocytic precursors nucleated red cells can be readily identified. Not shown here but of extreme diagnostic usefulness is the presence of megakaryocytes. *(H&E)*

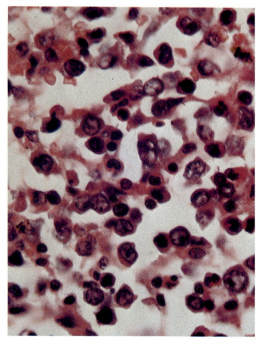

**666** **Malignant lymphoma, diffuse lympho-cytic poorly differentiated (lymphoblastic), convoluted cell type** Convoluted lympho-cytic lymphomas are a recently defined entity which affects males more often than females. They arise most commonly in the mediastinum (thymus) and may be associated with an acute lymphocytic leukaemic-like picture, either from the start of the disease or developing during the course of the illness. Unlike ALL of childhood, convoluted cell lymphomas are most common around puberty and they are rarer than other types of lymphoblastic lymphoma. Marker and histochemical studies have defined them as of T-lymphocytic origin. This example was from an 11-year-old child with massive involvement of the

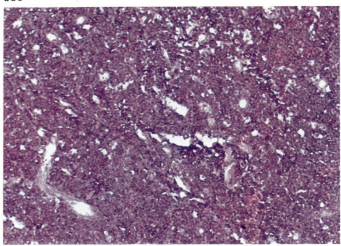

**666**

thymus and mediastinum, with direct extension of the tumour into the neck. The response to treatment with prednisone was dramatic and characteristic. *(H&E)*

**667**

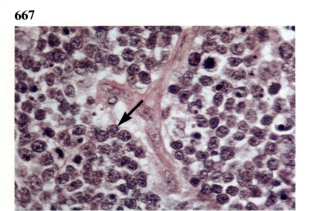

**668**

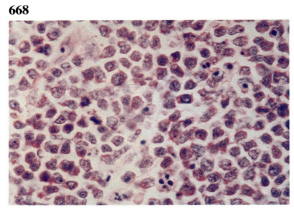

**667 and 668** **Malignant lymphoma, diffuse lymphocytic poorly differentiated (lymphoblastic), convoluted cell type** At this magnification it can be seen that the small to medium sized lymphoid cells in the vicinity of a small vessel are non-cohesive, being well separated from one another, **667**. The nuclei are generally rounded in shape – though some show an irregular cerebroid or convoluted contour – and finely dispersed chromatin. The presence of strands of chromatin intersecting the nucleus produces in a few cells the appearance of the imprint of a chicken's foot *(arrow)*. Note the considerable mitotic activity and the presence of pyknotic cells and a few reactive macrophages. Figure **668** emphasises the sparsity of cytoplasm which is only moderately pyroninophilic, and the inconspicuous nucleoli. *(667 H&E; 668 MGP)*

**669** **Malignant lymphoma, lymphocytic poorly differentiated (lymphoblastic), convoluted cell type, semi-thin section** Plastic embedding of T-cell tumours is a good method by which the cerebroid or convoluted nature of the malignant lymphocytes can be visualised. The nuclei never appear, however, as irregular as those of the cutaneous T-cell lymphomas (see **842**), though they do share with them the presence of focal tartrate labile acid phosphatase activity. *(Toluidine blue)*

**669**

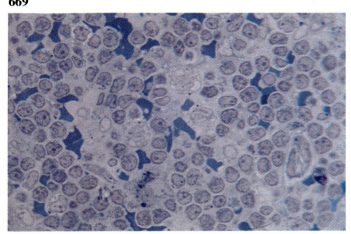

**670**

**671**

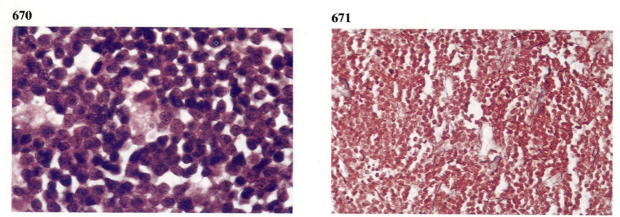

**670 and 671   Malignant lymphoma, diffuse lymphocytic poorly differentiated (lymphoblastic), convoluted cell type** In this example of a lymph node in a young boy with a mediastinal tumour, **670**, the infiltrating cells are more monomorphous and less obviously convoluted – though it is still possible to recognised a few 'chicken foot' cells. A very useful feature shown by silver impregnation techniques, **671**, is the very sparse and fine reticulin fibre content in this group of lymphomas. It is in this type of lymphoblastic lymphoma that there may be some retention of normal architecture in the early stages of lymph node involvement and, again, reticulin stains are useful. *(670 H&E; 671 Gordon & Sweets)*

**672   Malignant lymphoma, diffuse lymphocytic poorly differentiated (lymphoblastic), non-convoluted T-cell type, ultrastructure** Not all proven T-cell lymphoblastic lymphomas demonstrate nuclear convolutions at light microscopical level: a fact which is becoming increasingly recognised. The ultrastructural appearances of such a lymphoma of thymic origin shown to be of T-cell type on the basis of marker studies is shown here. Only occasional nuclei show some irregularity, most being ovoid with broad indentations. The nuclear chromatin is dispersed and two nucleoli (Nu) are included. In this field no lysosomal structures are evident. *(× 9,400)*

**672**

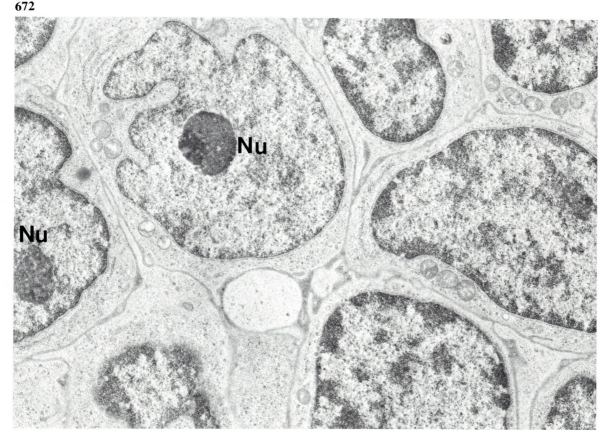

**673 Malignant lymphoma, diffuse poorly
differentiated (lymphoblastic), convoluted
cell type** The distinction between a T-cell
acute lymphoblastic leukaemia and a T-cell
lymphoblastic convoluted lymphoma may be
impossible since the morphology is often
identical, and in both conditions there may
be partial preservation of the architecture of
involved lymph nodes. Equally, in some
cases, although the neoplastic lymphoid cells
(seen here infiltrating bone marrow in an
infant) show the typical appearances of
convoluted cells most apparent in the larger
cells (*arrow*), marker studies have failed to
confirm their T-cell nature. (*H&E*)

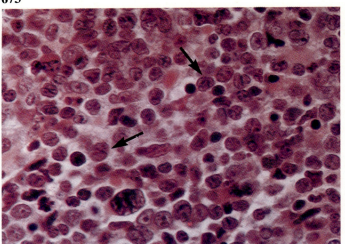

**674 Malignant lymphoma, lymphocytic poorly differentiated (lymphoblastic), convoluted cell type, ultra-
structure** Three deeply folded or cerebroid nuclei of the non-cohesive cells are seen here. Ribosomes in the
form of polyribosomes may be very numerous and there are also a few profiles of rough endoplasmic
reticulum. A few electron dense lysosomal structures are present; these tend to be most numerous in the
Golgi zones (not shown here). Same case as **666**. (× *8,400*)

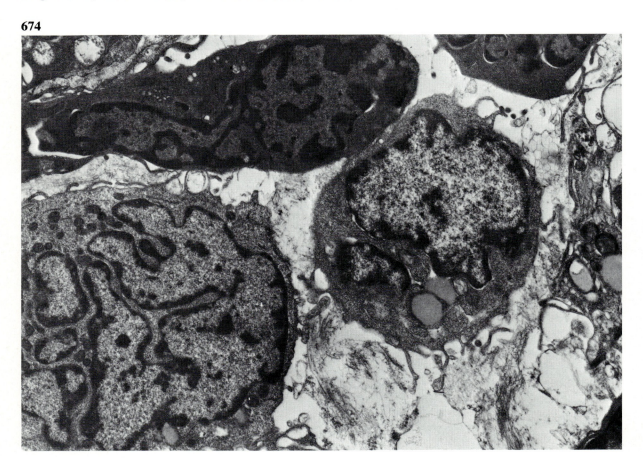

**675 Malignant lymphoma, diffuse lymphocytic poorly differentiated (lymphoblastic) T-cell type without convolutions**
As already stated there is a group of poorly differentiated or lymphoblastic lymphomas which lack nuclear convolutions or a 'chicken foot' appearance but which have been interpreted as of T-cell largely on the basis of focal acid phosphatase positivity. In this lymph node the tumour cells are medium sized and discrete, and contain round, ovoid or indented nuclei with a very finely dispersed or granular heterochromatin and small inconspicuous nucleoli numbering from one to five. The cytoplasm consists of a narrow rim showing moderate pyroninophilia. Other lymphomas of a similar appearance lack even acid phosphatase activity, and are best categorised as poorly differentiated lymphocytic or lymphoblastic lymphomas of undesignated type. Bone marrow involvement and a leukaemic blood picture are common, and there is an overlap with ALL of null type with tissue involvement. *(H&E)*

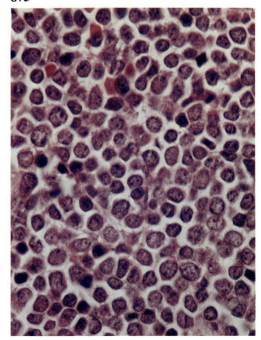

## Lymphocytic lymphoma, mixed small and large cell type (mixed follicle cell)

The term mixed lymphoma is restricted in the BNLI classification to tumours composed only of mixtures of small and large follicle centre cells, which thus are viewed as the diffuse counterpart of the mixed follicular lymphomas. Mixed lymphomas are not mixed, therefore, in the sense of containing cells of different origin. The large follicle centre cell component ranges from 30–60 per cent of the total. With more numerous large follicle centre cells, which may be of either regular or irregular nucleated type, the lymphoma is classified as a large (lymphoid) cell lymphoma. Like other B-cell lymphomas they may also show plasmacytoid differentiation. Lymphomas showing a mixed appearance due to the presence of reactive cellular elements, such as Lennert's lymphoma, **687**, are excluded by definition. One of the few differences in categorisation of the non-Hodgkin's lymphomas shown by the BNLI classification and Stanford formulation is the acceptance by the latter of lymphomas containing reactive histiocytic elements within the mixed category. True mixed lymphomas are uncommon in lymph nodes, forming only 2·4 per cent in the BNLI series. Like their follicular lymphoma counterpart they occur predominantly in the elderly, though their prognosis is generally worse. However, they appear to have a better prognosis than the large (immunoblastic) lymphoid cell tumours, plasma cell lymphomas and histiocytic lymphomas.

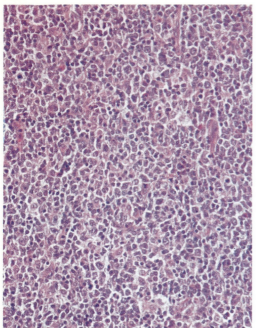

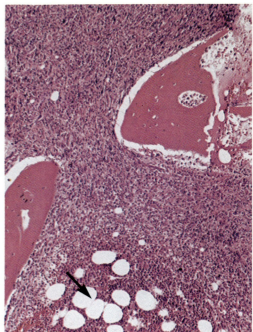

**676 and 677  Malignant lymphoma, diffuse lymphocytic mixed small and large cell (mixed follicle cells)** A mixed lymphoma is now believed to represent the diffuse counterpart of a follicular lymphoma of mixed cell type and therefore is composed of mixtures of large and small follicle centre type lymphocytes, resulting in a pleomorphic appearance which is apparent even at low magnification. The term 'mixed lymphoma' should not be used to describe a lymphoma in which there are reactive lymphocytes or reactive histiocytes, or both, and which can also result in a pleomorphic appearance. Figure **676** shows a nodal mixed cell lymphoma; and **677** shows a bone marrow deposit adjacent to an area of uninvolved marrow (*arrow*). *(H&E)*

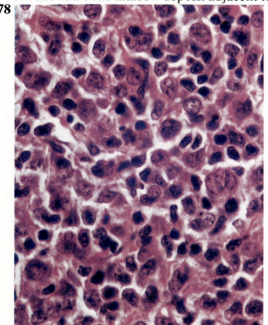

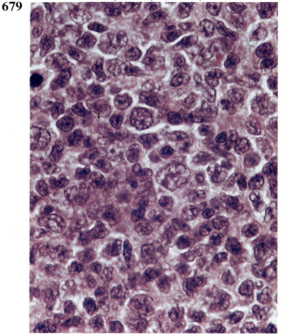

**678 and 679  Malignant lymphoma, diffuse lymphocytic mixed small and large cell (mixed follicle cell)** As in the diffuse lymphoma of intermediate type, lymph node architecture is generally completely effaced. The proportion of large to small cells is variable and usually falls within the range of 30–60 per cent of the total. Figure **678** shows a typical mixture of small irregularly nucleated cells and large lymphoid cells of both regular and irregular (large cleaved cells, large centrocytes) nucleated type; **679** shows the effects of poor fixation, which produces an even more marked irregularity of nuclei and vacuolation of cytoplasm. *(H&E)*

**680a**

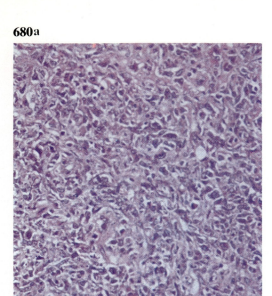

**680b**

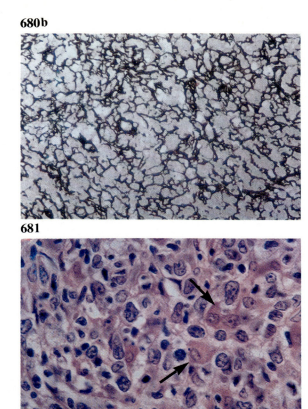

**681**

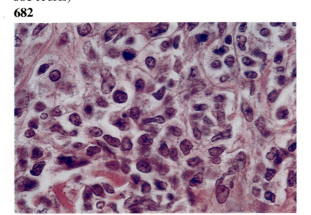

**680a, 680b and 681  Malignant lymphoma, diffuse lymphocytic mixed small and large cell (mixed follicle cell)** Banded fibrosis is sometimes a feature, but more typically there may be a diffuse fine sclerosis, **680a**, which can result in a somewhat packeted appearance with silver impregnation techniques, **680b**. The diagnostic difficulty then arises as to whether the lymphoma truly represents a mixed or a histiocytic lymphoma – since the latter type may also show a diffuse, fine sclerosis. Helpful distinguishing features from histiocytes, malignant or reactive, as in **681** (*arrows*), are the less abundant cytoplasm, less vesicular nuclei and the more peripherally placed nucleoli of the large irregularly nucleolated follicle centre lymphocytes, and the invariable presence of small intermediate lymphocytes and large regularly nucleated 'blasts'. In lymph nodes eosinophils and necrosis are usually absent. (**680a** *H&E;* **680b** *Gordon & Sweets;* **681** *H&E)*

**682**

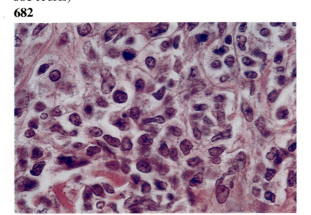

**683**

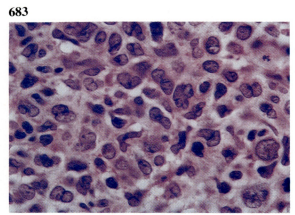

**682 and 683  Malignant lymphoma, diffuse lymphocytic mixed small and large cell (mixed follicle cells)**
These uncommon tumours may arise in extra nodal sites: **682** shows a mixed cell lymphoma arising in the gastrointestinal tract. The helpful feature of an absence of eosinophils, does not always hold in this location where eosinophils, together with plasma cells and proliferating fibroblasts, frequently accompany the neoplastic proliferation, causing an even more pleomorphic appearance. Tumours at this site are often poorly fixed. Diagnosis on morphological grounds must then depend solely on the recognition of both small irregular and large irregular follicle centre type cells in addition to larger immunoblast type cells. Figure **683** shows a mixed lymphoma presenting as a localised skin tumour. *(H&E)*

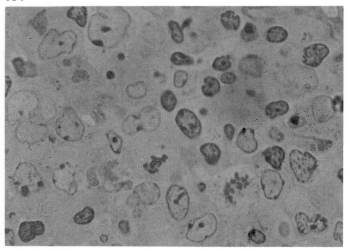

**684 Malignant lymphoma, diffuse lymphocytic mixed small and large cell type (mixed follicle cells) – semi-thin section** Processing through plastic greatly facilitates the recognition of mixed lymphomas. The mixture of follicle centre type cells shown here in a diffuse lymphoma are indistinguishable from those of a follicular lymphoma of mixed cell type. Note the finely dispersed nuclear chromatin of the large cells and the affinity of many nucleoli to the nuclear margins. *(Toluidine blue)*

685

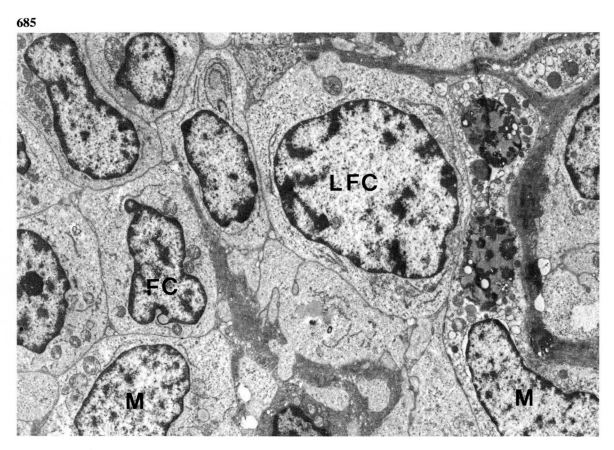

**685 Malignant lymphoma, diffuse lymphocytic mixed small and large cell type (mixed follicle cells), ultrastructure** In this low power electron micrograph of a mixed lymphoma involving testis, the lymphoid cells range from small follicle cells (FC) to large follicle cells (LFC). Parts of two macrophages (M) are included, one with phagocytic material. *(× 4,800)*

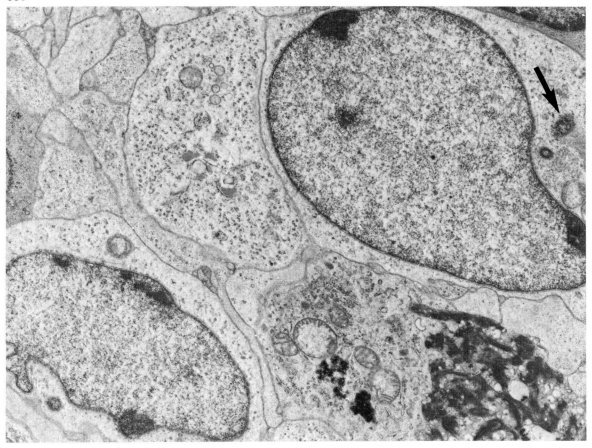

**686 Malignant lymphoma, diffuse lymphocytic mixed small and large cell type (mixed follicle cells), ultrastructure** The large irregularly nucleated or cleaved lymphocytes show the presence of coarse nuclear indentations and protrusions, finely dispersed nuclear chromatin, and peripheral nucleoli which show a tendency to be associated with the nuclear protrusions. The cytoplasm contains fewer ribosomes and polyribosomes than immunoblasts or centroblasts and rough endoplasmic reticulum is very scanty. As in the diffuse lymphoma of intermediate type, processes of dendritic cells may be seen in between the follicle centre type population. The upper cell contains a centriole (*arrow*). (× 8,750)

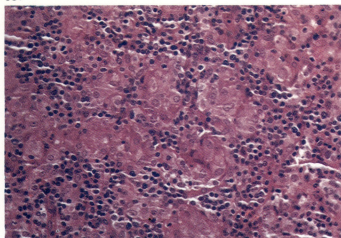

**687 Lennert's lymphoma (lymphoma with high epithelioid cell content)** Certain lymphomas, particularly diffuse lymphocytic well differentiated with or without plasma cell differentiation, and large lymphoid cell (immunoblastic) lymphomas may contain large numbers of epithelioid cells. The importance of this finding is in not allocating tumours with this cellular combination to the mixed *or* histiocytic lymphoma categories, and in recognising the neoplastic nature of the lymphoid cells between the reactive epithelioid cells. *(H&E)*

# Diffuse lymphoma, large (lymphoid) cell

Like the majority of non-Hodgkin's lymphomas, a large cell lymphoma predominantly occurs in the elderly and is often widely disseminated at the time of presentation. It is not a morphologically homogeneous entity. The majority however approximate to the immunoblast, few being composed solely of large irregularly nucleated (cleaved) cells. Most of these tumours represent the 'histiocytic' lymphoma of Rappaport, and in the old terminology they formed the majority of the reticulum cell sarcomas. The group as a whole forms a significant proportion of the non-Hodgkin's lymphomas (23 per cent) and the majority are of poor prognosis – though recent studies have indicated that those composed of large follicle centre type cells behave in a more benign fashion. For this reason the Stanford formulation separates them into two prognostic categories – a large cell type showing features of follicle centre cells being placed in the intermediate prognostic category, and the immunoblastic type of B- or T-cell origin in the high grade category. In practice, this separation is not always easy or possible on morphological grounds alone.

On the basis of marker studies approximately 50 per cent are null and of the remainder, the majority are B-lymphocytic rather than T-lymphocytic type. However, newer T-cell entities such as the pleomorphic leukaemic T-cell lymphoma (adult T-cell leukaemia) and some of the T-zone lymphomas (Kiel) have been defined recently. Plasma cell differentiation is quite common in the B-lymphocytic type and in those composed of large follicle centre cells, the presence of fine sclerosis may be prominent and can lead to confusion with a histiocytic lymphoma.

On the basis of their *morphological* features they may be separated into five main groups:

1 Predominantly large regularly nucleated lymphoid cells (B- or T-immunoblasts, centroblasts). Those showing a rather clear cytoplasm are likely to be of T-lymphocytic type (see **699**)

2 Large regularly nucleated lymphoid cells (B-immunoblasts, centroblasts) with evident plasma cell differentiation

3 Large irregularly nucleated follicle centre (large cleaved) cells

4 Mixtures of large regularly and irregularly nucleated follicle centre cells
Groups 3 and 4 may also show plasma cell differentiation but this feature is seldom so pronounced as in group 2.

5 Large 'undifferentiated' cells thought to be lymphoid in origin but with few distinguishing features

Inevitably some true histiocytic and other large cell tumours of lymph node origin will be included in the large lymphoid cell category. Another source of confusion is provided by anaplastic carcinomas and amelanotic melanomas.

**688 and 689  Malignant lymphoma, diffuse large cell type** This heterogeneous group of tumours which consists mainly of neoplasms composed of large lymphoid cells, may occur at any age but are most common in the elderly. They are important because they form a significant proportion of the non-Hodgkin's lymphomas, are aggressive in behaviour and often have disseminated widely at the time of presentation. In lymph nodes, **688**, effacement of architecture is complete and there is replacement with a monomorphous population of large cells, among which there are a few residual small lymphocytes. Figure **689** shows bone marrow involvement by a large cell lymphoma with the morphological features of immunoblasts. Mitotic activity is marked and there is no reactive or residual cellular component. *(H&E)*

**688**

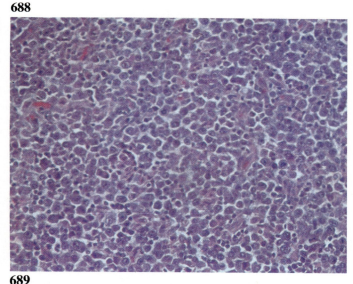

**689**

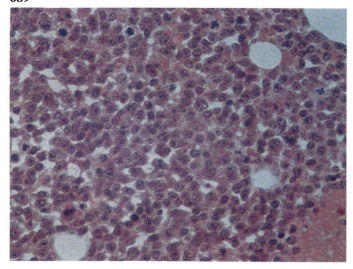

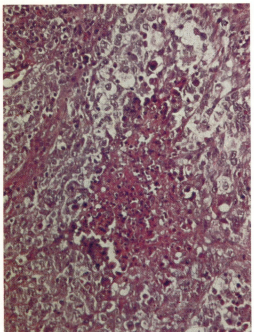

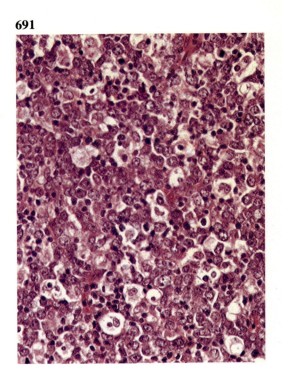

**690 and 691   Malignant lymphoma, diffuse large lymphoid cell** A characteristic of this group of tumours as a whole is the tendency for it to undergo necrosis. The areas of necrosis may be quite extensive as in **690** or may be small and focal. Mitotic activity is prominent, and a not infrequent finding, **691**, is the appearance of a 'starry sky' due to the presence of numerous reactive tingeable body macrophages. *(H&E)*

**692 Malignant lymphoma, diffuse large lymphoid cell** The cytoplasm of these large lymphoid cells is markedly pyroninophilic due to the high content of free RNA (see **697**, **698**) and is not abundant in relation to the nuclear size. *(MGP)*

**692**

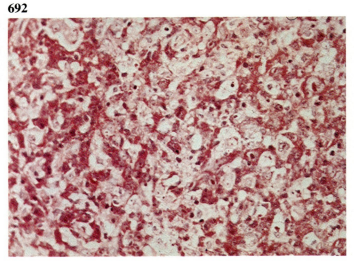

**693**

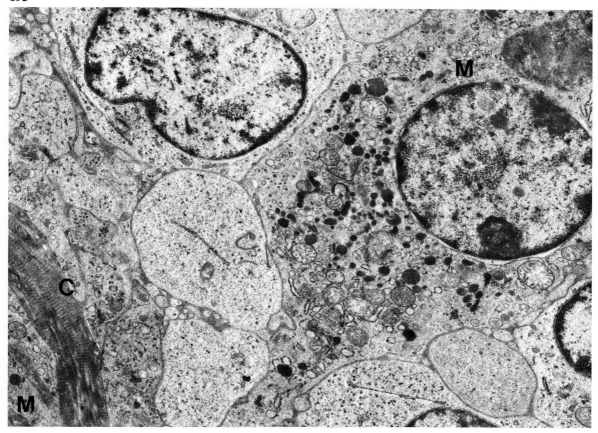

**693  Malignant lymphoma, diffuse large lymphoid cell, ultrastructure** There may be large numbers of tingeable body macrophages, and also other macrophages and histiocytes in intimate contact with the tumour cells may be very numerous and lead to diagnostic confusion with a histiocytic lymphoma. Two such reactive macrophages (M) are seen here, one lying between parts of four large lymphoid cells, and the other below the long-spacing collagen (C). *(× 8,650)*

**694**

**695**

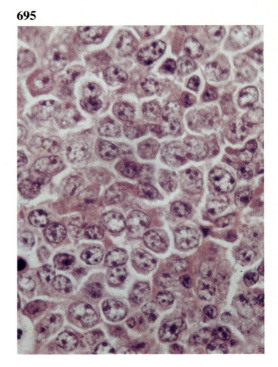

**694 and 695  Malignant lymphoma, diffuse large lymphoid cell regularly nucleated type** Both of these examples show large lymphoid cells with nuclei that are generally round or ovoid and larger in volume than that of a normal histiocyte. The cells in **694** approximate to immunoblasts; nuclear chromatin is dispersed but shows peripheral accentuation and the large prominent nucleoli are situated either centrally or at the nuclear membrane. The cytoplasm is somewhat variable in amount but is not abundant in relation to nuclear size and the cytoplasmic boundaries are well defined. Scattered throughout are small differentiated lymphocytes. Figure **695** shows large lymphoid cells with the nuclear features of centroblasts, which are not quite so large as immunoblasts and contain several peripheral nucleoli. *(H&E)*

**696**

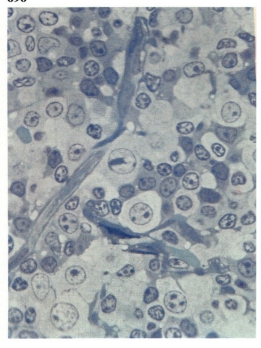

**696  Malignant lymphoma, diffuse large lymphoid cell (regularly nucleated type) semi-thin section** Plastic processing is very helpful in defining the morphological characteristics of the large lymphoid cells of both immunoblastic and centroblastic type since preservation of cellular detail is usually optimum. The nucleoli are darkly stained and stand out strongly against the pale background of the nuclei, and the cytoplasm is well defined. A number of small residual lymphocytes are intermingled with the large lymphoid cells. *(Toluidine blue)*

697

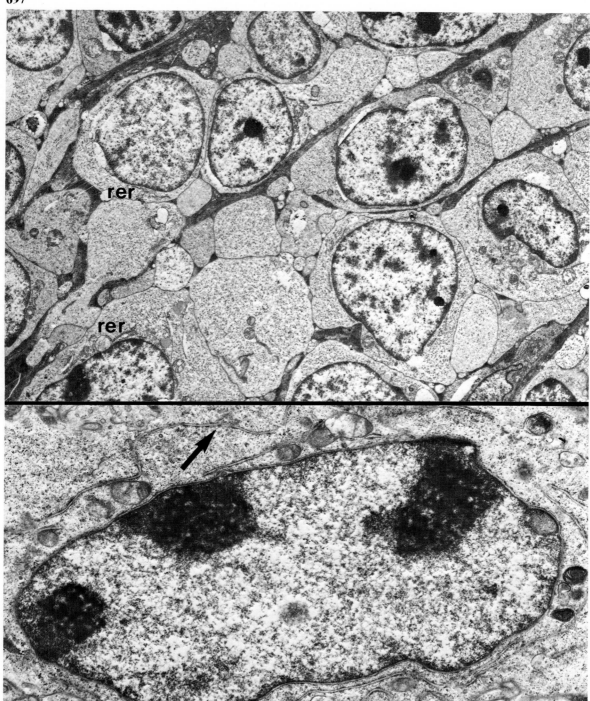

698

**697 and 698  Malignant lymphoma, diffuse large lymphoid cell (regularly nucleated type), ultrastructure** These are representative electronmicrographs from two large regularly nucleated lymphoid cell tumours. Figure **697** shows a lymphoma in which the individual cells contain rounded or only slightly indented nuclei, a finely dispersed nuclear chromatin and large nucleoli which are either central or situated at the nuclear membrane. The well-defined cytoplasm contains abundant ribosomes (the basis for the pyroninophilia exhibited by these cells) but rough endoplasmic reticulum (rer) is extremely sparse. Note the presence of electron dense material between the cells. Figure **698** shows a typical cell from a predominantly centroblastic type of large cell tumour. The nuclei may be ovoid as shown here, or rounded, but the distinctive feature is the nuclear appearance with the several peripheral nucleoli applied to the nuclear margin. The cytoplasm is rich in ribosomes – single or grouped – and there are a few strands of rough endoplasmic reticulum (*arrow*). (**697** × *4,150;* **698** × *21,000*)

**699**

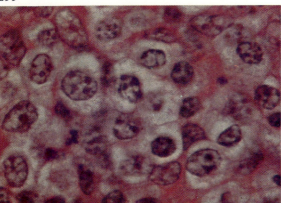

**699 Malignant lymphoma, diffuse large lymphoid cell (regularly nucleated of possible T-cell type)** In less well-fixed preparations the nuclear shape appears much more varied and the cytoplasm is often very poorly visualised. It is possible, therefore, that some tumours placed in the large lymphoid cell category may represent malignancies of other types, such as the histiocytic lymphomas or metastatic carcinoma, since in the absence of special techniques it is not always possible to achieve a definitive diagnosis. In this example the nuclei are well-defined and 'blastic' but the cyto-plasm is more abundant and unusually clear. Tumours composed of this type of immunoblast are likely to be of T-cell origin. There may or may not be complete destruction of architecture and some T-cell lymphomas have a very pleo-morphic appearance (see also **791**, **792**). *(H&E)*

**701**

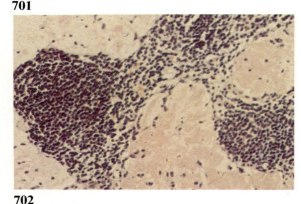

**702**

**700**

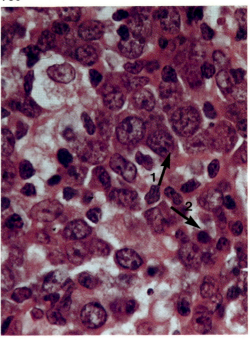

**700 Malignant lymphoma, diffuse large lymphoid cell (regularly nucleated type with plasma cell differentiation)** The infiltrating large cells in this lymph node show plasma-cytoid differentiation. Many of the nuclei are slightly eccentric; there is a suggestion of a perinucleus halo in some *(arrow 1)* and the cytoplasm is darkly staining. There are also a few smaller plasma cells *(arrow 2)*. *(H&E)*

**701 and 702 Malignant lymphoma, diffuse large lymphoid cell (regularly nucleated type with plasma cell differentiation)** The spleen is rarely the primary site of involve-ment in the non-Hodgkin's lymphomas, though it is frequently involved during the course of the disease. Any type of lymphoma may occur but, as in lymph nodes, the majority are B-cell lymphomas. In this example the spleen was the primary site of a large cell lymphoma associated with the production of IgM. The abdominal nodes showed no evidence of lymphoma but many, **701**, showed the presence within sinuses of pink proteinaceous material (negative for amyloid). The splenic tumour cells in **702** in a semi-thin plastic section are very large and plasmacytoid with prominent nucleoli and cytoplasm in which there are more densely staining areas *(arrow)*. *(**701** H&E; **702** Toluidine blue)*

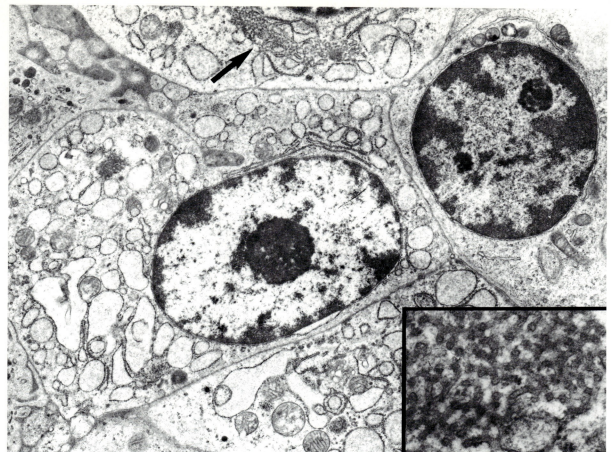

**703 Malignant lymphoma, diffuse large lymphoid cell (regularly nucleated type with plasma cell differentiation), ultrastructure** These are representative cells of the lymphoma in **702**. The central nucleus is of plasmablastic type and its cytoplasm, together with that of neighbouring cells, is filled with dilated rough endoplasmic reticulum containing moderately electron dense granular material (immunoglobulin). Following splenectomy there was disappearance of the monoclonal IgM. The upper cell (*arrow*) contains a tubular profile seen in greater magnification in the *inset*. Such tubular profiles were related to the rough endoplasmic reticulum and were a very striking feature in this lymphoma. They bear a distinct morphologic resemblance to some animal RNA virus-associated structures. (× 9,650; inset × 42,000)

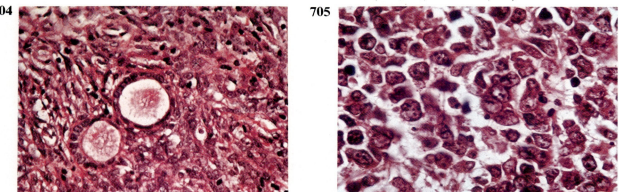

**704 and 705   Malignant lymphoma, diffuse large lymphoid cell (regularly and irregularly nucleated types)** Large cell lymphomas composed almost exclusively of the large irregularly nucleated follicle centre lymphocytes (large cleaved cells, large centrocytes) occur as in this ovarian lymphoma, **704**. Others are composed of mixtures of large regular and irregularly nucleated follicle centre lymphocytes, **705**. They are important to recognise since current experience suggests that large cell lymphomas of evident follicular centre origin are associated with a better response to treatment. When they show fine sclerosis it may be difficult to separate them from the well differentiated histiocytic group of lymphomas. The two round structures in **704** are primordial follicles. *(H&E)*

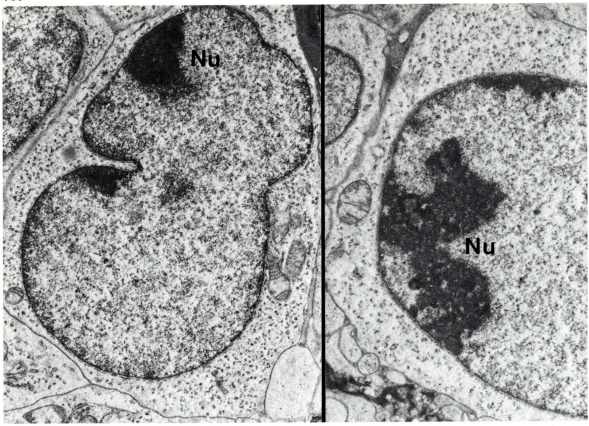

**706 Malignant lymphoma, diffuse large lymphoid cell (regularly and irregularly nucleated type), ultra-structure** The ultrastructural appearance of the large irregularly nucleated follicle centre lymphocytes (shown on the left) is in every way similar to those seen in the follicular lymphomas and in the mixed cell lymphomas. Note the tendency for the nucleoli (Nu) to be situated at the nuclear membrane. The cell on the right is a developing immunoblast with a very large single nucleolus (Nu) at the nuclear margin. Both cells show an absence of rough endoplasmic reticulum and numerous polyribosomes. *(× 11,500)*

**707**

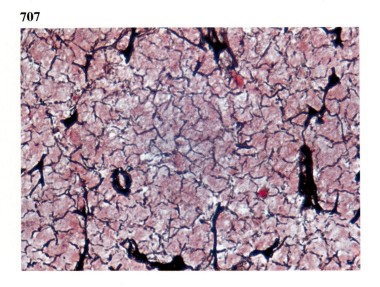

**707 Malignant lymphoma, diffuse large lymphoid cell** The amount of reticulin fibre is very variable. In some there is a virtual absence but in others there is sometimes abundant reticulin which appears to enclose groups of cells and even single cells – an appearance which in the past led to the concept of reticulin production by the tumour cells and, hence, the term reticulum cell sarcoma. *(Gordon & Sweets)*

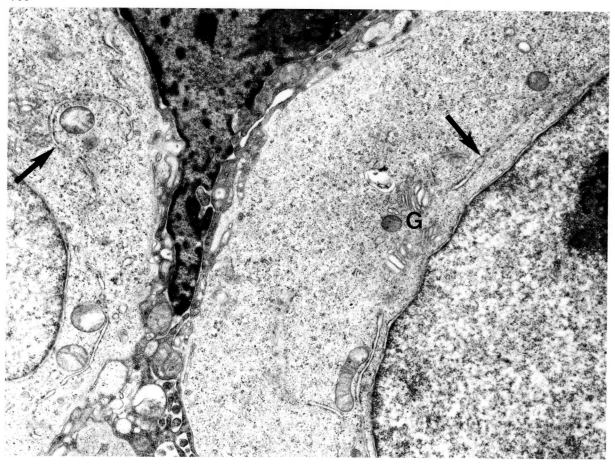

**708 Malignant lymphoma, diffuse large lymphoid cell, ultrastructure** At ultrastructural level such reticulin-producing tumours show the presence of attenuated fibroblasts sandwiched between the large lymphoid cells. It is the fibroblasts which are responsible for the reticulin production. The cytoplasmic detail of the immunoblasts is visualised with great clarity. Note the abundant ribosomes either singly or as polyribosomes, the small Golgi apparatus (G) and the scanty rough endoplasmic reticulum (*arrows*) which shows no evidence of secretory products. *(× 22,320)*

## Plasma cell lymphomas (extramedullary plasmacytomas) and heavy chain diseases – in particular alpha-chain disease

Plasma cell lymphomas (extramedullary plasmacytomas) are generally regarded as being uncommon or rare. Even when this diagnosis is made such tumours have not been included formerly in any classification of the non-Hodgkin's lymphomas. In fact, plasma cell lymphomas are not so rare as is suggested by the literature and in certain sites, such as Waldeyer's ring and the gastro-intestinal tract, salivary gland, breast and testis, they are not infrequently encountered. Other sites at which plasma cell tumours have been recognised are the respiratory tract, skin and sub-cutaneous tissue, orbit and central nervous system. In the BNLI series, which excludes children, plasma cell lymphomas form less than 2 per cent of primary nodal non-Hodgkin's lymphomas, but their incidence rises when extra-nodal sites are included. Reasons for their apparent rarity include unfamiliarity with the less differentiated forms and failure to recognise them when they occur in extramedullary sites unless composed of mature plasma cells.

Plasma cell lymphomas on the basis of our studies may be divided into four types:

1 Well differentiated plasma cell tumours composed of mature plasma cells showing the classical eccentric nucleus with a well-developed perinuclear halo of hof. Such well differentiated plasmacytic lymphomas present the least diagnostic difficulty but are uncommon in lymph nodes and spleen. It is only this type which is accepted as an extramedullary plasmacytoma in the Kiel classification. They are also, with the exception of alpha-chain disease, the least common type of plasma cell proliferation involving the gastrointestinal tract.

2 Lymphoplasmacytoid tumours which are composed of small lymphoid cells showing at light microscopical level the nuclear appearance of lymphocytes or plasma cells, but with a less abundant cytoplasm than that of mature plasma cells. Pyroninophilia is present, however, and at ultrastructural level the majority of cells show secretory activity. It is this type which is most frequently seen in association with primary Waldenström's macroglobulinaemia. In some classifications of lymphomas it is designated an immunocytoma of the lymphoplasmacytoid subtype (see **615 – 625**).

3 Plasmablastic plasma cell tumours composed *largely* of plasmablasts with variable numbers of differentiated plasma cells, immunoblasts and lymphocytes. These are also seldom recognised and usually are called lymphoblastic or poorly differentiated lymphocytic lymphomas or, if the cells are slightly larger, large lymphoid cell lymphomas or immunoblastic sarcomas.

4 Pleomorphic plasma cell tumours containing many multinucleated plasma cells in addition to varying numbers of differentiated and poorly differentiated plasma cells, lymphocytes and immunoblasts; these are likely to be called Hodgkin's disease, histiocytic lymphoma, reticulum cell sarcoma or immunoblastic sarcoma.

Some examples of our types 3 and 4 are categorised as the polymorphic variant of an LP immunocytoma (Kiel).

The well differentiated plasmacytic lymphomas and those of the lymphoplasmacytoid type (1 and 2) are considered to carry a relatively good prognosis in contrast to pleomorphic and plasmablastic tumours (3 and 4) which are high grade malignancy. Because of conceptual difficulties and reluctance to accept plasma cell lymphomas as forming one of the categories of the diffuse non-Hodgkin's lymphomas, the Stanford 'formulation' allocates them to the miscellaneous category. Lymph nodes may be involved in patients with multiple myelomatosis and the appearances are usually those of an infiltrate composed of well differentiated plasma cells, though plasmablastic and pleomorphic forms are recognised. In contrast to multiple myeloma, extramedullary plasma cell lymphomas other than those associated with Waldenström's macroglobulinaemia are rarely associated with paraprotein production on presentation; in this respect, they resemble the solitary plasmacytoma of bone.

Heavy chain diseases are a group of unusual plasma cell proliferative disorders characterised by the monoclonal production of the Fc fragment of the heavy chains of the different sub-classes of immunoglobulin. They are thus devoid of light chains. The three types so far recognised are alpha-chain disease, gamma-chain disease (Franklin's disease) and mu-chain disease. Of these, alpha-chain disease is by far the most common and, with rare exceptions, affects predominantly the alimentary tract. The patients are generally young adults who present with symptoms of severe malabsorption. Initially, the disease was thought to be confined to the Mediterranean areas and to form part of the spectrum of the so-called Mediterranean lymphoma. Since then, however, many cases have been described in patients of diverse geographical and ethnic origins from the Middle East, Greece, Southern Italy, South Africa and Bangladesh. Nevertheless, the majority of cases are still seen in patients of Sephardic Jewish origin. The clinical diagnosis is confirmed by the demonstration of the anomalous protein in serum, urine and sometimes duodenal juice and saliva, and the histological appearance of the small intestinal biopsy. In the early phase of the disease the plasma cell proliferation is confined to the lamina propria of the small intestine and can be arrested (temporarily) with broad spectrum antibiotics but, later, most patients so far documented have developed localised tumours throughout the gastrointestinal tract with a much more variable morphology. According to some workers the majority of these tumours are immunoblastic sarcomas. In our view they represent extramedullary plasmacytomas usually of types 3 and 4 (see above).

**709**

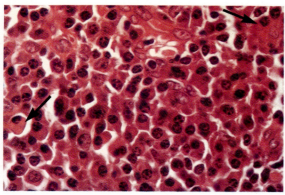

**710**

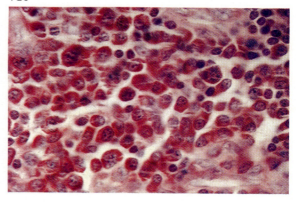

**709 Plasma cell (extramedullary) lymphoma well differentiated** Although rare in lymph nodes primary plasma cell tumours do occur but are seldom recognised unless composed of well differentiated (Marschalko-type) plasma cells. Furthermore, in some classifications of the non-Hodgkin's lymphomas only tumours composed entirely of *mature* plasma cells are accepted as examples of extramedullary plasmacytomas. This cervical lymph node was greatly enlarged and replaced with a population of mature and readily recognised plasma cells. Binucleate forms are not evident and mitotic activity was minimal. No circulating paraprotein was present and the bone marrow was uninvolved. Note the

retained cytoplasmic secretory products (*arrow*) resulting in a globular cytoplasmic appearance. *(H&E)*

**710 Plasma cell (extramedullary) lymphomas well differentiated** These are rather less rare in extranodal sites than lymph nodes. One such site is skin, when they may occur as single or multiple lesions. Generally, they are deeply located and extend down into the subcutis, often hugging closely the skin appendages. Here, the majority of the cells are well differentiated plasma cells but there are also some more immature forms. *(MGP)*

**711 and 712 Plasma cell (extramedullary) lymphoma well differentiated** The gastrointestinal tract is a not so uncommon site of plasma cell tumours. In this patient only the mesenteric nodes at laparotomy were found to be involved. The tumour cells were mature plasma cells and a common finding, **711**, was the eosinophilic crystalline inclusions present in a proportion of the cells. These crystals stain dark red with Masson's trichrome, (*arrow*), **712**, but were PAS negative indicating that the immunoglobulin is likely to be light chains. Toluidine blue stained plastic sections are another excellent method for visualising crystals, and other plasma cell features (see **843** or **844**). *(711 H&E; 712 Masson's trichrome)*

**711**

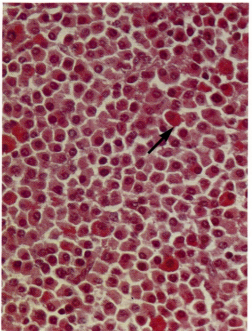

**712**

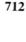

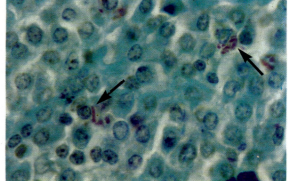

713

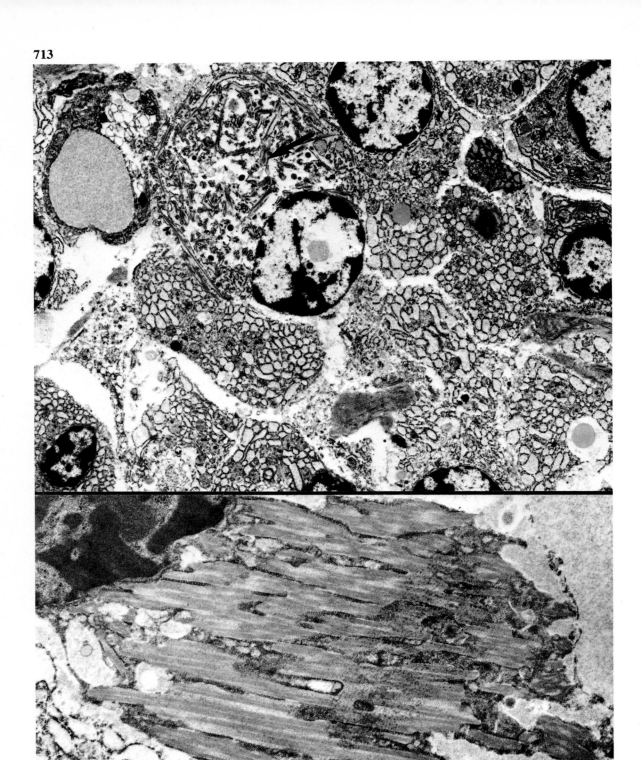

**713 Plasma cell (extramedullary) lymphomas well differentiated, ultrastructure** A large gastric tumour resected in an emergency had shown features diagnosed at light microscopical level as a 'lympho-sarcoma' on the basis of the nuclear appearances. At ultrastructural level, however, virtually all the cells are manifestly engaged in the production of immunoglobulin. The cytoplasm contains abundant rough endoplasmic reticulum and many dilated cisternae, some of which contain rod-shaped inclusions (*arrow*) which are seen at higher magnification to consist of crystals. Intranuclear inclusions or Dutcher bodies are also evident (see **623**). The immunoglobulin proved to be IgM. *(upper × 5,800; lower × 27,000)*

266

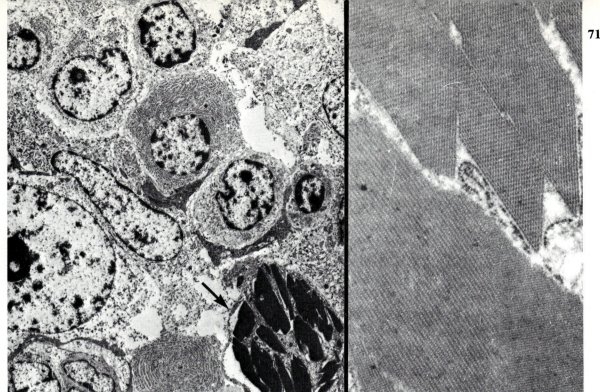

**714 Plasma cell (extramedullary) lymphomas well differentiated** In this gut lymphoma the majority of component cells are mature plasma cells, many of which showed intracytoplasmic crystals. At ultrastructural level the crystalline inclusions appear as electron dense spicules *(arrow)*, often filling the cytoplasm. The large cell to the left is an immunoblast. Despite delay in fixation and the use of formalin, cytological preservation is surprisingly good. The right-hand field shows the paracrystalline structure of the immunoglobulin with great clarity. *(right × 3,800; left × 37,000)*

**715 Multiple myeloma** The involvement of lymph nodes or other extra-nodal sites by multiple myelomatosis rarely provides a diagnostic problem. It generally occurs after the initial diagnosis has been made, and the infiltrating myeloma cells are usually well differentiated. Occasionally one encounters more primitive tumours, as in this patient treated for multiple myeloma (IgG), whose enlarging testis on excision showed a virtually pure infiltrate of plasmablasts. *(H&E)* **716 Multiple myeloma** Another problem hindering the recognition of plasma cell tumours – which of course applies to all tumours – is poor fixation. Shown here is a multiple myelomatous infiltrate in which the majority of cells seen in the upper field are very poorly preserved and their cytoplasm appears syncitial. *(H&E)*

**715**

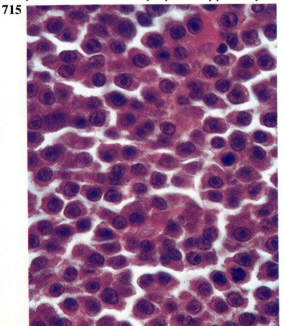

**716**

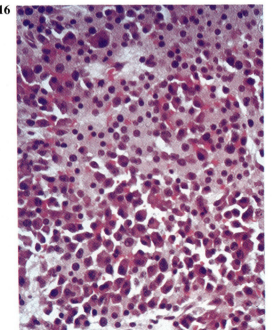

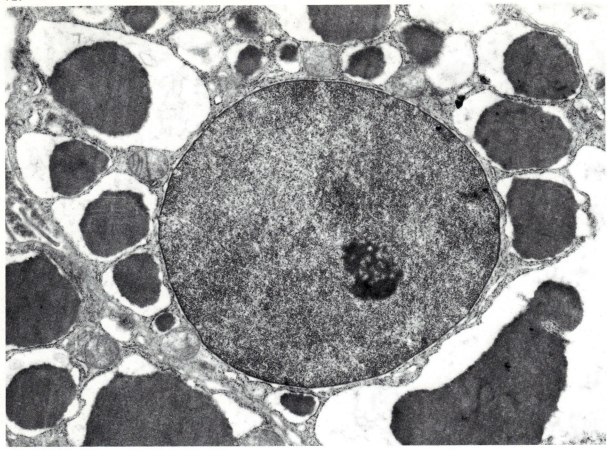

**717  Multiple myeloma, ultrastructure** In some patients, as shown here, although the bone marrow and osseous involvement is typical of multiple myelomatosis, there is no accompanying serological gammopathy. The tumour cells show the presence of abundant Ig contained within the rough endoplasmic reticulum suggesting that the anomaly is not one of synthesis of protein but of defect of export; or that the protein itself is anomalous. A similar situation occurs in some of the extramedullary plasma cell lymphomas. (× 15,000)

**718 and 719  Plasma cell (extramedullary) lymphoma plasmablastic** The gastrointestinal tract is one of the more common sites to show involvement with a predominantly plasma cell tumour. The majority are of plasmablastic or pleomorphic type and consequently they are usually designated as lymphocytic poorly differentiated (lymphoblastic) lymphoma or (immunoblastic) large cell lymphoma. If reactive cellular elements are numerous then a diagnosis of Hodgkin's disease may be made. In this small intestinal tumour, **718**, the plasmablastic nature of the cells with their round, usually centrally placed nuclei and often single central nucleoli (*arrows*) together with their rather irregular cytoplasmic contour and visible hof, is apparent. Immunoblasts contain less nuclear chromatin, show a regular rim of cytoplasm and lack perinuclear haloes of hofs. Figure **719** shows the intense pyroninophilia of plasmablast cytoplasm and nucleoli. Note the multinucleate cell with round similarly sized nuclei, and the huge plasmablast (*arrow*).

**718**                     **719**              (*718 H&E; 719 MGP*)

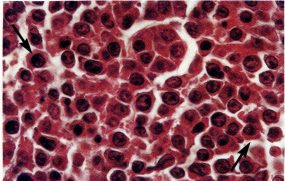 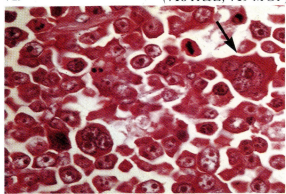

**720**

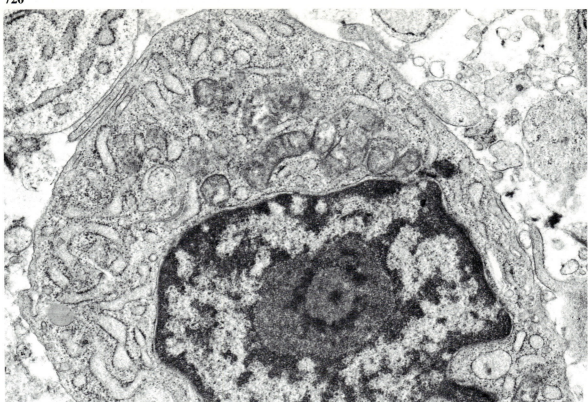

**720  Plasma cell (extramedullary) lymphoma, ultrastructure** This cell is intermediate between a plasma-blast and a mature plasma cell. The nucleus contains a very large central ring-shaped nucleolus but the heterochromatin is assuming a more radial or peripheral arrangement and the cytoplasm contains an abundance of secretory rough endoplasmic reticulum. No Golgi is visible in this field. The patient had macroglobulinaemia with skin infiltration (see **843**). *(× 12,800)*

**721 and 722  Plasma cell (extramedullary) lymphoma plasmablastic** In this primary small intestinal lymphoma, **721** shows the way in which the lamina propria is diffusely infiltrated but the crypts are still pre-served. There was no ulceration and no extension of tumour beyond the submucosa. At higher magnifica-tion, **722**, the majority of cells are immature plasma cells or plasmablasts, though there are also some more mature forms. The very large cell (*arrow*) might be interpreted by many as an immunoblast. *(H&E)*

**721**

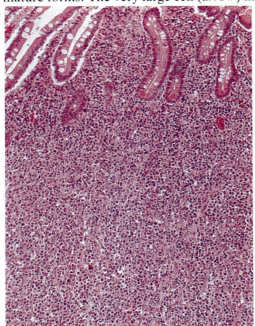

**722**

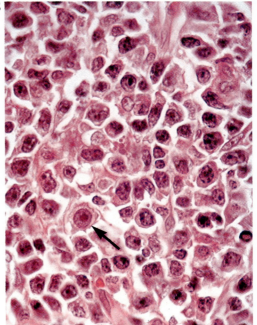

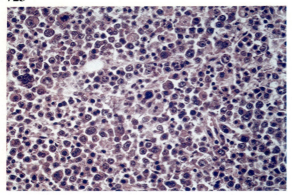

**724**

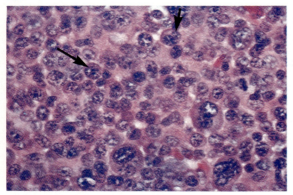

**725**

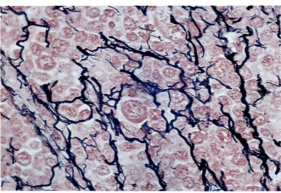

**726**

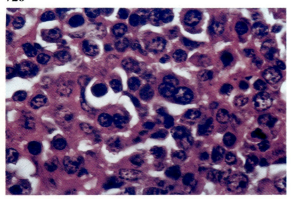

**723, 724, 725 and 726  Plasma cell (extramedullary) lymphoma pleomorphic** This variant of a plasma cell lymphoma is seldom recognised in extramedullary sites in the absence of a paraprotein. The giant and multinucleate forms are likely to lead to a consideration of Hodgkin's disease or, if these are less conspicuous, to a diagnosis of a pleomorphic reticulum cell sarcoma or immunoblastic lymphoma. Figure **723** shows an inguinal node removed from an elderly woman. The range in cell size is considerable and there are many multinucleate forms with up to 4 or more nuclei. The patient did not have multiple myelomatosis or abdominal or gastrointestinal tract involvement at the time of presentation. Figure **724** is from a recurrence in cervical lymph nodes (diagnosed and treated 2 years previously as a reticulum cell sarcoma); it shows a much more pleomorphic appearance than the original. The pleomorphism is due not only to the range in cell size but to the frequent multinucleate forms. On close inspection it is apparent that the nuclear configuration of all the cells is that of the plasma cell series and not immunoblasts or histiocytes. Furthermore the abundant cytoplasm, although not well delineated in all cells, shows the presence of hofs (*arrows*), and is markedly pyroninophilic. On review, the original neck node also showed a plasma cell tumour, and immunoglobulin studies showed the *in situ* production of IgM heavy ($\mu$) chain. The reticulin fibre content and pleomorphism, **725**, had contributed to the original diagnosis of a reticulum cell sarcoma.

Primary gastrointestinal tract lymphomas not uncommonly are of plasmablastic or pleomorphic plasma cell type whether associated with alpha-chain disease or not (see **728–736**). Most frequently they are encountered in the terminal ileum and caecum but they are also seen in colon and stomach, **726**. Unlike alpha-chain disease there is no sex predominance or peak age incidence, and their importance lies in their likelihood of being diagnosed as Hodgkin's disease. One of the most helpful morphological characteristics is, in fact, the nuclei of the multinucleate cells which, in addition to the clumped chromatin pattern, generally rounded contour and equality in size, do not possess the large eosinophilic nucleoli of Reed-Sternberg cells. Mitotic activity is usually prominent, and in well fixed material the limits of the eosinophilic cytoplasm well defined. (**723, 724, 726** *H&E;* **725** *Gordon & Sweets/neutral red*)

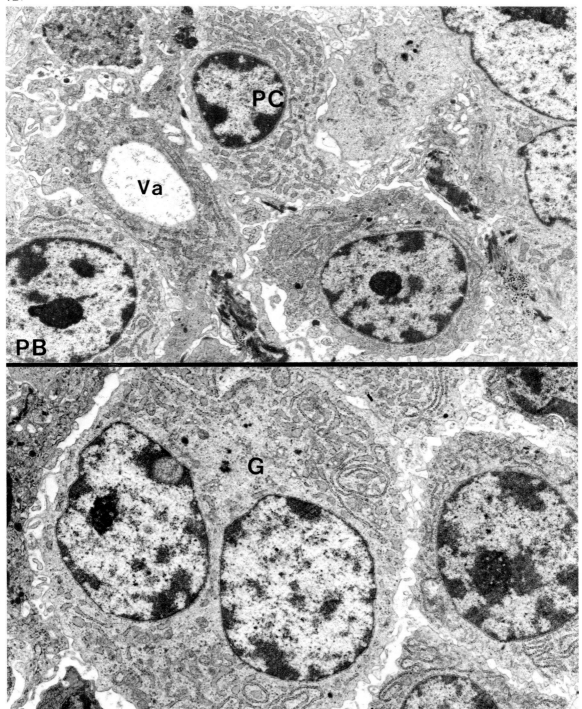

**727 Plasma cell (extramedullary) lymphoma pleomorphic, ultrastructure** Any doubt as to the nature of the proliferating cells shown at light microscopical level in **724, 725** is removed by the ultrastructural findings. Apart from a few reactive histiocytes all the cells including the multinucleated cells showed abundant rough endoplasmic reticulin containing secretory (immunoglobulin) material, and a range in nuclear appearances from well differentiated plasma cells (PC) to plasmablasts (PB). A feature noted in some plasma cell lymphomas particularly those associated with $\mu$ chain and in upper EM (Va), is the presence of cytoplasmic vacuoles containing finely divided electron dense material. Golgi zones (G) are prominent and present in mononucleated as well as multinucleated cells. *(upper × 6,000; lower × 8,110)*

**728**

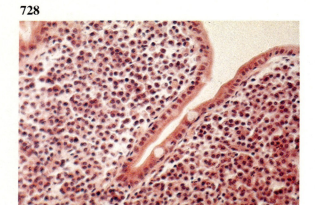

**729**

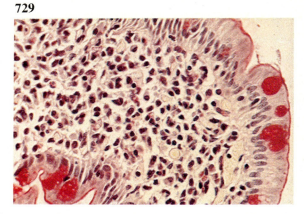

**728 and 729  Alpha-chain disease** This heavy chain disease is characterised by the production of the Fc fragment of IgA. Clinically the patients are usually young males who present with severe malabsorption – often accompanied by clubbing and abdominal pain. At one time thought to be confined to Mediterranean areas, the disease is now recognised in many parts of the world and in different ethnic groups. In its early stages it may be suspected on the appearances of the jejunal biopsy alone, when there is the highly distinctive combination of abnormal villous morphology, crypt sparsity, relatively normal enterocytes and a striking mononuclear cellular infiltrate more or less confined to the lamina propria. The appearances of the cellular infiltrate is somewhat variable in different patients, and ranges from well differentiated plasma cells, **728**, to a more lymphoplasmacytoid appearance, **729**. Note the normality of the epithelial cells in contrast to coeliac disease. *(728 H&E; 729 PAS)*

**730  Alpha-chain disease, ultrastructure** That the abnormal proliferation of plasma cells in the early stages of the disease can be suppressed by treatment with broad spectrum antibiotics alone, supports the theory that at first there is a non-malignant proliferation of plasma cells – probably in response to low grade intestinal pathogens in susceptible individuals. The proliferating cells in a typical case show well developed rough endoplasmic reticulum filled with electron dense secretory products, and prominent Golgi zones (G). This marked secretory activity is somewhat at variance with immunoglobulin studies, since only a small proportion of cells can be shown to be synthesising alpha-chain. *(× 8,000)*

**730**

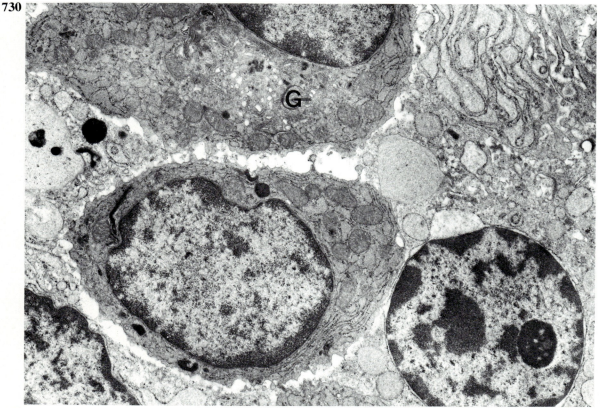

**731 Alpha-chain disease** Despite initial response to therapy patients usually relapse with localised gastrointestinal tumours in addition to the diffuse mucosal infiltrate. These tumours may be sited anywhere in the GI tract. The lymphoma shown here from a young Bangladeshian man was in the rectum but there were also polypoid duodenal, jejunal, ileal and caecal tumours. In addition an enlarged cervical lymph node (see **735**) had been excised prior to the terminal illness.

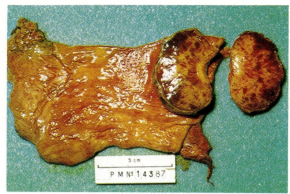

731

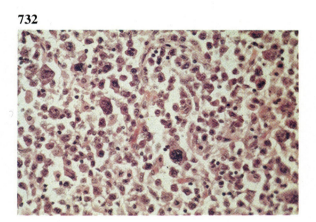

732

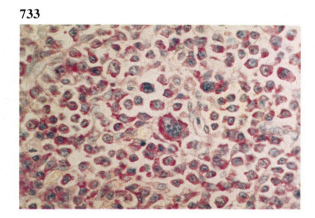

733

**732 and 733 Alpha-chain disease** Representative fields from two gastrointestinal tumours are shown – the caecal tumour in **732** and the rectal tumour in **733**. Both are composed of pyroninophilic plasma cells of variable size and include giant and multinucleate forms. There were no features to suggest a histiocytic (mononuclear phagocytic) origin or Hodgkin's disease; nor is the label immunoblastic lymphoma justified or appropriate. (*732 H&E; 733 MGP*)

**734 Alpha-chain disease** In contrast to the well differentiated plasma cell infiltrate localised to the lamina propria of the proximal small intestine in the early stages of the disease, the terminal phase of the illness in this patient was characterised by the presence of a pleomorphic plasma cell infiltrate in the submucosae, in addition to localised tumour formation. Note the numerous plasmablasts and multinucleated plasma cells (*arrows*). Similar plasma cells were present also in the sinuses of the mesenteric lymph nodes. (*H&E*)

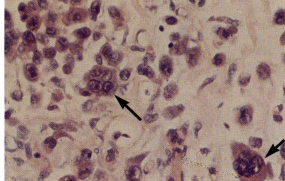

734

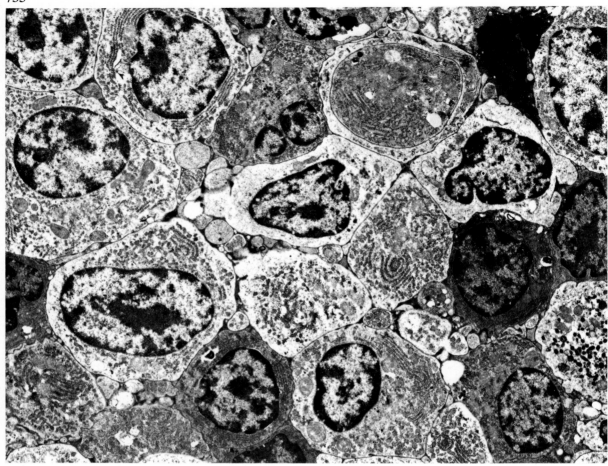

**735 Alpha-chain disease, ultrastructure** The enlarged cervical lymph node excised from a patient with alpha-chain disease was involved by a plasma cell lymphoma composed of a mixture of relatively well differentiated actively secreting plasma cells and plasmablasts. There were also a few lymphocytes and reactive histiocytes. It has been stated that in alpha-chain disease (with the exception of the rare respiratory form) in contrast to the other heavy chain diseases, the plasma cell proliferation is confined to the abdomen. (× 4,800)

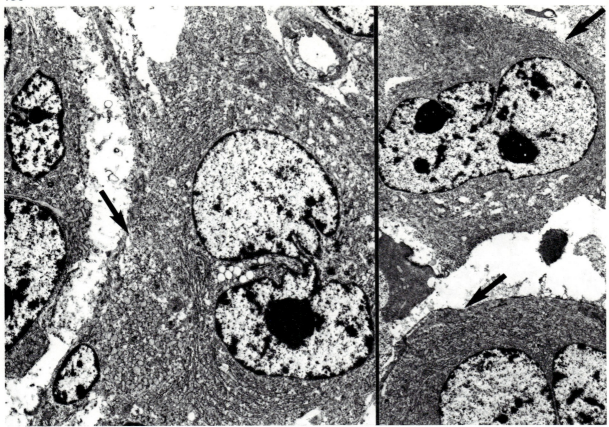

**736  Alpha-chain disease, ultrastructure** Despite poor fixation of post-mortem material obtained from the duodenal (left field) and rectal (right field) tumours, the plasmacytic nature of the variable sized and multi-nucleated cells is still evident. The cytoplasm is filled with stacks of rough endoplasmic reticulum containing immunoglobulin (*arrows*). (× 4,000)

**737  Plasma cell lymphoma** A number of intestinal pathogens has been identified both in patients with alpha-chain disease and in those from Mediterranean and Middle Eastern countries without alpha-chain production. None of these pathogens has been consistent and ranged from giardia lamblia to an intestinal coccidian organism. In this patient from the Middle East with a well differentiated gastric plasma cell lymphoma cytomegalovirus inclusions were present in the residual epithelial cells (*arrows*). (*H&E*)

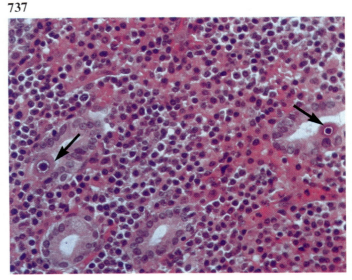

# Histiocytic lymphoma

The term histiocytic lymphoma is used here to describe a solid tumour arising in peripheral lymphoreticular tissue but derived from cells of the mononuclear phagocytic cell system. It is not to be confused with Rappaport's 'histiocytic' lymphoma which is now considered to represent a proliferation of large lymphoid or immunoblastic-like cells; nor with the systemic malignant histiocytoses typified by histiocytic medullary reticulosis.

Most workers consider true histiocytic lymphomas to be a rarity or, that if they do occur, they should not be included within any classification of malignant lymphoma. This latter view derives, of course, from the belief that the term lymphoma should be restricted to those tumours of lymphoid tissue *arising only from lymphoid cells*. Since, however, it has been established that mononuclear phagocytes are derived from monocytes but are capable of local division before developing into mature end cells, and since they collaborate so intimately with cells of the lymphoid series, it seems to us illogical to exclude histiocytic lymphomas from the lymphomas as a whole. In the Stanford 'formulation' histiocytic lymphomas are put in the miscellaneous category.

Before applying the term histiocytic lymphoma it is of course important to exclude involvement of peripheral lymphoreticular tissue either during the course of a malignant histiocytosis or in a differentiated histiocytoses such as histiocytosis X, or in certain reactive histiocytoses. Histiocytic lymphomas form 5 per cent of all lymphomas other than Hodgkin's disease (BNLI) and, in a smaller personal series, 10 per cent of diffuse large cell lymphomas – a not insignificant number. These neoplastic histiocytic lymphomas may be divided into three broad categories:

*1* a well differentiated type approximating quite closely to mature tissue histiocytes
*2* tumours composed of histiocytes of varying degrees of differentiation – including many multinucleated forms – the pleomorphic type
*3* a blast cell type in which the tumours are composed predominantly of 'histioblasts'

In any of these types eosinophils or plasma cells may be quite conspicuous, in addition to residual lymphocytes. Phagocytosis is an inconstant feature; so is the demonstration of lysosomal activity, since this feature is dependent on rapid and suitable fixation as well as the degree of differentiation in the tumour cells. Ultrastructural morphology, in our hands, has been a more accurate method of establishing the diagnosis of this group of tumours. The solid histiocytic lymphoma arising in lymph node is unlikely to be confused with histiocytic medullary reticulosis or Letterer Siwe disease (see **450**) unless much architecture is destroyed in the latter two conditions. A *histiocytic lymphoma* arising in tissue such as the gastrointestinal tract, however, must be carefully distinguished from a *malignant histiocytosis*. Other tumours arising in lymph nodes which at light microscopical level may simulate a histiocytic lymphoma are the very rare examples of dendritic cell tumours and fibro- and myofibrosarcomas.

**738a**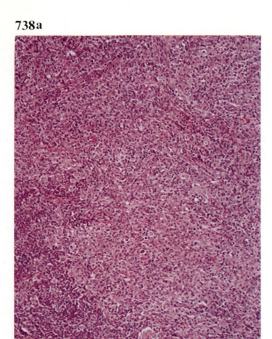

**738b**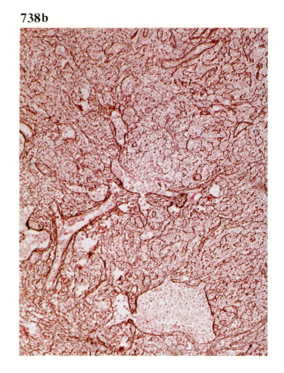

**738a and 738b  Histiocytic lymphoma** A localised tumour derived from mononuclear phagocytic cells arising in peripheral lymphoreticular tissue is by no means rare. Males are more frequently affected than females, with peak incidences in childhood and late in life. True histiocytic lymphoma is to be distinguished from the majority of Rappaport's 'histiocytic' lymphomas, since these are now believed to be lymphoid tumours, and from peripheral lymphoreticular tissue involvement by a systemic malignant histiocytosis (see **788, 789**). Lymph nodes may be extensively replaced by the malignant cells but there may be also focal areas of uninvolved tissue, **738a**. When the tumours are cohesive the distinction from a lymphoid tumour on the one hand and metastatic carcinoma on the other may be difficult. Stains for reticulin, **738b**, are useful in delineating residual sinuses filled with tumour. *(738a H&E; 738b Gordon & Sweets)*

**739  Histiocytic lymphoma well differentiated** In this cervical lymph node the proliferating cells are mostly relatively well differentiated histiocytic cells with an abundant pink cytoplasm, and vesicular nuclei which are ovoid or slightly indented and contain a single centrally placed nucleolus. There are usually some residual small lymphocytes (helpful as a marker of size), and variable numbers of eosinophils. Note the erythrophagocytosis *(arrow)*. *(H&E)*

**739**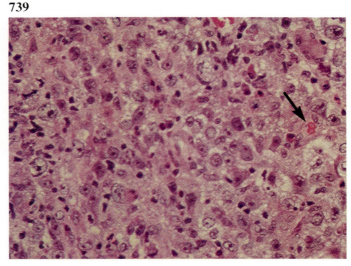

**740 Histiocytic lymphoma well differentiated**
Other tumours may show a nodular aggregation of
cells or a rather characteristic pattern of cells
streaming in from the capsule, as seen here,
together with fibroblasts. Fibroblasts, like
eosinophils and plasma cells, are in fact a common
component of histiocytic tumours and are responsible for the sometimes very abundant reticulin
fibre content. *(H&E)*

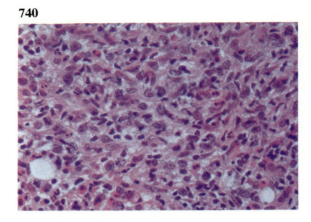

740

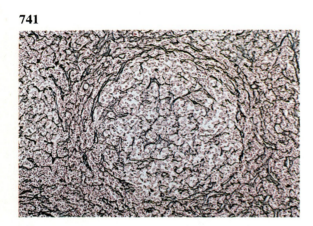

741

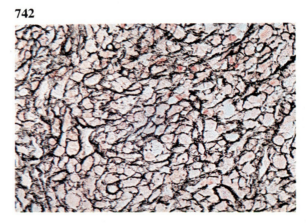

742

**741 and 742  Histiocytic lymphoma** In some tumours, **741**, the nodular pattern is better appreciated by
reticulin preparations, and appears to be related to small vessels. In diffuse areas, **742**, the reticulin fibre
present is usually abundant and encloses groups of cells in a manner somewhat similar to the large
irregularly nucleated lymphoid tumours. *(Gordon & Sweets)*

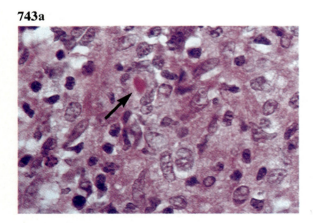

743a

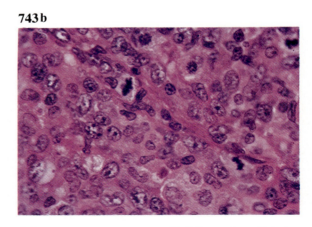

743b

**743a and 743b  Histiocytic lymphoma well differentiated** These two examples of well differentiated histiocytic lymphomas show the deceptively bland appearance of the neoplastic cells. Figure **743a** shows
phagocytosis including erythrophagocytosis *(arrow)*, while **743b** shows prominent mitotic activity. The
abundant ill-defined and foamy eosinophilic cytoplasm helps to distinguish the cells from an irregularly
nucleated large lymphoid (large cleaved) cell lymphoma or from a carcinoma. Histochemical techniques to
demonstrate the presence of lysozyme, acid-phosphatase and non-specific esterases (see **852–856b**) are
also useful, particularly in the better differentiated histiocytic malignancies. *(H&E)*

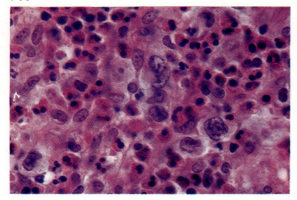

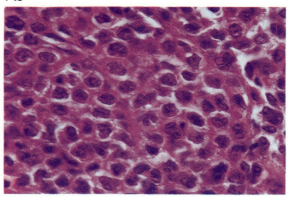

**744 Histiocytic lymphoma** Reactive eosinophils very frequently accompany the malignant histiocytic proliferations, though their numbers vary considerably. When they are very numerous, as here, Hodgkin's disease or the systemic histiocytoses may enter into the differential diagnosis. Their occurrence, which does not seem to be influenced by the presence or absence of necrosis, is a useful marker for distinguishing histiocytic nodal lymphomas from some of the large lymphoid cell lymphomas. *(H&E)*

**745 Histiocytic lymphoma well differentiated** Less commonly differentiated histiocytic lymphomas are composed of cells very similar to monocytes and then it is important to exclude tissue involvement by a monocytic leukaemia. This solitary tumour was involving skin in an adult male. It is arguable whether a cutaneous histiocytic lymphoma is not better included with the malignant histiocytosis. In our view, if there is no diffuse liver, spleen, or bone marrow involvement, and no abnormal circulating cells, the tumour is regarded as a peripheral histiocytic lymphoma, bearing in mind that the skin is considered as part of the peripheral lymphoreticular tissue. *(H&E)*

**746 Histiocytic lymphoma, ultrastructure** Ultrastructural examination of the well differentiated histiocytic lymphoma in **739** confirms the histiocytic nature of the proliferating cells. The abundant cytoplasm of this representative cell shows peripheral infoldings, and contains abundant vesicular structures and electron dense primary lysosomes. Note also the *short* profiles of rough endoplasmic reticulum (rer). No phagocytosed material is evident in this field. *(× 10,250)*

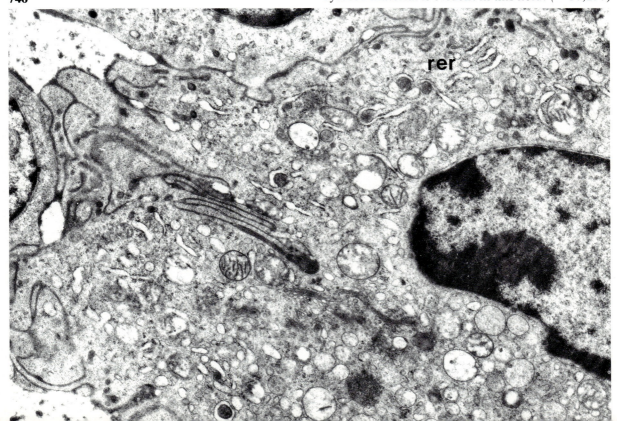

rer

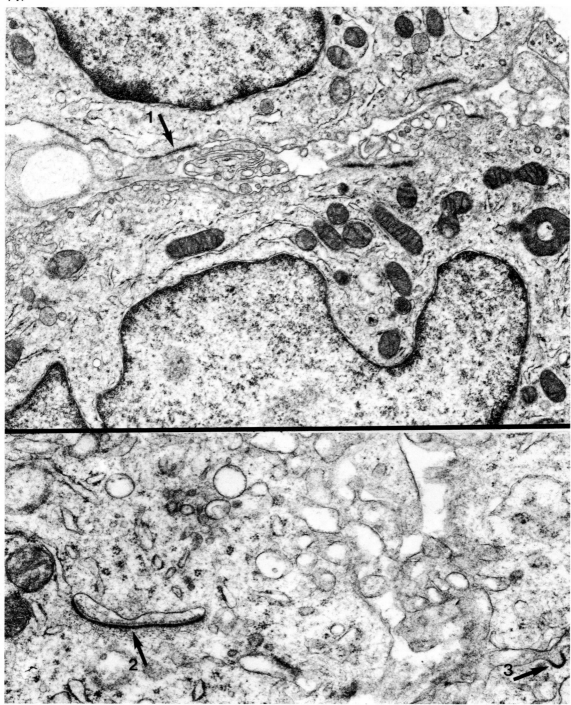

**747 Histiocytic lymphoma, ultrastructure** A useful ultrastructural marker present in many of these histiocytic tumour cells is the focal linear densities (*arrow 1*) seen at intervals along the cytoplasmic membrane, similar to those in reactive histiocytes (see **251**). These densities are also seen lining 'vesicles' within the cytoplasm (*arrow 2*) but which are interpreted as being in contact with the extra-cellular space. At higher magnification (lower field) it is possible to see that the densities consist of fibrillar material both internal *and* external to the cytoplasmic membrane, and although fine cytoplasmic fibrils are seen in their vicinity they are not inserted into the densities in the manner of hemidesmosomes. On the other hand these specialised structures are very similar and indeed resemble developing coated vesicles (*arrow 3*) to which they are considered to be related. (Same tumour as in **743**) . *(upper × 14,700; lower × 24,280)*

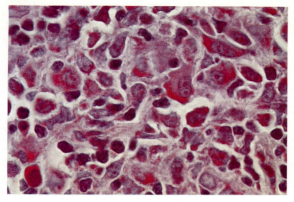

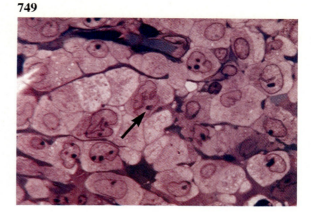

**748 Histiocytic lymphoma** Histiocytic cells may be quite rich in both free and fixed ribosomes and, therefore, quite pyroninophilic as seen here. There is, however, seldom the intense pyroninophilia characteristic of some lymphoid blast cells, but the MGP technique does serve to emphasise the voluminous cytoplasm and the sometimes pale paranuclear zone occupied by the Golgi apparatus. *(MGP)*

**749 Histiocytic lymphoma semi-thin section** In the absence of an electronmicroscope, plastic processing can be invaluable in separating this group of tumours from other large cell lymphomas. Not only are the characteristic angulated and pale nuclei with finely dispersed chromatin visualised, but the abundant cytoplasm is emphasised and phagocytosis *(arrow)* readily detected. Also by this technique, the material staining as reticulin in conventional paraffin processed sections is stained dark blue and is seen to enclose groups of cells. *(Toluidine blue)*

**750**

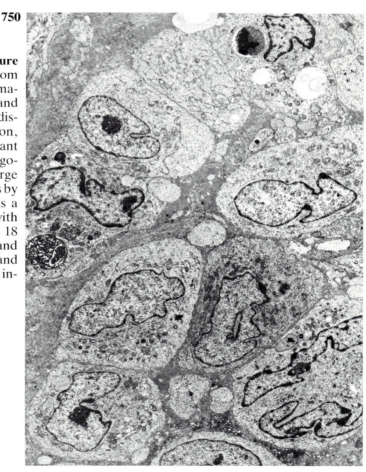

**750 Histiocytic lymphoma, ultrastructure** The cells illustrated in **749** range from relatively mature histiocytes to more immature forms. The irregular, angulated and lobated nuclei are emphasised; the dispersed chromatin with nuclear margination, central nucleoli, and the generally abundant cytoplasm containing lysosomes and phagocytosed material are unlike those of large lymphoid cells. Note the packeting of cells by electron dense material. The patient was a 14-year-old boy presenting initially with cervical lymphadenopathy but who died 18 months later with several skin deposits and *focal* deposits in kidney, liver, lung and myocardium. The bone marrow was not involved. *(× 2,450)*

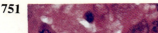

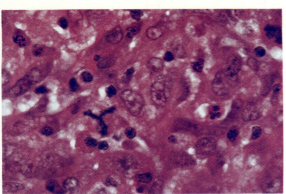

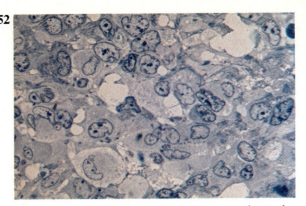

**751 and 752  Histiocytic lymphoma** This exhibits more nuclear pleomorphism with large more irregular nuclei and prominent nucleoli, **751**. The cytoplasm is still very characteristic, showing an eosinophilic and foamy appearance. Note the atypical mitosis and the presence of a few reactive plasma cells. Most of these features are even more clearly seen in the semi-thin plastic sections, **752**. *(751 H&E; 752 Toluidine blue)*

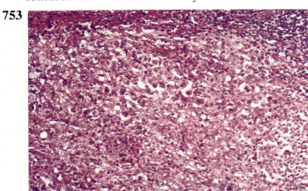

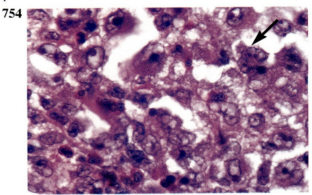

**753 and 754  Histiocytic lymphoma, pleomorphic** This lymphoma arises in a cervical lymph node; **753** shows the boundary zone between the lymphoma and the residual non-involved lymphoid tissue. There is a marked range in size of the malignant histiocytes and prominent multinucleate forms. Figure **754** is a high power view showing a multinucleated cell with peripherally arranged nuclei (*arrow*), and large lobated mononucleated cells with prominent nucleoli. Note the phagocytic activity of the tumour cells and the accompanying eosinophils. *(H&E)*

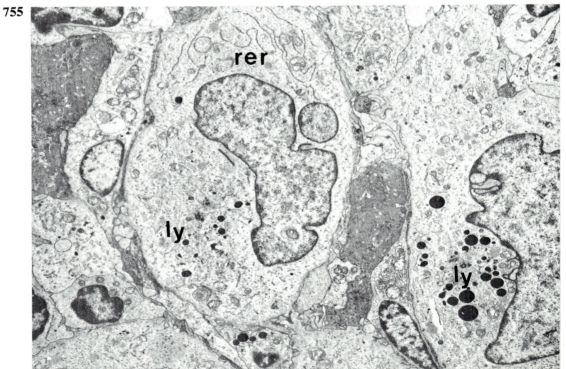

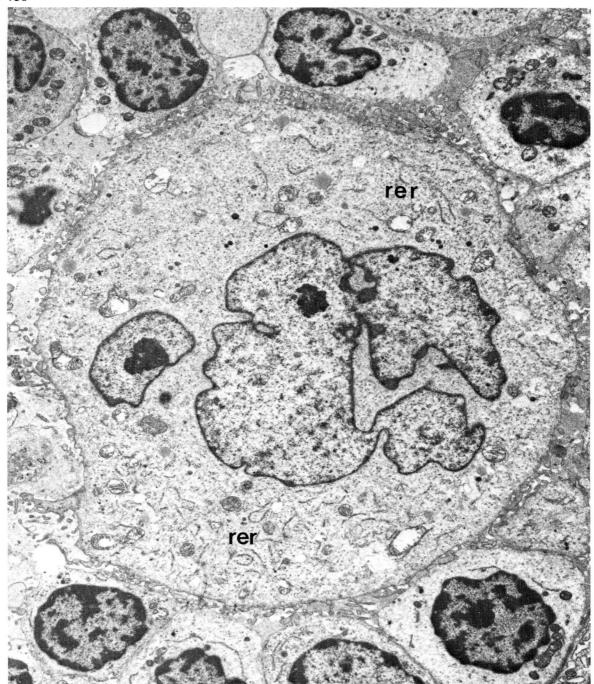

**755 and 756  Histiocytic lymphoma pleomorphic, ultrastructure** The mononucleated histiocytic cells of the lymphoma shown in **753** contain large lobated and irregular nuclei, with dispersed nuclear chromatin. The abundant cytoplasm contains numerous organelles including electron dense lysosomes and strands of rough endoplasmic reticulum (rer). In the histiocytic giant cell, **756**, note the very characteristic frilly cytoplasmic contour to which the surrounding rosette of small mature lymphocytes is making intimate contact. The abundant cytoplasm contains short runs of rough endoplasmic reticulum and numerous ribosomes. The nucleus appears multinucleated but in reality this is due to the hyperlobated nucleus being cut in different planes. Lysosomes-ly. *(755 × 5,800; 756 × 6,800)*

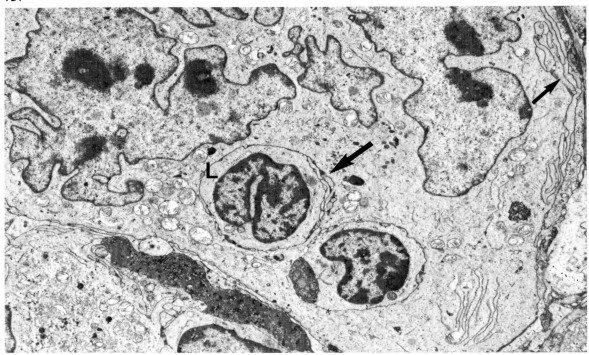

**757 Histiocytic lymphoma, pleomorphic; 758 Fixed paracortical histiocytes (interdigitating reticulum cells), ultrastructure** This malignant multinucleated histiocytic giant cell, **757**, shows a markedly infolded cytoplasmic contour (*arrows*) similar to that seen in epithelioid cells and the interdigitating so-called reticulum cells of the paracortex. The two lymphocytes (L) have not been phagocytosed but have merely invaginated the cytoplasm. This contains only a few dense granules, free ribosomes, fine filaments and a modicum of rough endoplasmic reticulum. Figure **758** shows interdigitating reticulum cells, believed to represent mononuclear phagocytic cells. These are characterised by highly irregular and angulated nuclear contour; the cytoplasm which is voluminous shows complex interdigitations with similar cells, and contains scattered electron dense lysosomal structures. Although no phagocytosed material is evident gradations are seen between this type of cell and actively phagocytic free macrophages. *(**757, 758** × 5,800)*

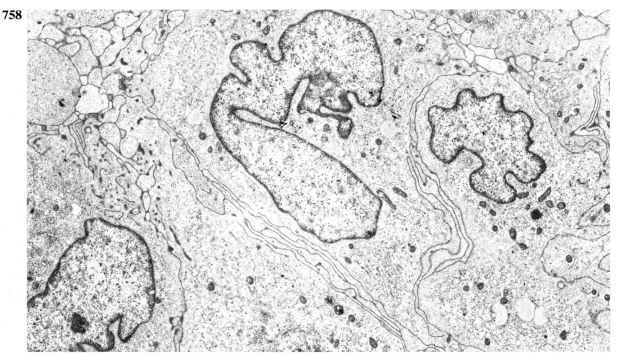

**759**

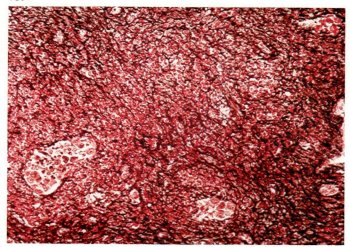

**759 Histiocytic lymphoma, pleomorphic** It is in this type of histiocytic lymphoma that the fibre content may be extremely abundant, a feature which taken together with the cellular morphology makes distinction from lymphocytic depletion type Hodgkin's disease difficult. A helpful finding is the preservation of a few sinuses. (*Gordon & Sweets*)

**760**

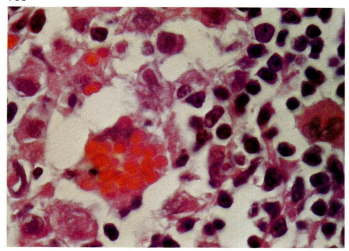

**760 and 761 Histiocytic lymphoma, pleomorphic** Although unusual, the large pleomorphic histiocytic cells may show striking phagocytosis, **760** – in this case erythrophagocytosis. The finding of phagocytosis is a helpful aid in the recognition of histiocytic lymphomas, but it should be borne in mind that phagocytosis is not always evident, that it may be shown by other malignant tumours, and that this feature must always be taken together with morphology. The histiocytic cells may be also strikingly pyroninophilic due to a high RNA content, **761**. This finding should not influence the observer towards making a diagnosis of a lymphocytic lymphoma. Note the Touton type giant cell (*arrow*). (**760** *H&E;* **761** *MGP*)

**761**

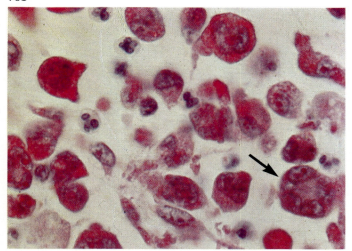

**762 Histiocytic lymphoma, histioblastic** A rare type of histiocytic lymphoma is that composed of predominantly large nucleolated 'blast' forms with very few well differentiated histiocytes or giant cells. The nuclei are rounded and vesicular but, in contrast to immunoblasts, the cytoplasm is abundant, eosinophilic and granular. Mitotic activity is high and nuclear pyknosis prominent. Note the presence of eosinophils. This type merges with the reticular form of lymphocytic depletion type Hodgkin's disease. *(H&E)*

**762**

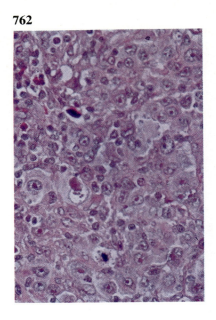

**763**

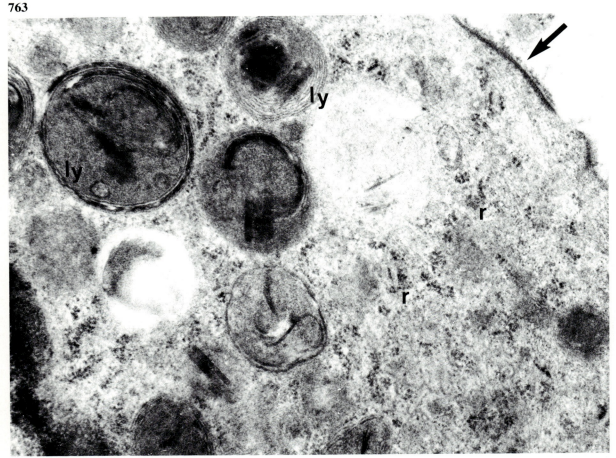

**763 Histiocytic lymphoma, histioblastic, ultrastructure** Despite the poorly differentiated nuclear appearance at light microscopic level, many of the cells show prominent cytoplasmic membrane bound electron dense lysosomal bodies(ly) with contained myelin-like figures. The cytoplasm is rich in fine filaments and polyribosomes (r) and cytoplasmic membranous densities are present *(arrow). (× 24,000)*

**764**

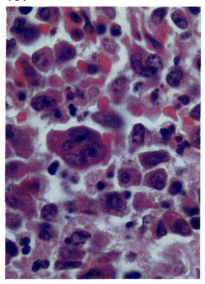

**764 Histiocytic lymphoma** These do occur in the gastrointestinal tract but are much less common than lymphocytic lymphomas. When these tumours are composed predominantly of histiocytic cells the diagnosis is not too difficult, but when there is marked pleomorphism, as seen here, together with residual or reactive cellular elements, a firm diagnosis based on morphology alone is difficult. Such tumours are likely to be labelled Hodgkin's disease, pleomorphic plasma cell tumour, immunoblastic lymphoma, reticulum cell sarcoma or large cell (undifferentiated) lymphomas. Histochemical and immunocytochemical techniques may be useful in demonstrating lysosomal enzymes – particularly the method now available to demonstrate lysozyme (see **856a**) and alpha 1 anti-trypsin and chymotrypsin. Plastic sections with or without proceeding to ultrastructural level are also invaluable. *(H&E)*

**765**     **766**     **767**

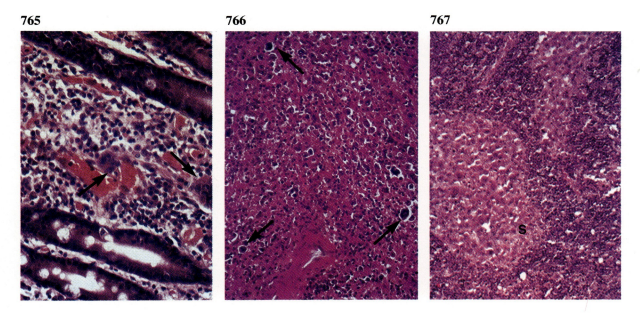

**765, 766 and 767   Malignant histiocytosis** The gut may be involved in the course of a malignant histiocytosis and should not then be labelled as a *primary* gastrointestinal histiocytic lymphoma. A characteristic finding in this condition is the sparsity of malignant histiocytic cells, **765**, *(arrows)* present in the granulation tissue of the ulcerating lesions or reactive inflammatory infiltrate. This finding contrasts with the numerous histiocytic cells found in other organs, such as spleen, **766**, *(arrows)* liver or bone marrow. In this elderly woman abdominal lymph nodes were involved also but the neoplastic infiltrate was confined to the sinuses(s), **767**. There was no history of coeliac disease, and the small intestinal morphology adjacent to the ulcer was normal. *(H&E)*

768

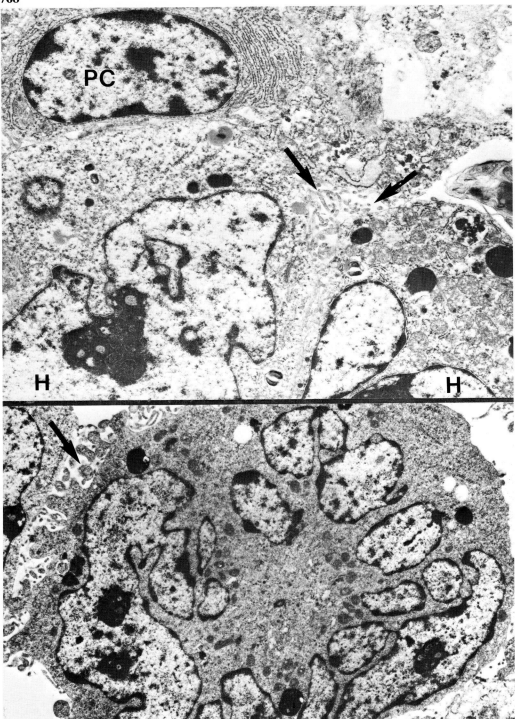

**768 Malignant histiocytosis, ultrastructure** The ultrastructural features of the malignant cells in **765–767** confirm a histiocytic origin. The upper field includes parts of two lobated histiocytic cells (H), with cytoplasm showing villiform projections (*arrow*), and phagocytosed material, adjacent to a reactive plasma cell (PC). The lower field shows a multinucleated giant histiocyte with peripherally arranged nuclei and irregular cytoplasmic contour (*arrow*). (*upper × 8,640; lower × 5,800*)

# Miscellaneous neoplastic proliferations of the LRMPS

There are a number of neoplastic lymphoproliferative and mononuclear phagocytic proliferative conditions which may involve peripheral lymphoreticular tissue but which do not fit readily into a classification of the lymphomas because (1) they are essentially leukaemic in nature; (2) they are widely disseminated in both central *and* peripheral lymphoid tissue at the time of presentation; or (3) the primary target organ is extranodal and there may be also leukaemic manifestations, as in cutaneous T-cell lymphomas. The lymphocytic and myelomonocytic leukaemias, and multiple myelomatosis are not included in this section. Diseases which will be illustrated because of the diagnostic difficulty they may present when involving lymph nodes are the following:

## Cutaneous T-cell lymphomas *(The Sézary syndrome and mycosis fungoides)*
Although the clinical presentation of these two lymphoproliferative conditions is different and the Sézary syndrome is characterised by the circulation of T-cells with a highly characteristic morphology and frequent bone marrow involvement, the Sézary syndrome and mycosis fungoides are considered to represent different parts of a spectrum involving a neoplastic proliferation of peripheral T-cells which is located principally within the skin. These conditions are important to the histopathologist since the lymph nodes may be involved, when it is not always easy to identify the infiltrating lymphoid cells as the characteristic Sézary/Lutzner cells.

## Hairy cell leukaemia *(leukaemic reticuloendotheliosis)*
This chronic condition usually presents with anaemia and splenomegaly with or without lymph-adenopathy. The confirmation of the disease is made by the demonstration of the characteristic hairy cells in blood or bone marrow, and the treatment of choice is splenectomy. If, however, the histopathologist is unfamiliar with the morphological features of the involved spleen or if, occasionally, lymph nodes are biopsied *or* splenectomy carried out for diagnostic purposes because the disease has not been recognised, then there may be difficulties in the interpretation of the histopathology.

## Histiocytic medullary reticulosis *(HMR, malignant histiocytosis)*
The condition known as histiocytic medullary reticulosis (HMR) or malignant histiocytosis is a clinicopathological entity characterised by a progressive and malignant *systemic* proliferation of histiocytes. HMR predominantly involves the sinusoidal areas of lymph nodes, spleen, liver and marrow, and shows a high incidence of skin involvement. When in the early stages of the disease the neoplastic proliferation in lymph nodes is confined to the sinuses and architecture is preserved, diagnostic dificulties may result in differentiating HMR from prominent reactive sinus histiocytosis, including massive sinus histiocytosis or Dorfman's disease, and other histiocytic proliferative disorders.

## Leukaemic T-cell lymphoma *(pleomorphic type, adult T-cell leukaemia)*
The pleomorphic variant of the $T_2$-lymphocytic group of lymphomas which includes the adult form of T-cell leukaemia is a recently defined entity believed to derive from *peripheral* T-lymphocytes in contrast to the lymphoblastic (convoluted and non-convoluted) lymphomas of *central* $T_1$-lymphocytic origin. The majority of patients present with leukaemic manifestations usually accompanied by hepatosplenomegaly and lymphadenopathy, and the disease pursues a rapidly fatal or sub-acute course. Because the disease appears to be common in Japan, and because the histopathological features apparently can mimic a number of different lymphomas, including Hodgkin's disease, the entity is included here.

**769**

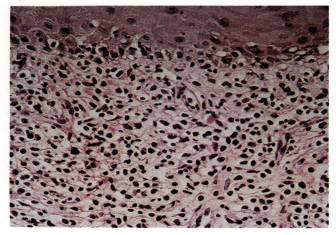

**769 Cutaneous T-cell lymphoma** This term includes mycosis fungoides and Sézary's syndrome. Although the clinical manifestations are different, the cellular components of the cutaneous infiltrate are characterised by proliferation of a specific T-derived lymphocyte – the Sézary/Lutzner cell. The Sézary syndrome is viewed as the leukaemic variant, but it should be stressed that a high percentage of patients with mycosis fungoides also show circulating Sézary cells. A feature of T-lymphocytic cutaneous infiltrations in contrast to B-cell cutaneous infiltrates is the manner in which the lymphoid cells extend right up and into the epidermis (epidermotrophism). The convoluted nuclear configuration is not particularly evident at this magnification. *(H&E)*

**770**

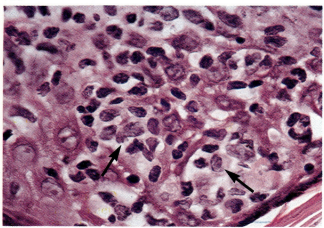

**770 Cutaneous T-cell lymphoma** In the absence of a clinical history and knowledge as to whether circulating cells are present, it is not always possible to distinguish between the two variants on morphological grounds alone. The infiltrating cells are similar though there tends to be a greater size range, greater nuclear pleomorphism, and more condensation of nuclear chromatin in mycosis fungoides. In this example of an intraepidermal Pautrier's microabscess in Sézary's syndrome the nuclear irregularity (*arrows*) of the infiltrating cells can best be appreciated by using the oil immersion lens and focusing up and down on the nuclei. It must be emphasised that the finding of convoluted cells within a skin infiltrate occurs in a variety of non-lymphomatous dermatoses and their presence is only of diagnostic importance if the cells occur in groups or sheets within the affected dermis and are present within the epidermis. *(H&E)*

**771**

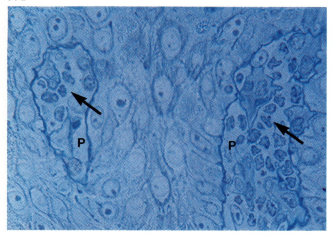

**771 Cutaneous T-cell lymphoma** Any doubt as to nuclear irregularity is immediately resolved by viewing the semi-thin plastic processed sections, which here show Sézary/Lutzner cells within two dermal papillae (P). When groups of such cells form within epidermolytic spaces they constitute the so-called Pautrier's microabscess. That Sézary cells represent a population of T-cells is confirmed by their property of forming *spontaneous* rosettes with sheep-red blood cells – the E rosettes (see **860**). They also react with anti-human T-cell antisera and respond to phytohaemoglutinin. Conversely, they lack B-cell markers. Evidence has been given that the cells represent a neoplastic proliferation of T helper cells. *(Toluidine blue)*

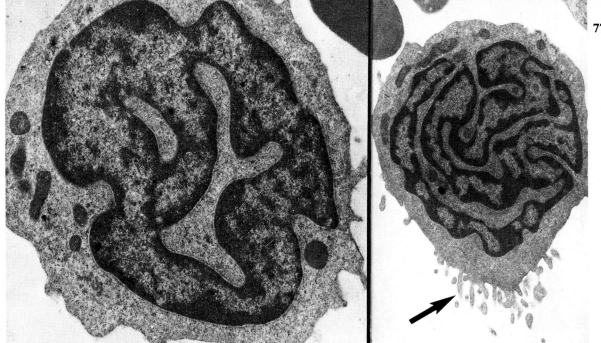

**772 and 773  Cutaneous T-cell lymphoma ultrastructure** The hallmark of Sézary cells is the highly convoluted or cerebriform nucleus, which is best appreciated in semi-thin plastic processed sections or in electron
micrographs. The size of the cell and degree of nuclear irregularity vary considerably: **772** shows a classical
Sézary/Lutzner cell while **773** shows the small cell variant which at light microscopical level is easily
mistaken for a small lymphocyte. Note the abundant cytoplasmic pseudopods (*arrow*). (× 7,500)

**774  Cutaneous T-cell lymphoma, ultrastructure** At this magnification of a Sézary/Lutzner cell from a
patient with mycosis fungoides, it can be seen that the features are similar to those of the circulating cells in
the Sézary syndrome. Organelles include variable numbers of lysosomes(ly), mitochondria and a modicum
of rough endoplasmic reticulum. Other constant features in all cells is the presence of fine filaments (*arrow*)
and glycogen (g) which is sometimes very abundant. Nucleoli when present tend to be rounded and
sometimes ring forms are evident. It is the lysosomal component which is responsible for the granular acid
phosphatase content, and which in contrast to that of hairy cell leukaemia is tartrate labile. (× 17,700)

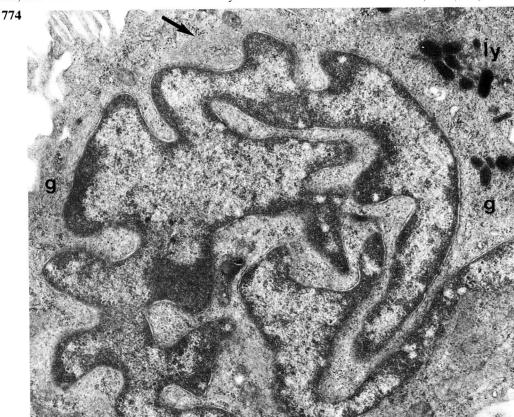

**775 Cutaneous T-cell lymphoma, lymph node** In both the Sézary syndrome and mycosis fungoides, lymph nodes may be affected during the course of the disease. The proliferating neoplastic cells involve initially the thymic dependent paracortex, and in nodes which are the site of dermatopathic lymphadenopathy early involvement is difficult to assess. In this patient with Sézary syndrome there were no dermatopathic features, and the features were typical of a T-cell lymphoma in that the paracortex was filled with proliferating lymphoid cells and showed prominent postcapillary venules. Note the residual lymphoid follicle, upper left. *(H&E)*

**775**

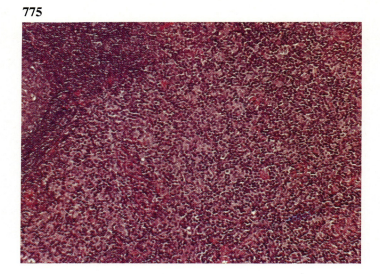

**776 Cutaneous T-cell lymphoma, lymph node** At higher magnification and with the oil immersion lens, the nuclei of the infiltrating cells in **775** reveal striae and a fine nuclear irregularity while still retaining a generally rounded contour. This crenellated appearance is very characteristic of Lutzner cells when viewed in paraffin sections. The cells also appear hyperchromatic and in this example exhibit wide variation in size, and the presence of nucleolated forms *(arrow)*. *(H&E)*

**776**

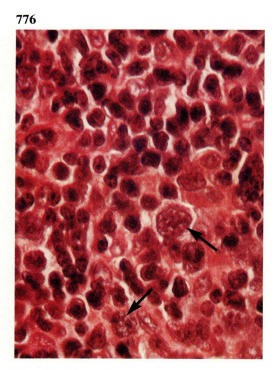

**777**

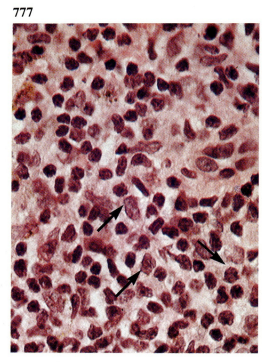

**777 Cutaneous T-cell lymphoma, lymph node** The diagnosis of early lymph node involvement in patients with dermatopathic lymphadenopathy sometimes can be difficult; not only may the infiltrating cells be few but it should be remembered also that irregularly nucleated (convoluted) T-cells may be seen in reactive conditions affecting the paracortex. In this lymph node from a patient with mycosis fungoides, also showing features of dermatopathic lymphadenopathy, there is no doubt as to involvement since numerous cells with the characteristic T-cell nuclear irregularity can be identified in the paracortex *(arrows)*. The nuclear striae are also evident. *(H&E)*

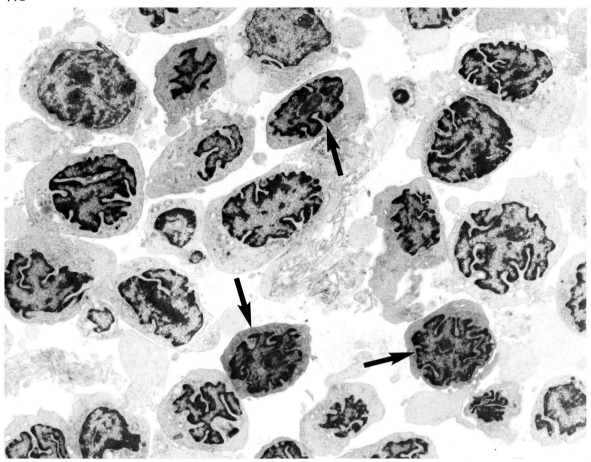

**778 Cutaneous T-cell lymphoma, lymph node, ultrastructure** Semi-thin sections of plastic processed material (see **842**) with or without electronmicroscopy are even more useful in confirming the diagnosis of infiltration with Sézary cells. In this electronmicrograph of the lymph node in **775** and **776**, not only are the majority of the cells shown to be Sézary/Lutzner cells but the markedly convoluted nature of the nuclei is emphasised, and it is also evident that there are a number of blast forms (*arrows*). *(× 2,900)*

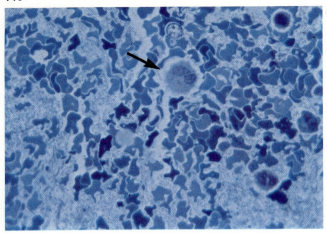

**779 Hairy cell leukaemia (leukaemic reticulo-endotheliosis** Patients with this rare chronic leukaemic lymphoproliferative disorder are usually slightly younger than those with CLL, and in addition to anaemia and often pancyto-paenia, present with massive splenomegaly. Lymphadenopathy is a late symptom. The diagnosis is generally made on finding the characteristic cells in peripheral blood. The thin cytoplasmic hair-like projections are not well visualised in routine preparations, but are seen easily with phase contrast microscopy and in plastic processed buffey coat material as shown here (*arrow*). The most useful cytological markers in imprint or smear preparations is the presence of tartrate resistant acid phosphatase activity (see **851**). (*Toluidine blue*)

**780**

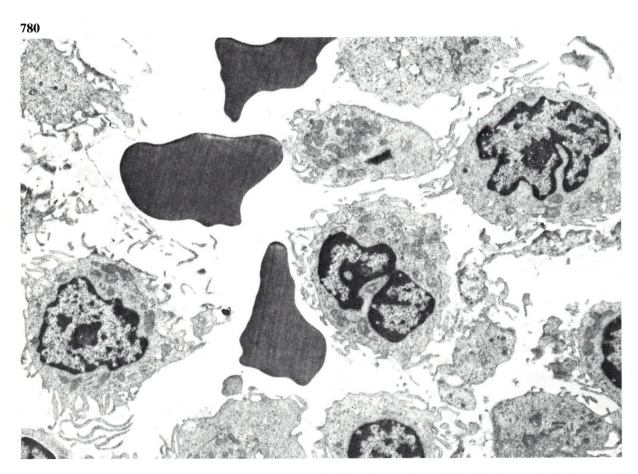

**780 Hairy cell leukaemia, ultrastructure** A group of hairy cells are shown lying free in a splenic sinus, and cytoplasmic processes are seen easily. When the cells are packed together in pulp cords the 'hairs' are not visible but there is cytoplasmic infolding and interdigitation between adjacent cells. The nuclei often appear irregular or lobated and contain more chromatin than histiocytic cells. The cytoplasm contains a number of organelles including electron dense lysosomal structures and the characteristic ribosomal lamellae complexes. (× 5,000)

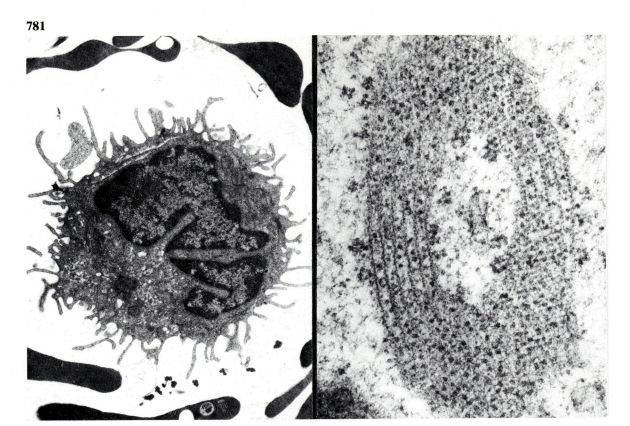

**781 Hairy cell leukaemia, ultrastructure** The peripheral blood hairy cell in **779** is seen here on the left at ultrastructural level, and the innumerable long thin cytoplasmic processes are emphasised. A ribosomal lamellae complex is shown on the right, and is essentially similar to those seen in macroglobulinaemia. There is now general acceptance that the hairy cells represent a special type of B-lymphocyte, but their precise origin and counterpart in normal tissue is unknown. (× *left 7,500;* × *right 63,500*)

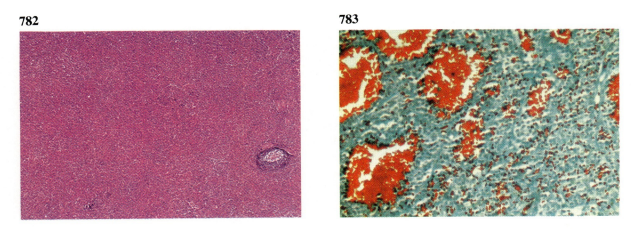

**782 and 783 Hairy cell leukaemia** The condition is believed to start in the spleen since this is the site of the earliest and most striking proliferation of cells, and may be massively enlarged on presentation. Splenectomy is also the treatment of choice. In late cases there is total effacement of normal architecture, but in earlier disease it may still be possible, **782**, to identify residual lymphoid follicles which are widely separated due to the proliferating cells in the pulp cords. Some spleens are very congested with the sinusoids filled with red cells. Trichrome stains are then very useful, **783**, in demonstrating the widened pulp cords between the distended sinuses. (**782** *H&E;* **783** *Masson's trichrome*)

**784  Hairy cell leukaemia** The blood 'lakes' derived from dilated sinuses have been named pseudo-sinuses by some workers. Reticulin preparations confirm the loss of normal pattern with increased fibre in the cords and loss of the normal ladder-like reticulin pattern enclosing the sinuses. *(Gordon & Sweets)*

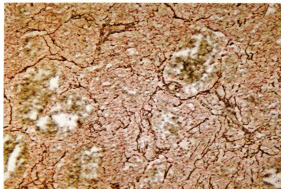

**785  Hairy cell leukaemia** The infiltrating cells here seen adjacent to a sinus present a very monomorphic appearance with nuclei appearing rounded or oval; though occasionally they may appear irregular and be eccentrically located. The chromatin is generally less dense than that of mature small lymphocytes, and the cytoplasm which in relation to the size of the nuclei is quite abundant, results in an appearance of well-defined and widely-spaced nuclei. The overall appearance can be confused sometimes with a monocytic leukaemic infiltrate. A noteworthy feature is the very low mitotic activity. *(H&E)*

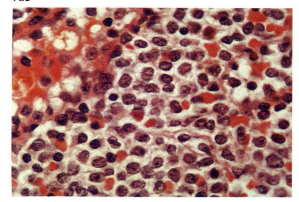

**786  Hairy cell leukaemia** In some examples, as in this spleen, plasma cells either singly or in groups are seen among the sheets of hairy cells. This finding is of considerable interest in view of the patients who have been described with features borderline between hairy cell leukaemia and macroglobulin-aemia of Waldenström, and the ribosomal lamellae complexes which are common to hairy cells and the lymphoplasmacytoid cells of macroglobulinaemia. *(MGP)*

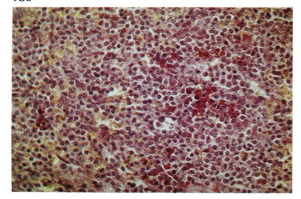

**787  Hairy cell leukaemia** The lymph nodes are usually only slightly enlarged at presentation. Such nodes show partial preservation of architecture but it is generally possible to identify groups of hairy cells in the B-lymphocytic zones – particularly the area subjacent to the subcapsular sinus. In this example a group of hairy cells is seen within the sinus of a lymph node and, because they are lying free it was just possible to discern the fine cyto-plasmic hairs with the oil immersion lens. *(H&E)*

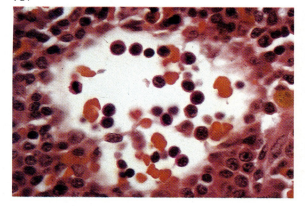

**788 Histiocytic medullary reticulosis (malignant histiocytosis)** This rather well defined clinico-pathological entity with a wide age range usually runs a rapidly fatal course. The dominating features include anaemia, jaundice, fever and hepato-splenomegaly. Lymph nodes are usually only moderately enlarged. In early nodal involvement the histiocytic proliferation is confined to the sinuses and the histiocytic cells appear relatively well differentiated. Plasma cells are an invariable accompaniment, particularly in the adjacent medullary cords and erythrophagocytosis is usually easily seen. Erythrophagocytosis by histiocytes can be seen, however, in many reactive conditions and should never be used as the sole criterion for the diagnosis of this disease. *(H&E)*

**789 Histiocytic medullary reticulosis** This condition appears not to be so rare as formerly supposed. Unfortunately, however, there seems to be a tendency to confuse it with histiocytic lymphoma arising in peripheral lymphoreticular tissue. As the histiocytic proliferation progresses there is gradual effacement of nodal architecture and replacement by malignant histiocytic cells which lack the cohesive pattern seen in the histiocytic lymphomas, and show prominent erythrophagocytosis *(arrows)*. By this stage there is usually extensive bone marrow involvement and lymphadenopathy, in addition to hepatosplenomegaly, fever and jaundice. *(H&E)*

**790 Histiocytic medullary reticulosis** This disease has been reported as affecting predominantly men, and in some countries such as China and Africa is a well recognised entity. If suspected, a diagnosis may be made on the liver biopsy appearances alone when the proliferating cells lying within the liver sinusoids are a prominent feature *(arrows)*. These too may show erythrophagocytosis. *(H&E)*

**788**

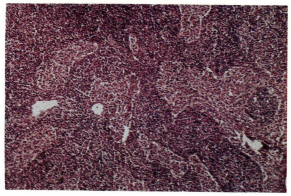

**789**

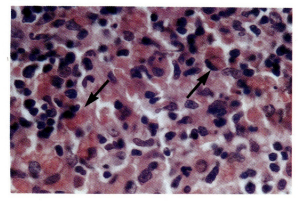

**790**

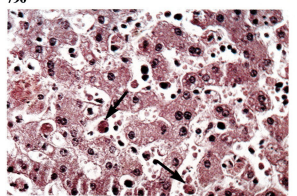

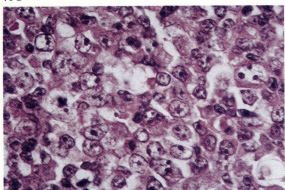

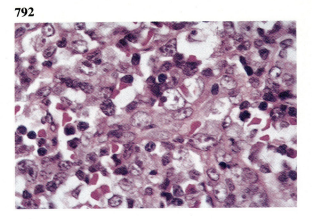

**791 and 792   Leukaemic T-cell lymphoma** This entity is well documented in Japan where it appears to be common. The patients generally present with leukaemic manifestations with circulating cells shown to be of T-cell origin. Lymphadenopathy and hepatosplenomegaly are usual. The importance of the condition appears to be in the wide range of histopathological appearances seen in biopsied lymph nodes, and its poor prognosis. In this example the predominating cell, **791**, is a large lymphoid cell similar to an immunoblast, but there were also bizarre giant forms and even multinucleated cells. A characteristic feature, shown in **792**, is the prominence of postcapillary venules. *(H&E)*

## Tumours and tumour-like conditions other than lymphoproliferative disorders affecting lymph nodes

Of the non-lymphoproliferative malignancies involving lymph nodes; by far the most common are metastatic carcinomas. Usually the nature of the infiltrating neoplastic cells is obvious. There are, however, certain situations where metastases may be *either* overlooked because they are very tiny or overshadowed by reactive processes, *or* misinterpreted as a reactive or malignant histiocytic process, various types of lymphomas, or even as benign epithelial inclusions. Tumours which are particularly liable to be confused with lymphomas are largely amelanotic melanomas, anaplastic carcinomas, and in the neck, metastases from nasopharyngeal carcinomas and ectopic thymomas. Oat cell carcinomas and metastases from Ewing's tumour may also pose problems.

In contrast, there are certain benign inclusions or malformations which may be misinterpreted as metastatic tumour. Important among these are epithelial inclusions and the rare blue naevi. Also included in this section is Kaposi's sarcoma which in African patients and children may particularly involve lymph nodes.

**793   Metastatic carcinoma** Lymph node biopsy is a frequent procedure since in the absence of histopathological examination diagnosis of the cause of lymph node enlargement can never be made with certainty. This is particularly true in the case of suspected metastatic carcinoma. Some enlarged lymph nodes in patients with carcinoma may be enlarged due to reactive hyperplasias. Conversely lymph nodes which are the site of metastasis need not be enlarged. Even in lymph nodes which are massively replaced by carcinoma and where a primary carcinoma has not been diagnosed, metastatic carcinoma cannot be recognised with certainty on the macroscopic features; the nodes may be extremely hard due to a desmoplastic response but equally they may be soft and resemble a lymphoma, as in this example of abdominal nodes excised for frozen section with a presumptive diagnosis of Hodgkin's disease before the carcinoma in the gall bladder was found.

**793**

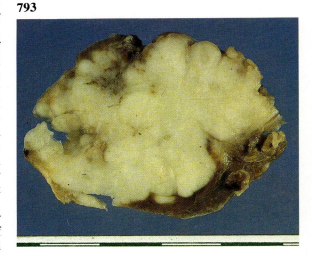

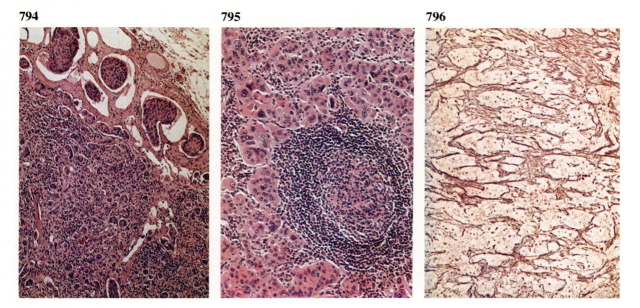

**794, 795 and 796   Metastatic carcinoma** In most examples of metastatic carcinoma there is no diagnostic problem. Often the carcinoma cells are found lying in groups within the sinuses, **794**, or arranged in irregular islands, **795**, throughout the substance of the node. It is most unusual for the nodal tissue to be replaced completely by carcinoma. When however there is widespread involvement, reticulin stains, **796**, can be useful by delineating the epithelial islands; the cancerous tissue itself, in contrast to most lymphomas, shows a virtual absence of reticulin fibre. When there is a more diffuse infiltrate by non-cohesive carcinoma cells and a resulting fibrocytic response, reticulin fibre may be increased. (**794, 795** *H&E;* **796** *Gordon & Sweets*)

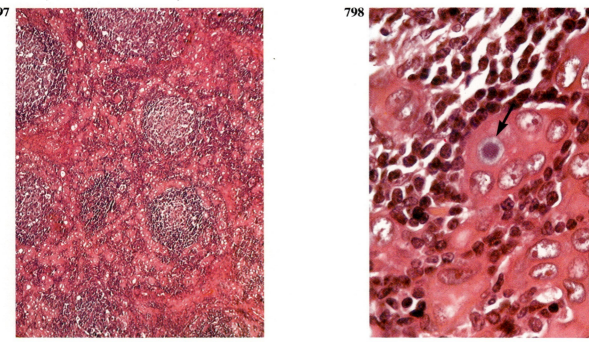

**797 and 798   Metastatic carcinoma** Lymph nodes which are the site of a florid reactive sinus response to the drainage of tumour products but which do not contain metastases, may be wrongly interpreted as showing evidence of carcinoma. Conversely, lymph nodes in which the infiltrating carcinoma is restricted to the sinusoidal system may simulate at low magnification, **797**, a sinus histiocytosis. At higher magnification, **798**, the epithelial nature of the cells is evident, and in adenocarcinomas, as in this example, mucin secretion (*arrow*) often can be identified. (*H&E*)

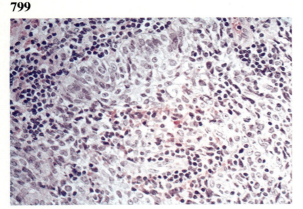

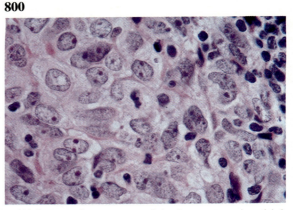

**799 and 800   Metastatic carcinoma** A useful feature in identifying carcinoma as such is the manner in which the peripheral cells of an island of carcinoma assume a polar or pallisade arrangement, **799**, with sharp demarcation from the residual lymphoid tissue. It is also important to appreciate that in well fixed material the nuclear features of epithelial cells differ from those of lymphomas, the most obvious difference being the finely distributed chromatin resulting in a stippled appearance in carcinoma cell nuclei, **800**. Nucleoli are very variable in size. *(H&E)*

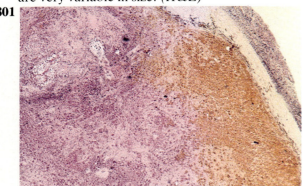

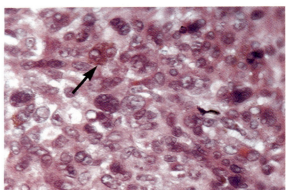

**801 and 802   Metastatic melanoma** Lymph nodes which are the site of metastasis from a malignant melanoma, do not usually present problems when melanin production is obvious. In **801**, most of the lymph node is replaced by melanin-containing cells, the pigment being so extensive that cellular detail is largely obscured. Diagnostic difficulties are liable to arise with mainly amelanotic melanomas presenting as an enlarged lymph node due to metastases. If a melanoma is not considered and melanin pigment not therefore carefully looked for, such metastases may be misinterpreted – quite frequently as large cell lymphomas. In the field selected in **802**, occasional melanin-producing cells can be identified *(arrow)*. *(H&E)*

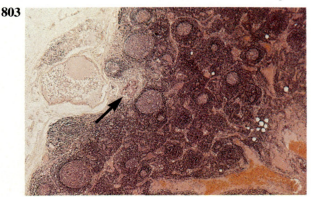

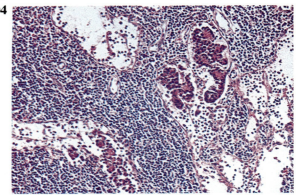

**803 and 804   Metastatic carcinoma** In lymph nodes which are the site of early metastases, the foci of carcinoma may be so small that they are overlooked, misinterpreted or obscured by reactive features. Figure **803** shows microscopic foci of carcinoma in the subcapsular sinus *(arrow)* which has been permeated via the afferent lymphatic; **804** reveals small groups of carcinoma cells within dilated medullary sinuses. *(H&E)*

**805**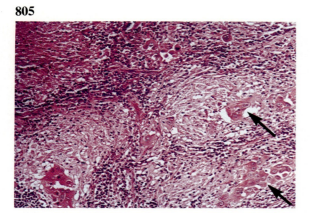

**806**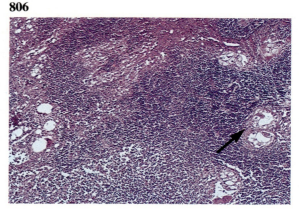

**805 and 806   Metastatic carcinoma** Occasionally the presence of carcinoma within a lymph node evokes a granulomatous response which may be so extreme as to obscure the metastases, as in **805**, with the carcinoma cells (*arrows*) merging with the epithelioid and histiocytic cells. This problem is further aggravated by the knowledge that granulomatous epithelioid foci may be found in lymph nodes draining tumour products. In other examples of early metastatic lesions, the epithelial foci are noted, but their deceptively benign appearance may lead them to be interpreted as benign epithelioid inclusion. This is particularly the case in lymph nodes related to the salivary glands and thyroid, and in the inguinal region. The benign looking glandular structures (*arrow*), **806**, were in the cystic node from a patient with carcinoma of the gall bladder and represent metastases. *(H&E)*

**807**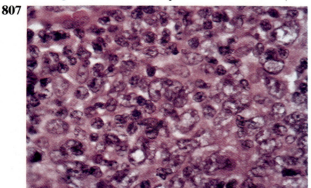

**808**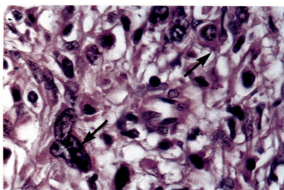

**807 and 808 Metastatic carcinoma** This condition can simulate a lymphoma and is particularly prone to do so in the cervical metastases from an occult nasopharangeal carcinoma, **807**. A similar problem exists with some of the infrequently encountered ectopic cervical thymomas. Lymph nodes in which the infiltrating carcinoma cells (*arrow*) are non-cohesive, exhibit marked nuclear pleomorphism and reveal an atypical pattern, **808**, are also likely to be misinterpreted as a lymphoma in the absence of a known primary carcinoma. *(H&E)*

**809   Metastatic carcinoma** Less well differentiated carcinomas may display marked pleomorphism with frequent giant cell forms. In this field the binucleate giant cell with its large eosinophilic nucleoli surrounded by haloes could be mistaken by the inexperienced for a Reed-Sternberg cell. *(H&E)*

**809**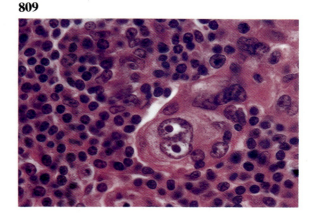

**810**

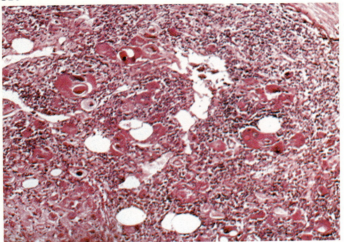

**810 Metastatic carcinoma** Radiotherapy may also considerably modify the appearance of malignant cells. In this irradiated axillary lymph node from a patient with breast carcinoma, the large malignant cells with their abundant cytoplasm exhibiting phago-cytosis somewhat resemble malignant histio-cytes. *(H&E)*

**811**

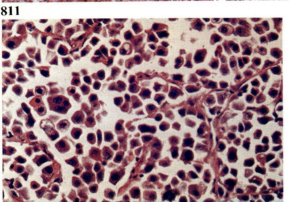

**812**

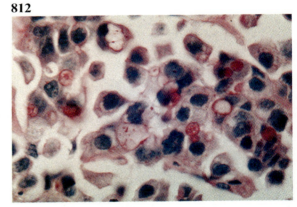

**811 and 812 Metastatic carcinoma** This node was virtually replaced by non-cohesive malignant cells including multinucleate forms, **811**, which at this level superficially resemble plasmacytoid cells. With PAS staining, **812**, many of the cells can be seen to contain mucin droplets which render the diagnosis of a lymphoproliferative tumour untenable. Also the chromatin pattern of the nuclei, when viewed at high power, is not that of the plasma cell series. *(811 H&E; 812 PAS)*

**813**

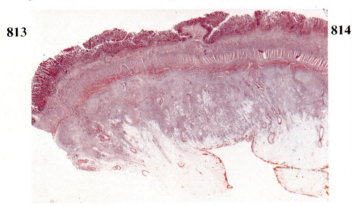

**814**

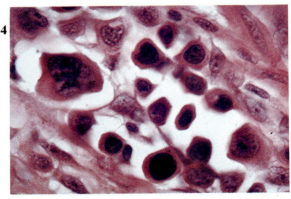

**813 and 814 Metastatic carcinoma** This specimen, **813**, is part of a resected segment of small intestine in which there was a diffuse infiltrate of serosa, muscularis propria and submucosae, but little involvement of the mucosa. The way in which the infiltrating cells lack cohesion and are spreading apart muscle fibres rather than destroying them is characteristic of a lymphomatous infiltrate. However, at high magnification, **814**, the nuclear chromatin pattern is atypical of lymphoma cells, and some cells also showed the presence of tiny PAS positive intracytoplasmic droplets. Electron microscopy (see **815**) confirmed the diagnosis of adenocarcinoma. *(H&E)*

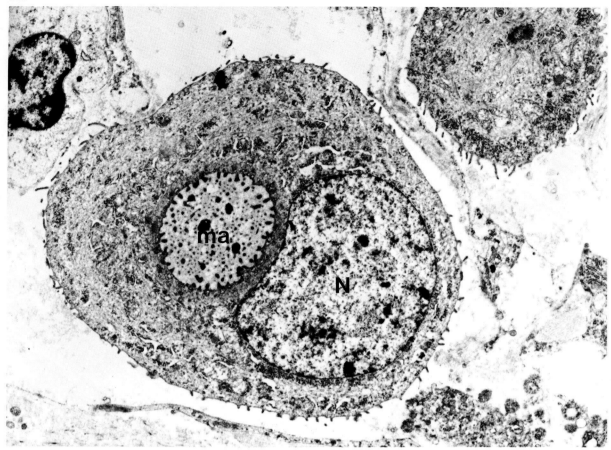

**815 Metastatic carcinoma, ultrastructure** In this electron micrograph two malignant cells from the tumour in **813/814**, and an adjacent lymphocyte are included. The material has been formalin fixed. The larger of the two cells contains a microacinus lined by microvilli and containing mucin – the structure responsible for the PAS positive globules seen at light microscopical level. Both cells show numerous microvilli at their periphery. These features and the nuclear chromatin arrangement confirm the diagnosis of a carcinoma. (Microacinus – ma; Nucleus – N) *(× 4,800)*

**816** 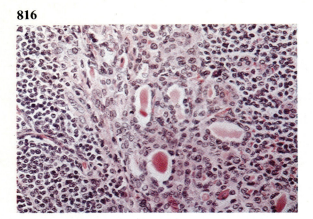 **817**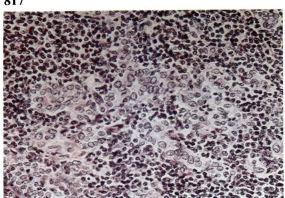

**816 and 817   Epithelial inclusions in lymph nodes** Benign epithelial inclusions occur in lymph nodes excised from many different locations – particularly those adjacent to salivary glands or thyroid glands. In these cervical lymph nodes, **816** shows formation of acini and small cysts containing proteinaceous material with a resemblance to parathyroid tissue; in **817** the epithelial cells are aggregated into tubular structures which superficially may resemble hyperplastic postcapillary venules. *(H&E)*

**818   Epithelial inclusions in lymph nodes**
Epithelial tubules lined by tall columnar cells resembling non-secretory proliferative endometrial glands may be found within lymph nodes in the iliac and inguinal regions. These endometrioid foci are not considered to represent endometriosis and their origin is obscure. Awareness of the existence of such epithelial inclusions is important since, to the uninitiated, they may be mistaken for foci of metastatic carcinoma. *(H&E)*

**818**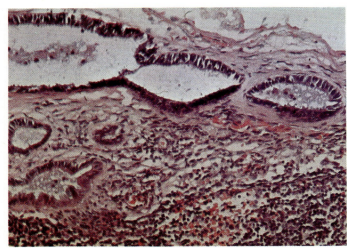

**819** 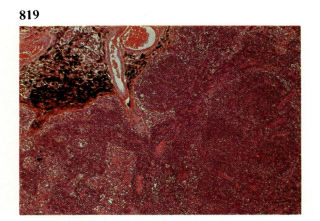 **820**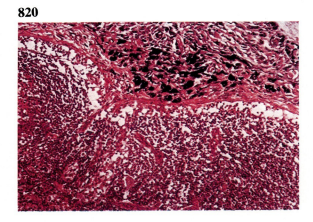

**819 and 820   Blue naevi of lymph nodes** A rare but distinctive finding in lymph nodes is the presence of pigment laden cells in relation to the fibrous tissue of the capsule and hilum, **819**. The majority of these pigment laden cells, seen in **820** in the capsule, are melanophages although some melanocytes are also present. Their origin is not established; existing evidence favours a developmental arrest of migrating melanocytes. *(H&E)*

**821** Kaposi's sarcoma Outside Africa Kaposi's
sarcoma is a relatively rare entity though one
of world-wide distribution. Its comparatively
high incidence in Africans (5 per cent of all
tumours in some African countries) is reflected
by an increased incidence of lymph node and
visceral involvement. There is also a rare but
rapidly progressive variant of the disease
occurring mainly in children, in which lymph
nodes are involved in the absence of any skin
lesions. The classical appearance of Kaposi's
sarcoma in a lymph node is a combination of
spindle cells and vacuolated cells blending
with variably formed vascular spaces. *(H&E)*

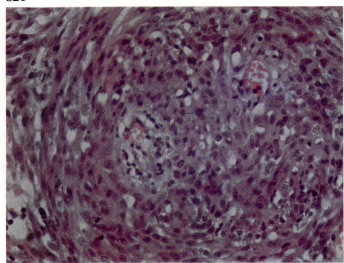

**822** Kaposi's sarcoma The specific changes usually
develop first in the sinuses and then spread to involve
the remainder of the node. In cases with skin involvement groups of tumour cells sometimes can be seen in
lymphatics. However, in patients with purely nodal involvement the process is thought to arise primarily in
lymph nodes. The morphology of the tumour cells is
well seen at higher magnification. Spindle cells are
present (*arrow 1*), there are small poorly formed
spaces some of which contain red cells, and a red cell
has been phagocytosed by one of the foamy cells
(*arrow 2*). Haemorrhage is a conspicuous feature in
some affected nodes, and it is also common to find
deposits of haemosiderin. *(H&E)*

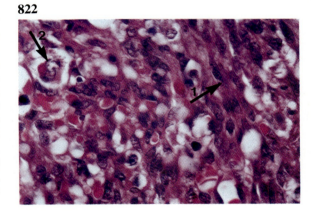

**823** Kaposi's sarcoma There is good statistical
evidence that there is an increased incidence of
lymphoma in Kaposi's sarcoma, particularly follicular
lymphoma and Hodgkin's disease, though the association is much rarer in Africans. The lymphoma may
precede or follow the onset of Kaposi's sarcoma. In
this example in an African child, the lymphoma
adjacent to the Kaposi's sarcoma in **822** is diffuse and
of poorly differentiated lymphocytic (lymphoblastic)
type. Tingeable body macrophages are very numerous
and an interesting feature is the numerous red cells
ingested by the macrophages. *(H&E)*

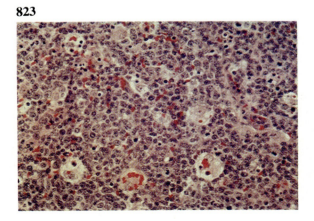

# Lymph nodes and thymus – some technical aspects

The interpretation of thymus and lymph nodes is greatly hindered by delayed or poor fixation, by faulty processing, cutting and staining, by inappropriate sectioning (sampling) and by surgical artefacts. Some of these aspects have been touched upon in the earlier sections of this Atlas. The choice of stains is also important. We recommend, in addition to good haematoxylin and eosin stained sections, the routine use of Gordon and Sweets reticulin stain with a nuclear red counterstain, the periodic-acid Schiff technique (McManus) for lymph nodes and a combined alcian blue/ PAS method for thymus followed by a haematoxylin nuclear counterstain, and methyl green-pyronin (Unna Pappenheim's stain). This last method demonstrates not only the various pyronin-ophilic cells of reactive and neoplastic conditions but is also invaluable as a routine mast cell stain. A trichrome stain such as Masson's trichrome is often extremely useful as is the phosphotungstic acid haematoxylin method (Anderson's modification) in thymic tissue. Romanovsky stains such as May-Grünwald-Giemsa and Papanicolaou's stain are recommended for the touch preparations. Useful histochemical techniques used in our laboratory to demonstrate enzyme activity are Barka and Anderson's method for acid phosphatase, Holt's indoxyl acetate method and Leder's naphthyl acetate esterase method for non-specific esterase, Leder's naphthol-AS-D-chloro-acetate esterase method, and Leder and Stutte's method for tartrate-resistant acid phosphatase. The immunoperoxidase (enzyme-bridge) method is used for the demonstration of lysozyme (muramidase) and other lysozymal enzymes. This latter method may be applied to paraffin processed sections, but the other enzyme techniques require frozen sections or imprint/smear preparations.

Frozen sections as a method for histopathological interpretation of the majority of conditions affecting lymph nodes and thymus are unsuitable, and there are very few instances when a request for a frozen section is justified. Exceptions to this rule are lymph nodes or thymic tissue which are sent to the laboratory during parathyroid exploration of the neck, when the problem is simply to identify whether the tissue is parathyroid or not, and in certain situations when the surgeon needs confirmation that a lymph node is the site of metastasis. If frozen sections are undertaken these should be cut with the cryostat and not the freezing microtome.

Another technique which usefully may be used in conjunction with conventional paraffin processing, is the plastic processing of thymic and lymph node material from which semi-thin sections may be cut; for in certain conditions the morphological features permit a definitive diagnosis not possible in the paraffin sections. Electronmicroscopy also is sometimes essential – particularly in some forms of lymphoma and thymoma and in distinguishing anaplastic carcinoma, thymoma or melanoma from a lymphoma. If material has not been prepared in advance for electron-microscopy, it is still possible to achieve good results with *formalin*-fixed material, provided there was minimum delay before fixation, and the material selected for processing is taken from a cut surface which would first have come into contact with the fixative. Even with less optimal fixation, material may still be salvaged for useful electronmicroscopy, particularly when it is a question of carcinoma versus lymphoma.

Methods aimed at differentiating T- from B-lymphoid cells, and lymphoid cells from macrophages, and which depend upon cell surface markers, are available but are usually beyond the scope of a routine histopathological laboratory. The demonstration of monoclonality of immunoglobulin secretion by B-lymphoid cells can also be demonstrated by immunoperoxidase (enzyme-bridge) techniques and may be applied to paraffin sections, but the method is capricious and stringent precautions and attention to detail are necessary to obtain consistent results. The most commonly available techniques for the differentiation of T- and B-lymphocytes and macrophages and their results are as follows:

| | T | B | M |
|---|---|---|---|
| Prominent membrane bound IgG | − | + | − |
| Sheep RBC rosettes | | | |
| E (spontaneous) | + | − | − |
| EA*C (IgM + complement) | − | + | + |
| EA* (IgG) | − | − | + |
| Cytoplasmic secretory immunoglobulin (CIg) | − | + | ±** |
| T-associated antigens e.g. HTLA | + | − | − |
| EBV antigen | − | true Burkitt tumour | − |
| Prominent non-specific esterase, acid phosphatase, lysozyme, alpha 1, anti-trypsin and chymotrypsin | − | − | + |

*A = antibody

**by ingestion

Finally, it should be stressed that despite the battery of sophisticated techniques now available for the identification of cells of the LRMPS, there remain neoplastic cells with no apparent identity as, for example, the 'null' cells which cannot be shown to possess surface markers, and cells which at ultrastructural level possess the apparatus and evidence of secretion but which cannot be shown to be producing any Ig. This should not surprise us unduly since most of these tests have been developed as extensions from the normal situation, and neoplastic cells may have lost these characteristics or acquired new ones which require the development of other techniques for their demonstration. The most exciting developments of the future, however, surely must lie in the refinement of techniques for specific tumour-associated-antigens, by means of monoclonal antibodies such as those defined in the leukaemias; and viral antigens such as the EBV-DNA antigen and EBNA — the Epstein-Barr nuclear antigen — in Burkitt's tumour.

**824** **825**

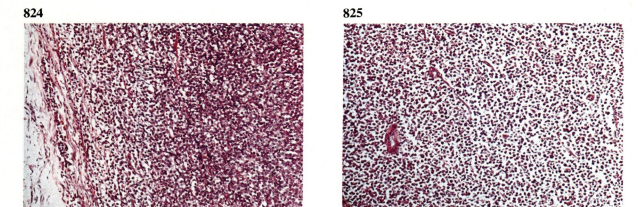

**824 and 825  Lymphoid tissue, fixation** Rapid and adequate fixation is of prime importance for the best results in interpreting lymph node histopathology. Because the capsule provides a barrier to the penetration of fixative, it is advisable in all but the smallest nodes to bisect the lymph node in its long axis in the plane of the hilum before placing it in the fixative. With very large nodes several slices may be necessary. In the case of thymus the upper and lower poles should first be identified, and the lobes or tumour sliced transversely. The fixative of choice is 10 per cent buffered neutral formalin, but another suitable fixative which results in little shrinkage artefact and is also suitable for subsequent histochemical studies is cold formal calcium. Mercury containing fixatives should be avoided. The final trimming of the slice(s) for routine paraffin processing should not be undertaken until the material is completely fixed. If such precautions are observed then the zonal fixation artefact shown here in a malignant lymphoma will be avoided. In the area just deep to the capsule, **824**, it can be seen that the lymphoma cells immediately below the capsule are not adequately fixed; neither are the cells, **825**, lying more deeply within the substance. *(H&E)*

**826** **827**

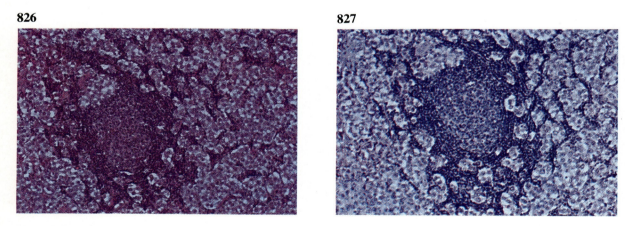

**826 and 827  Lymphoid tissue, staining** Optimum staining is another essential requirement in thymus and lymph node interpretation. To achieve the best results not only must fixation be adequate but the sections, which should never be thicker than 8 μm (or slightly thinner but not too thin), should be well cut and properly dried before staining. It is important also not to overheat the sections in the drying process. The choice of the haematoxylin and eosin used is a matter of personal preference, but it is important that the haematoxylin is well differentiated and that there is sufficient eosin for good contrast. Equally, over differentiating and overstaining with eosin result in too red a section which again lacks contrast. Figure **826** shows a good H&E stained section using Harris' haematoxylin; **827**, a section from the same area, is stained with Ehrlich's haematoxylin. There is insufficient eosin and the section is too blue. *(H&E)*

**828**

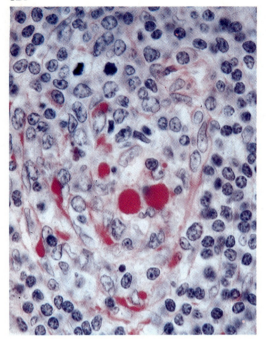

**829**

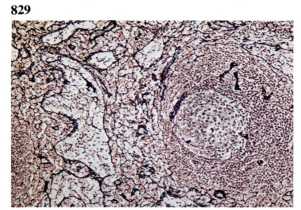

**828 and 829  Lymphoid tissue, routine staining** In addition to routine staining with MGP, two stains which are considered routine for the adequate interpretation of many conditions affecting thymus and lymph nodes are the PAS and silver stains. The PAS technique will demonstrate mucins, certain immunoglobulin inclusions, other protein-aceous material – including basement membrane protein – and various infectious agents. Silver stains for reticulin are necessary for the interpretation of architecture as well as in delineating certain structures such as sinuses, follicles and vessels. The Masson's trichrome stain has also been found to be increasingly useful (see **505** and **783**). Figure **828** shows PAS+ve intracytoplasmic and intercellular material in a poorly defined germinal centre; **829** shows the reticulin fibre pattern associated with normal sinuses and follicles. (**828** *PAS;* **829** *Gordon & Sweets*)

**830**

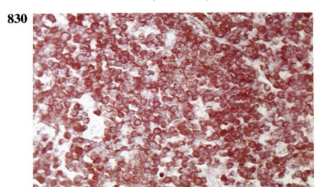

**831**

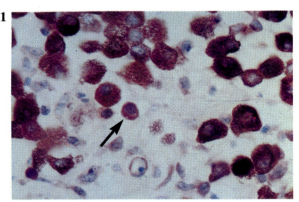

**830 and 831  Lymphoid tissue, routine staining** Mast cells may be very numerous in thymus and a variety of different conditions affecting lymph nodes as in Waldenström's disease, as well as in the very rare lymph node involvement in malignant mastocytosis and mast cell leukaemia. With the routine use of methyl green-pyronin mast cells are easily and consistently demonstrated as shown in these mastocytomas from dogs. Mast cell granules stain a reddish-orange brown, **830**, due to the affinity of pyronin to certain mucopoly-saccharide compounds contained in the granules. In contrast pyroninophilic cells such as plasma cells (*arrow*) stain a diffuse pink, **831**. Mast cells may also be demonstrated histochemically by the naphthol-AS-D chloroacetate esterase, a property shared with cells of the myelomonocytic series, and best shown in smear/imprint preparations. Even if the observer suffers from red/green colour blindness the mast cells can be recognised in both techniques by their granularity. (*MGP*)

**832 Lymphoid tissue, staining** Useful adjuncts to the routine stains advocated are the Perls Prussian blue technique for haemosiderin and Masson's fontana stain for melanin when the differential diagnosis lies between a malignant melanoma and a lymphoma. The Prussian blue reaction also has another application in mapping out the iron-containing cells of the mononuclear phagocytic system in haemosiderosis or haemochromotosis. In this example of a liver from a patient with haemosiderosis due to multiple blood transfusion, the Kupffer cells lining the liver sinusoids are clearly delineated by their blue staining cytoplasm. *(Perls stain)*

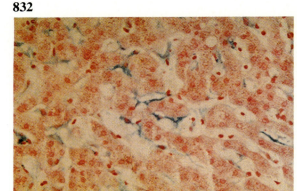

**833 Lymphoid tissue, frozen section** There are very few situations when it is justifiable for a surgeon to request a frozen section on a lymph node. Cellular detail is poor in cryostat sections and even worse in freezing microtome preparations. The area sampled is also limited. Thus the distinction of a reactive or inflammatory process from a neoplastic one is not usually possible; and is even more difficult should there be only focal involvement. Furthermore by taking material for a frozen section where tissue is in limited supply, the subsequent interpretation of the remaining tissue can be adversely affected. One of the few occasions when frozen section is justified is when moderately enlarged nodes are found during resection of a carcinoma, as shown here, the question being 'is the node simply reactive or is there a metastasis'? Although detail is not good, it is usually possible to confirm or refute the presence of metastatic carcinoma. Frozen sections on thymic (mediastinal) masses are more rewarding since it is usually possible to identify the dual cell population of lymphocytes and epithelial cells present in the majority of thymomas. *(H&E)*

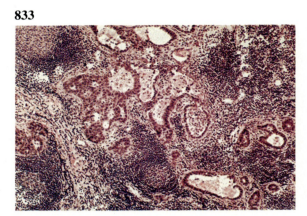

**834 Lymph node, imprint (touch) preparations** It is very convenient on receipt of the fresh lymph node and following section gently to press a *clean* dry slide down on to the cut surface. It is very important not to press too hard or too long and to avoid any type of rotary or smearing movement prior to lifting off the slide. An alternative method is to press the lymph node surface gently on to the glass slide. There is little indication for imprint preparations in thymus. This example of an enlarged abdominal lymph node taken for frozen section during cholecystectomy for what later proved to be carcinoma of the gall bladder, shows the value of the technique in demonstrating carcinoma cells – in this case a papillary adeno-carcinoma. *(H&E)*

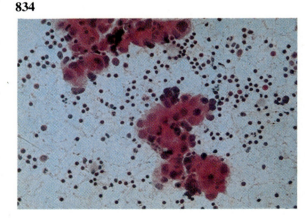

**835**

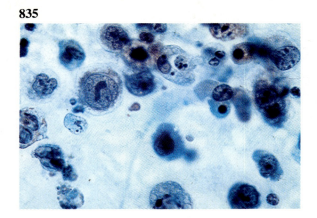

**836**

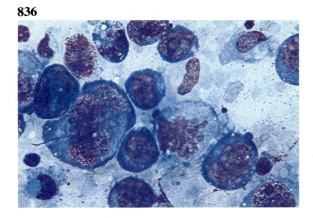

**835 and 836 Lymph node, imprint and smear preparations** Imprint preparations are less useful in differentiating reactive from malignant lymphoproliferative conditions, but their interpretation depends very much on individual experience and on the choice of fixation and subsequent staining. Shown here are two preparations from the cervical lymph node of a boy with a histiocytic lymphoma. One imprint has been fixed immediately and stained with Papanicolaou's stain, **835**, while the other, **836**, has been air-dried and stained with May-Grünwald-Giemsa. Despite the apparent differences in appearance the cells show the characteristic cytological features associated with malignant histiocytes in the two different types of preparations. (*835 Papanicolaou; 836 May-Grünwald-Giemsa*)

**837, 838 and 839 Lymph node, imprint preparations** The choice of stains is wide. It is our custom to employ May-Grünwald-Giemsa, and sometimes Papanicolaou's stain in addition to routine haematoxylin and eosin, methyl green-pyronin, and PAS stains. Touch preparations are also very useful for subsequent enzyme- or immunocytochemistry. In **837**, a mucus secreting metastatic carcinoma, the emprinted cells show good preservation of mucin secretion as demonstrated by the PAS technique, **838**. There were also cells with large pyroninophilic nuclei, **839** – a feature not uncommon in poorly differentiated and anaplastic cancer cells – and not to be confused with Reed-Sternberg cells. (*837, 838 PAS; 839 MGP*)

**837**  **838**  **839**

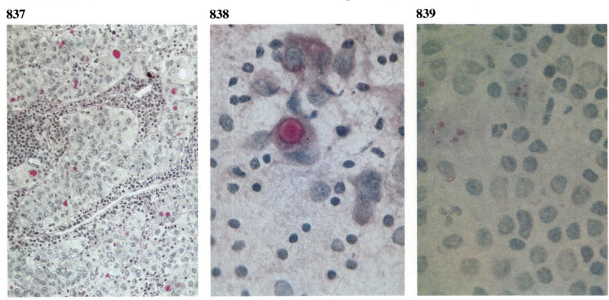

**840**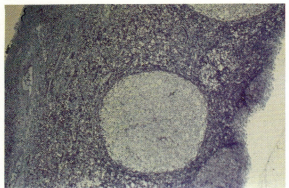

**841**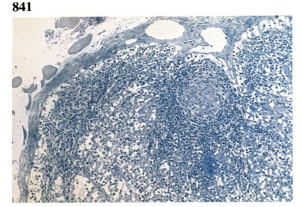

**840 and 841 Lymphoid tissue, semi-thin plastic sections** A very much underutilised method as applied to thymus and lymph nodes but one which is now generally available to all histopathology laboratories is the preparation of semi-thin sections from plastic processed material. Blocks are prepared from a fresh cut surface, the mirror image of which is processed in the conventional manner through paraffin. The size of the blocks is limited by the fixative used, and by the width of the effective cutting edge of the knife. If the intention is to proceed down to ultrastructural level, smaller blocks or tissue slices are required, but we have not found that the choice of fixative is so important as prompt fixation. Any type of ultramicrotome using glass knives is satisfactory and slices several millimetres in length are easily handled. Alternatively, with larger blocks the newer types of microtomes specifically designed to carry the large Ralph knives may be used. In **840**, from the cortex of a tonsil, and **841**, from a lymph node, the block area is quite large but fixation and permeation by the plastic is good, and subsequent staining with toluidine blue optimum. *(Toluidine blue)*

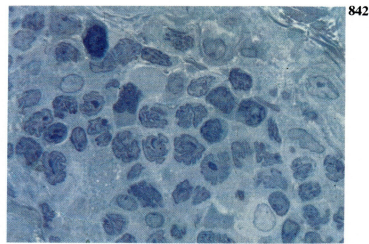 **842**

**842 Lymphoid tissue, semi-thin plastic sections** Certain cell types are shown to great advantage by this method and permit a definitive diagnosis without the need to progress to ultrastructural level or for other special techniques. One such example is in the early stages of the lymph node involvement which may complicate cutaneous T-cell lymphomas. In this lymph node from a patient with mycosis fungoides a group of cells with the characteristic and pathognomic ceribriform nuclei are seen below the capsule. *(Toluidine blue)*

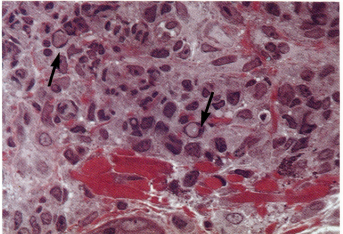 **843**

**843 Lymphoid tissue, semi-thin plastic sections** Toluidine blue is a satisfactory stain for the vast majority of conditions affecting lymph nodes. It suffers, however, from lack of colour contrast, a feature which can be accentuated by too *thin* a plastic section. Rendering the toluidine blue metachromatic, or using a commercial dye such as paragon may be preferred. In this field of lymphoid cells infiltrating skin in a patient with macro-globulinaemia, intranuclear inclusions or 'Dutcher' bodies are well visualised *(arrow)*. The reddish staining material is collagen. *(Paragon)*

**844 Lymphoid tissue, semi-thin plastic sections** Not only may cell types be recognised but it is possible also to identify certain structures helpful in establishing the diagnosis. In this lymph node initially called a lymphoma, blue staining filamentous aggregates characteristic of tonofilaments (keratin) can be identified in the cytoplasm of the epithelial cells (*arrows*) of what proved to be a metastasis from a nasopharyngeal carcinoma. It is also possible sometimes to identify desmosomal connections, a useful finding in both metastatic carcinoma and thymoma. (*Toluidine blue*)

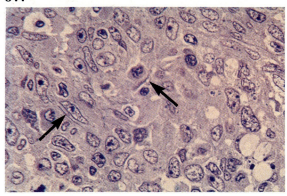

**845 and 846 Lymphoid tissue, semi-thin plastic sections** The choice of epoxy resin (plastic) used depends upon how urgently the sections are needed, since some have a much shorter polymerisation time than others, and whether special stains are envisaged. It is our practice to use araldite, and to stain with toluidine blue. It has seldom been necessary to use other stains. It is also an important practical point that for easier interpretation of the sections, these should not be too *thin*; 0.75–1.0 mu rather than 0.5 mu is preferred. The thinner sections lack contrast, whatever the stain used. In these examples of two different formalin fixed plasma cell lymphomas, nuclear and cytoplasmic detail are very clear. Figure **845** of a rather thick section shows the clumped chromatin arrangement characteristic of the nuclei of plasma cells and **846** from a thinner section of less well fixed material plainly shows the accumulated immunoglobulin (Ig) within the cytoplasm in the form of crystals (*arrow*). (*Toluidine blue*)

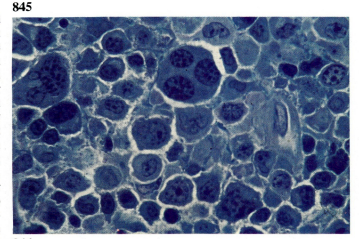

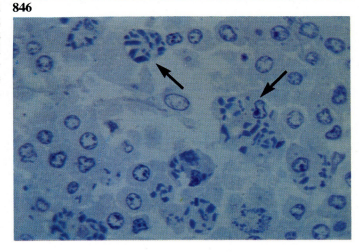

**847**

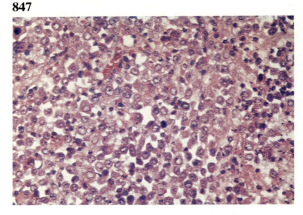

**847 and 848  Lymphoid tissue, electronmicroscopy** It has long been our practice to process when available, fresh thymus, nodal and other lymphoid tissue for electronmicroscopy. While, as already mentioned, it may not be necessary to proceed to ultrastructural study to achieve a diagnosis, since this can be made either on the conventional material or semi-thin plastic sections, material is available for research purposes. Also there are occasions when electronmicroscopy is necessary in routine pathology practice either to confirm a diagnosis or to identify the neoplastic process. Regrettably, material is not always processed for electronmicroscopy, particularly when derived from extra-nodal sites. It is worth emphasising that in such cases material may still be salvaged from the formalin fixed specimen when, provided there has been little delay in fixation and the tissue selected for E.M. processing is taken from a cut surface, results are excellent. In **847**, the initial diagnosis favoured a large cell lymphoma rather than a carcinoma but at ultrastructural level, **848**, the tumour cells were shown to be epithelial and not lymphoid. Tonofilaments – t, desmosomes (*arrow*).
*(847 H&E; 848 × 19,700)*

**848**

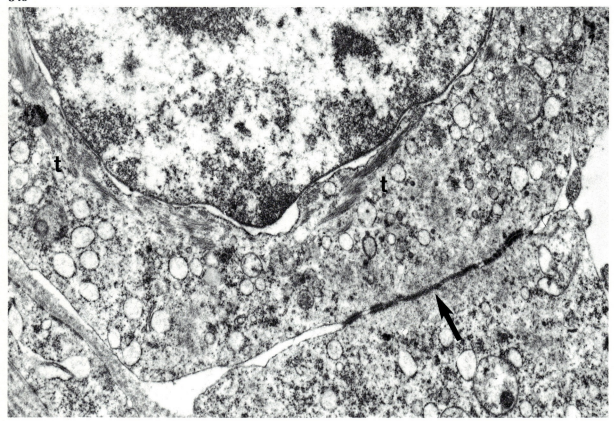

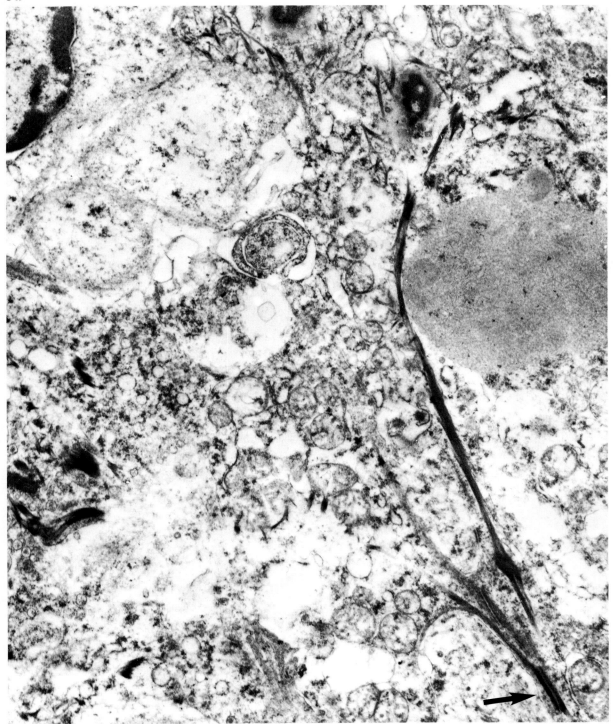

**849   Lymphoid tissue, electronmicroscopy** Even when there has been delay in fixing surgical material, formalin-fixed tissue may still be helpful since, although there is much artefact of cellular organelles, certain structures useful as cytological markers are well preserved. This is particularly true of the sclero-proteins, and desmosomes. This electronmicrograph from the cervical lymph node shown in **807** demonstrates abundant tonofilaments and desmosomes (*arrow*), characteristic of epithelial cells, and enabled a diagnosis to be made of a metastatic carcinoma rather than lymphoma. The patient was later found to have a nasopharyngeal carcinoma. *(× 36,000)*

**850**

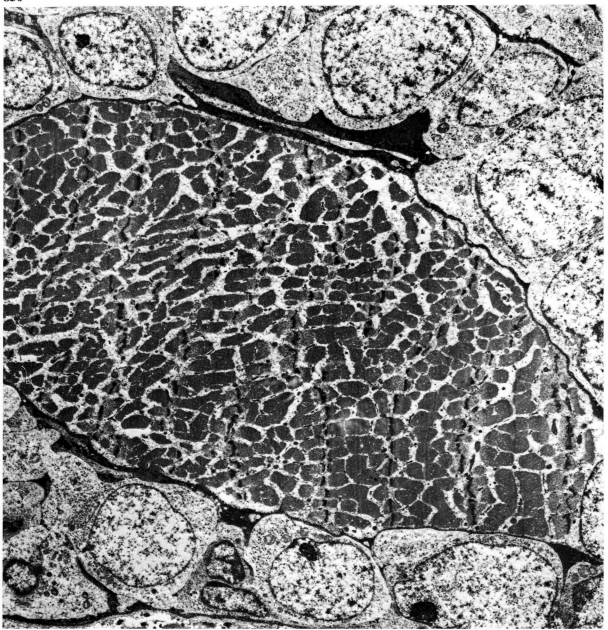

**850 Lymphoid tissue, electronmicroscopy** A biopsy of a large soft tissue tumour invading muscle in a young child showed at light microscopical level features which only permitted a diagnosis of 'malignant round cell tumour' to be made. The ultrastructural features, however, were those of a malignant lymphoma of large cell type. *(× 5,250)*

**851 Lymphoid tissue, enzyme histochemistry** A number of cyto-chemical techniques are available, useful in the identification of specific cell types, which can be applied to frozen sections or imprint preparations. One such method is the technique for the demonstration of acid phosphatase which is tartrate resistant. Cells which possess a high content of tartrate resistant acid phosphatase activity are hairy cells, here seen in an imprint preparation, with the granular enzyme activity revealed as a red staining reaction product. The only other cells which possess this property to some degree, are some chronic lymphocytic and prolymphocytic leukaemia cells. Certain T-cell malignancies, including cutaneous T-cell lymphomas, also possess acid phosphatase activity but this is generally tartrate labile. *(Tartrate resistant acid phosphatase)*

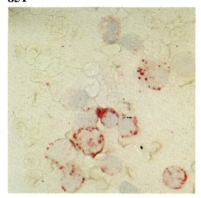

**852 and 853 Lymphoid tissue, histochemistry** Cells of the mononuclear phago-cytic system contain a number of different digestive enzymes necessary for the degrada-tion of phagocytosed material. These enzymes, acid phosphatase, non-specific esterase and lysozyme (muramidase), can be demonstrated at light microscopical level by specific techniques which are thus useful in the identification of phagocytic cells. Free macrophages (histiocytes) contain the largest amount of these enzymes. The dendritic cells of the follicles and sinus lining cells also contain generous amounts of non-specific esterase, but negligible acid phosphatase. On the other hand some lymphoid cells contain appreciable amounts of acid phosphatase and non-specific esterase. In these sections of tonsil the macrophages *and* dendritic fol-licular cells are revealed by their non-specific esterase content (stained red, **852**) and the macrophages by their lysozyme content (stained brown, **853**). *(852 non-specific esterase; 853 lysozyme (enzyme-bridge technique))*

**852**

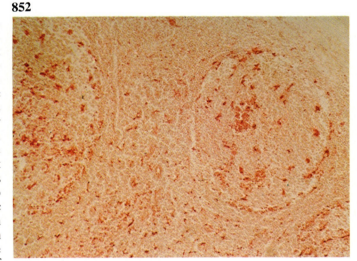

**853**

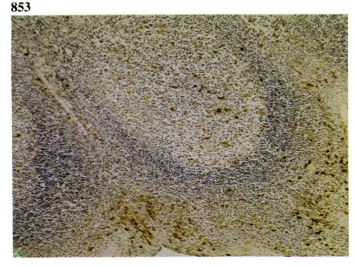

**854**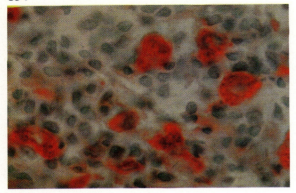

**855**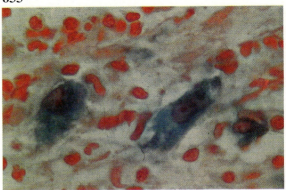

**854 and 855   Lymphoid tissue, histochemistry** Reactive mononuclear phagocytic cells (histocytes) may be very numerous in some lymphomas. Since they are not always present as tingeable-body macrophages a histiocytic neoplastic proliferation may be considered. If histochemical stains are then carried out to demonstrate non-specific esterase or acid phosphatase activity, **854**, and thus confirm the histiocytic nature of the cells, the strongly staining cells here appearing red look even more prominent. A histiocytic component is also common in Hodgkin's disease, **855**, but does not generally lend to diagnostic errors. The two histiocytes are stained blue due to their non-specific esterase content. (**854** *acid phosphatase;* **855** *indoxyl acetate non-specific esterase*)

**856a**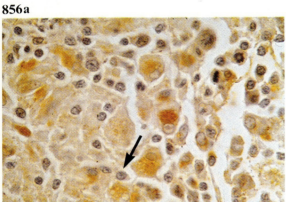

**856b**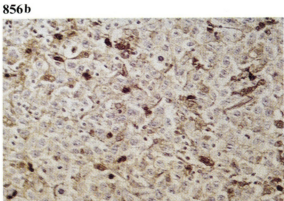

**856a and 856b   Lymphoid tissue, histochemistry** The demonstration of lysozyme (muramidase) and alpha 1 anti-trypsin and chymotrypsin activity is sometimes very useful in confirming the histiocytic nature of a lymphoma. The amount of lysozyme is very variable and not all lymphomas considered to be histiocytic give a positive reaction, particularly the pleomorphic variety. Figure **856a** shows a relatively well differentiated histiocytic lymphoma with prominent lysozymal activity. Note how the brown reaction product is concentrated in the vicinity of the Golgi apparatus, and the absence of staining in the few residual lymphocytes (*arrow*). Caution must always be exercised in the utilisation of these techniques in the diagnosis of lymphomas, in not mistaking previously unnoted *reactive* histiocytic cells as malignant histiocytes. Such an example is shown in **856b**, with numerous reactive histiocytes lying between the unstained lymphoma cells. In contrast to neoplastic histiocytes note the diffuse staining of the cytoplasm. (*immunoperoxidase stain for lysozyme*)

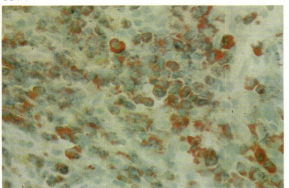

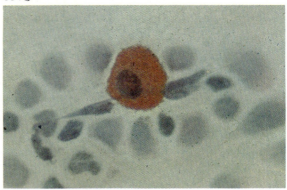

**857a and 857b Lymphoid tissue, histochemistry** Sometimes there are difficulties in differentiating myelo, myelomonocytic or monocytic leukaemic infiltrates from lymphomas. A useful histochemical technique in making the differentiation is the naphthol-AS-D chloroacetate esterase method, for the more mature cells of the myelopoetic series are usually positive – although to a variable degree – in **857a** from a child with acute myeloid leukaemia. Another cell which stains intensely for chloroacetate esterase is the mast cell. In **857b**, a splenic implant from a patient with hairy cell leukaemia, the hairy cells are negative but the mast cell granules appear bright red. *(857a/b Naphthol-AS-D chloroacetate esterase)*

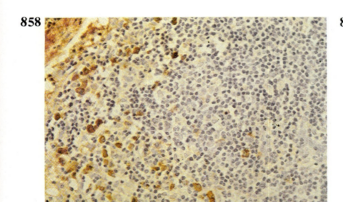

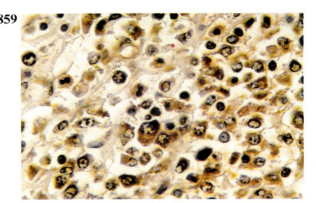

**858 Lymphoid tissue, immunocytochemistry** With the advent of the sensitive immunoperoxidase techniques, not only can cytoplasmic immuno-globulins be reliably demonstrated in either frozen or fixed tissue, but the cells containing immuno-globulin can be visualised. In this lymph node from a patient with Waldenström's macroglobulinaemia the plasma cells producing monoclonal IgM are stained brown. The basis of this method is the application of antibody to immunoglobulin reacted with a complex of peroxidase and antiperoxidase antibodies (PAP). The bound PAP is then visual-ised by a histochemical method to demonstrate peroxidase. Nuclear detail can also be observed by counterstaining with haematoxylin. *(immuno-peroxidase stain for immunoglobulin)*

**859 Lymphoid tissue, immunocytochemistry** One of the great advantages of the enzyme-bridge/PAP technique is that paraffin processed sections may be utilised and, therefore in theory, retrospective studies of immunoglobulin synthesis in stored blocks of lymphoid tissue can be carried out in addition to analysis of current material. In this gut lymphoma of plasma cell type the synthesising cells – in this case producing IgG – are revealed. Monoclonality is demonstrated by the application of anti-kappa and anti-lambda sera to serial sections. We have not always found the method reliable in the diagnosis of an immunocytoma. For example, in some lymphomas composed of immuno-globulin synthesising cells as demonstrated by electronmicroscopy, with the PAP technique no cytoplasmic immunoglobulin production of any of the major currently defined Ig classes can be demonstrated. Furthermore in some lymphomas, polyclonal immunoglobulin production has been found. *(immunoperoxidase stain for immuno-globulin)*

**860**

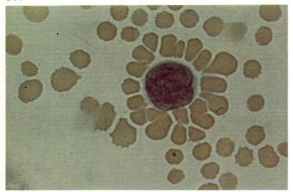

**860 Lymphoid tissue, cell surface markers** One of the most useful techniques used in identification of cell surface markers is the formation of rosettes with sheep red blood cells. This method may be adapted to reveal receptors to complement, a property shown by B-lymphocytes and macrophages, and receptors to surface IgG (Fc fragment) shown by macrophages. The formation of *spontaneous* rosettes with sheep red blood cells is a feature of T-lymphocytes, here demonstrated by a Sézary/Lutzner cell. *(E-rosette/May-Grünwald-Giemsa)*

**861**

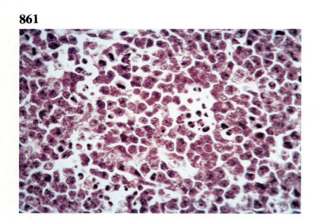

**862**

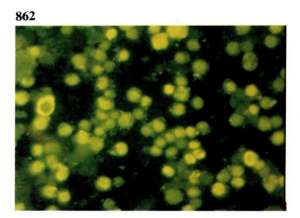

**861 and 862 Lymphoid tissue, tumour associated antigens** An exciting area of development mainly in the leukaemias has been the recognition of tumour associated antigens. In the field of lymphomas Burkitt's tumour also has been shown to possess specific antigens, but in this case related specifically to the EB virus, the causal agent in susceptible individuals. Of the methods to demonstrate the several antigens present in Burkitt's lymphoma cells, **861**, containing the EB viral genomes, probably the most reliable and specific is that demonstrating the Epstein-Barr nuclear antigen (EBNA), **862**. This is applied to methanol fixed slides by means of anti-complementary immunofluorescence. **(861** *H&E;* **862** *EBNA, immunofluorescence)*

# Recommended reading

With the exception of the references relating to the *classification* of malignant lymphoma, the following list is in no way intended to be comprehensive but merely to act as background to the terminology and conditions described in this Atlas and to serve as a further source of references.

A Histochemical Society Symposium (1980). Immunohistology of Human Lymphoma. *J. Histochem. Cytochem.* **28**, 731–791.

Carr, I. (Ed.) (1977). *Lymphoreticular Disease*. Blackwell Scientific Publications, Oxford.

Goldstein, G. and Mackay, I. R. (1969). *The Human Thymus*. Warren H. Green, St. Louis.

Henry, K. The Thymus Gland. In *Systemic Pathology*. Vol. 2, pp. 894–924. Churchill Livingstone, Edinburgh, London, New York.

Henry, K. and Goldmann, J. (1975). The Lymphocyte. In *Recent Advances in Pathology*. 9th edn., pp. 39–72. Harrison, C. V. and Weinbren, H. K. (Eds.). Churchill Livingstone.

Jelliffe, A. M. and Vaughan Hudson, G. (Eds.) (1981). A British National Lymphoma Investigation Symposium – the first ten years. *Clin. Radiology* **32**.

Kaplan, H. S. (Ed.) (1981). *Hodgkin's Disease*. 2nd edn. Harvard University Press, Cambridge, Mass.

Kendall, M. (Ed.) (1981). *The Thymus Gland*. Academic Press Inc (London) Ltd.

Lennert, K. (1978). *Malignant Lymphomas – other than Hodgkin's disease*. Springer-Verlag, Berlin, Heidelberg, New York.

Mathé, G. Seligmann, M. and Tubiana, M. (Eds.). Vol. 64. (1978). *Recent Results in Cancer Research*. Springer-Verlag.

Peckham, M. J. (Ed.) (1975). Symposium on non-Hodgkin's lymphomata. *British J. Cancer* **31**, Suppl. 11. H. K. Lewis & Co. Ltd., London.

Rosai, J. and Levine, G. (1975). Tumours of the Thymus. *Atlas of Tumour Pathology*. 2nd series, fascicle 13. Armed Forces Institute of Pathology, Washington D.C.

Smithers, D. (Ed.) (1970). *Hodgkin's Disease*. Churchill Livingstone.

Symmers, W. St. C. (1978). Lymphoreticular System. In *Systemic Pathology*. Vol. 2, pp. 563–893. Churchill Livingstone.

van Furth, R. (Ed.) (1975). *Mononuclear Phagocytes in immunity, infection and pathology*. Blackwell Scientific Publications, Oxford.

## Classification of lymphomas – key references
### Hodgkin's disease
Lukes, R. J. and Butler, J. J. (1966). *Cancer Res.* **26**, 1063.

Lukes, R. J., Craven, L. F., Hall, T. C., Rappaport, H. and Rubin, P. (1966). *Cancer Res.* **26**, 1311.

### Lymphomas other than Hodgkin's disease
*B.N.L.I.* – Bennett, M. H., Farrer-Brown, G., Henry, K. and Jelliffe, A. (1974). *Lancet* **ii**, 405.

Henry, K., Bennett, M. H. and Farrer-Brown, G. (1978). *Recent Advances in Histopathology*. 10th edn., pp. 275–302. P. P. Anthony and N. Woolf. (Eds.). Churchill Livingstone.

*Dorfman* – Dorfman, R. F. (1974). *Lancet* **ii**, 1295.

Dorfman, R. F. (1977). *Am. J. Surg. Path.* **1**, 167.

*Kiel* – Gerard-Marchant, R., Hamlin, I., Lennert, K., Rilke, F., Stansfeld, A. G. and Van Unnik, J. A. M. (1974). *Lancet* **ii**, 406.

Lennert, K., Stein, H. and Keiserling, E. (1975). *Brit. J. Cancer* **31**, Suppl. 2, 29.

*Lukes & Collins* – Lukes, R. J. and Collins, R. D. (1974). *Cancer* **34**, 1488.

Lukes, R. J. and Collins, R. D. (1975). *Brit. J. Cancer* **31**, Suppl. 2, 1.

*Rappaport* – Rappaport, H. (1966). Tumours of the hematopoietic system. *Atlas of Tumour Pathology*. Section iii, fascicle 8. Armed Forces Institute of Pathology, Washington D.C.

*Stanford Formulation* – *National Cancer Institute Sponsored Study of Classifications of non-Hodgkin's lymphomas: summary and description of a working formulation for clinical use*. From the non-Hodgkin's Lymphoma Pathological Classification project, 1980 (in preparation).

*Traditional* – Gall, H. and Mallory, J. B. (1942). *Amer. J. of Pathology* **18**, 381.

*W.H.O.* – Mathé, G., Rappaport, H., O'Connor, G. T. and Torloni, H. (1976). Histological and cytological typing of neoplastic diseases of hematopoietic and lymphoid tissues. *International Histological Classification of Tumours*. No. 14. World Health Organisation, Geneva.

# Index

Figures in light type refer to pages; those in **bold** type refer to illustrations.

322

323

328